Myles **Midwifery**
Anatomy and **Physiology**
Workbook

Myles **Midwifery** **Anatomy** and **Physiology** Workbook

Second Edition

Jean **Rankin**

BSc(Hons) MMedSci PhD PGCE RM RGN RSCN

Professor (Maternal, Child and Family Health),
Head of Division (Midwifery and Specialist Nursing),
School of Health and Life Sciences,
University of the West of Scotland, Paisley, United Kingdom;
Adjunct Professor of Midwifery,
Auckland University of Technology,
Auckland, New Zealand.

With contributions by

Thomas **McEwan**

Lecturer in Midwifery, University of the West of Scotland & Honorary
Advanced Neonatal Nurse Practitioner, NHS Greater Glasgow & Clyde.

ELSEVIER

Edinburgh London New York Oxford Philadelphia St Louis Sydney 2020

First edition 2013

The right of Jean Rankin to be identified as author of this work has been asserted by her in accordance with the Copyright, Designs and Patents Act 1988.

Notices

Practitioners and researchers must always rely on their own experience and knowledge in evaluating and using any information, methods, compounds or experiments described herein. Because of rapid advances in the medical sciences, in particular, independent verification of diagnoses and drug dosages should be made. To the fullest extent of the law, no responsibility is assumed by Elsevier, authors, editors or contributors for any injury and/or damage to persons or property as a matter of products liability, negligence or otherwise, or from any use or operation of any methods, products, instructions, or ideas contained in the material herein.

ISBN: 978-0-7020-7648-0

Content Strategist: Alison Taylor
Content Development Specialist: Sheila Black/Kirsty Guest
Project Manager: Julie Taylor
Design: Amy Buxton
Illustrator: Narayanan Ramakrishnan

Printed in Poland

Last digit is the print number: 9 8 7 6 5 4

Contents

Developing the activities

This anatomy and physiology activity book is aimed at student midwives. The purpose is to provide a range of activities to assist them in the revision of their knowledge related to pregnancy, labour, childbirth, puerperium and the neonate. The two key textbooks used to inform the activities include Marshall and Raynor (2014) *Myles Textbook for Midwives* and Rankin (2017) *Physiology in Childbearing with Anatomy and Related Biosciences*. Where appropriate, updated information for specific activities is based on RCOG and NICE guidelines. The way midwives practice in specific areas can vary across the United Kingdom and internationally. Examples include the different approaches to manoeuvres or named movements used in obstetric emergencies. To some extent this is addressed as relevant activities deal with underlying principles.

In this second edition, the range of updates reflects feedback from United Kingdom and international students.

What students preferred:
Labelling diagrams: more diagrams requested (with a few labels to provide prompts).
Activities: match and connect; true or false and identify correct response.
More tables with questions requiring one word or short responses.
List of words and numerical values which assisted with completing the activities.
Crossing out incorrect words and statements.

What students did not like:
Too many MCQs because these were available to them on several websites.
Short answers where they needed to define or write a description.
Colouring figures was unhelpful.
Completing activities with no prompts (i.e., word lists or numerical values).

How to use this book
Icons and activities

Word lists and labels are provided with a number of the activities to prompt and guide students as they complete the activities. Students are referred to the textbook when completing those activities where no prompts are provided.

 Label: Identify and label structures on diagrams

 Shade/colour: Identify, shade or colour structures on diagrams (refer to an obstetric textbook if diagrams are coloured)

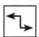 **Match:** Match statements in a variety of ways, e.g. structures with functions; structures with conditions; key choices with blanks in a paragraph, etc.

Combinations of these activities are also used to provide variety in the text for students.

 Complete: Identify the missing word(s) or remove incorrect word(s) to complete activities—when completing then students should carefully consider the information required to ensure the correct information is provided.

 True/false: Students are required to identify if statements are true or false. Again, these should be carefully considered and not be assumed to be correct. If the statement chosen is incorrect or false, then the student should refer to the textbook or relevant national guidelines for the correct response.

 Correct/incorrect: Similar to the aforementioned. Some students prefer to identify correct responses.

 Short answers: Students are required to refer to the textbook and provide short answers to complete the activities.

 Definitions: Explain the meaning of common obstetric, midwifery, neonatal terminology and anatomical and physiological terms.

 Multiple choice questions: Identify the correct answer from the list of options.

 Miscellaneous: A small number of activities are labelled 'miscellaneous' as they bring together a range of different topics within the same section.

Acknowledgements

Special thanks to two colleagues, School of Health and Life Sciences, University of the West of Scotland, United Kingdom:

- Thomas McEwan, Midwifery Lecturer, Advanced Neonatal Nurse Practitioner, for writing the chapters involving the fetus and neonate (Chapters 5, 6 and 17–20).
- Dr Lyz Howie, Midwife Lecturer and MSc (with registration) Midwifery Programme Leader, for her input to activities relating to midwifery and obstetric emergencies (Chapter 14).

Appreciation and special thanks to Sheila Black, Development Editor, for completing the extensive work required to update numerous activities in this workbook.

QUESTIONS

1 The female pelvis and pelvic floor

Detailed knowledge of the anatomy of the normal female pelvis is fundamental for midwifery practice. Progress in labour is estimated by assessing the relationship of the fetus to pelvic landmark. This knowledge is required to aid detection of deviations from normal. The following activities will test your knowledge of the related topics.

The pelvic bones

 Correct/incorrect

1. Consider the statements in Table 1.1 and tick the correct/incorrect statements about the pelvic girdle.

Table 1.1

	Statement	Correct	Incorrect
i.	The pelvic girdle is virtually incapable of independent movement except during childbirth		
ii.	The pelvic girdle is a funnel-shaped cavity		
iii.	The pelvic girdle provides the skeletal framework of the birth canal		
iv.	The pelvis is composed of four irregularly shaped bones: two innominate bones, the sacrum and the coccyx		
v.	The two innominate bones of the pelvis form the lateral and posterior walls		
vi.	Each innominate bone consists of three fused bones: ilium, ischium and pubic		
vii.	The coccyx and sacrum for the lateral and posterior wall of the pelvis		

 Complete

2. Table 1.2 provides a list of descriptive statements relating to the bones and structures of the pelvis. Complete Table 1.2 by ticking all the correct statements.

Table 1.2

	Descriptive statement	Correct
i.	The ischium, the thick lower part of the innominate bones, has a large prominence known as the *ischial tuberosity*	
ii.	The concave anterior surface of the sacrum is referred to as the *hollow*	
iii.	The pubis forms the posterior part of the ischium	
iv.	The upper border of the first vertebra of the sacrum juts forward and is known as the *promontory*	
v.	The ilium is the large flared-out part of the pelvis	
vi.	The anterior surface of the sacrum is roughened to receive muscle attachments	
vii.	The sacrum consists of five fused vertebra and the coccyx consists of four fused vertebrae	
viii.	The sacrum is pierced with four pairs of foramina through which nerves emerge to supply the pelvic organs	
ix.	The concave anterior surface of the ilium is known as the *iliac fossa*	
x.	The coccyx is a vestigial tail consisting of two fused vertebrae forming a small rectanglar bone	
xi	The coccyx articulates with the fifth sacral segment	

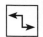 **Match and label**

3. Fig. 1.1 shows the lateral view of the innominate bone. The innominate bone contains a deep cup termed the *acetabulum* (receives the head of the femur). The acetabulum is composed of three fused bones (two-fifths ilium, two-fifths ischium and one-fifth pubis). Label the detailed landmarks of the innominate bone by matching to the key terms listed.

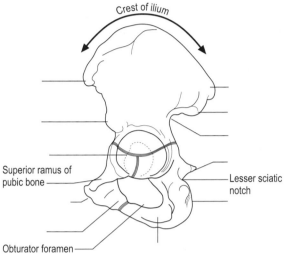

| Posterior superior iliac spine |
| Acetabulum |
| Anterior inferior iliac spine |
| Ischial tuberosity |
| Inferior ramus of ischium |
| Anterior superior iliac spine |
| Symphysis pubis |
| Ischial spine |
| Posterior inferior iliac spine |
| Inferior ramus of pubic bone |
| Greater sciatic notch |

Figure 1.1   Obturator foramen

Pelvic joints and ligaments

 Complete

4. There are four pelvic joints: one sacrococcygeal joint, one symphysis pubis joint and two sacroiliac joints. Anatomical structures involved in the sacroiliac joints are provided. Now complete the anatomical structures and details of the other two pelvic joints. An extended selection of anatomical-related terms are available to support you (some words may be used more than once).

Base	Pelvis	Sacrum	Rami	Left	Right	anterior	
Pubic bones	Ilium	Spine	Tip	Coccyx	articulates	cartilaginous	

  i. The **sacroiliac joints** join the <u>sacrum</u> to the <u>ilium</u> and as a result connect the <u>spine</u> to the <u>pelvis</u>.

 ii. The **symphysis pubis** is the midline cartilaginous joint uniting the _____ of the _____

     and _____ _____ _____.

iii. The **sacrococcygeal joint** is formed where the _____ of the _____ articulates with the

     _____ of the sacrum.

Match, label and colour

5. Fig. 1.2 provides a posterior view of the pelvis showing the ligaments. Match and label the appropriate landmarks and ligaments to the key choices provided. Colour the main ligaments.

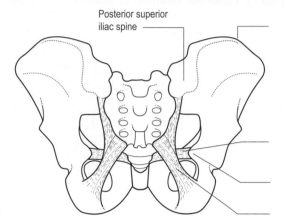

Ischial spine
Iliac crest
Sacrospinal ligament
Sacrotuberous ligament

Posterior superior iliac spine

Figure 1.2

Types of pelvis

 Labelling

6. There are four categories of pelves: gynaecoid, android, anthropoid and platypelloid. The gynaecoid pelvis is cited as the optimal type of pelvis for childbearing. Identify and label the other three types of pelves in Fig. 1.3.

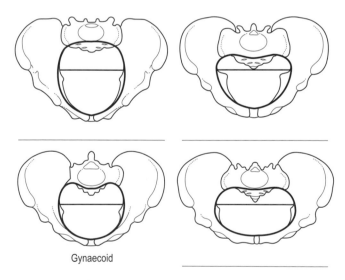

Gynaecoid

Figure 1.3

Completion

7. Consider the following list of descriptive words. Complete Table 1.3 by choosing the most appropriate words to describe the features of the different types of pelvis (some words may be used more than once).

Kidney-shaped	Narrow	Prominent	90 degrees	Straight
Convergent	Narrowed	20%	>90 degrees	Long oval
Wide	Divergent	<90 degrees	Generous	Rounded
Heart-shaped	50%	5%	Blunt	25% (50% non-Caucasian)

Table 1.3

Features	Gynaecoid	Anthropoid	Android	Platypelloid
Brim				
Forepelvis				
Side walls				
Ischial spines				
Sciatic notch				
Sub-pubic arch				
Incidence				

  Match and label

8. An extended list of descriptive terms relating to pelvic types is provided. In Fig. 1.4, match and label the terms that correctly refer to suitability of the gynaecoid pelvis for childbirth.

Sacral promontory is not prominent
Ischial spines are prominent
The sacrum is curved
Sciatic notch is narrow
The brim is rounded
Ischial spines are smooth
Sciatic notch is wide

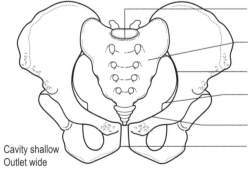

Cavity shallow
Outlet wide

Wide sciatic notch
Cavity shallow
Outlet wide
Sub-pubic angle 90 degrees
Sub-pubic angle is less than 90 degrees
Cavity is wide and divergent
Brim is long and oval

Figure 1.4

Complete

9. Table 1.4 provides descriptive statements related to the types of pelves. Consider each statement, correctly match and tick the appropriate pelvis by ticking the relevant box(es). Some statements may relate to more than one pelvis.

Table 1.4

	Statement	Gynaecoid	Android	Anthropoid	Platypelloid
a.	It has straight side walls				
b.	The anteroposterior diameter is reduced, and the transverse diameter increased				
c.	The anteroposterior diameter is longer than the transverse diameter				
d.	The side walls converge making it funnel-shaped				
e	The ischial spines are prominent and the sciatic notch is narrow				
f	There is a long oval brim				
g	It has a narrow forepelvis				
h	It has a deep cavity and straight sacrum				
i	The anteroposterior diameter is longer than the transverse diameter				
j	The transverse diameter is situated towards the back				
k	The sacrum is long and deeply concave				
l	The sacrum is flat and the cavity shallow				
m	It has a well-curved sacrum				
n	The forepelvis is narrow with the greater space found in the hindpelvis				

The pelvis in relation to pregnancy and childbirth

 Complete

10. Complete the activities by providing relevant information. The pelvis is divided into the true pelvis and the false pelvis.

1. The true pelvis is described as being the bony canal through which the fetus must pass during birth. Identify the three components of the true pelvis.

    a. _____ _____, b. _____ _____,

    c. _____ _____.

2. The false pelvis is the part of the pelvis which is situated above the pelvic brim.

    Anatomical structures forming the false pelvis include the _____

    _____

    The false pelvis protects the _____

The true pelvis

 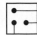 **Match and label**

11. The superior circumference forms the pelvic brim with the included space called the *inlet*. Fig. 1.5 shows the brim of the female pelvis. Match the landmarks a–h with the list provided. In addition, draw a line to represent the sacrocotyloid dimension.

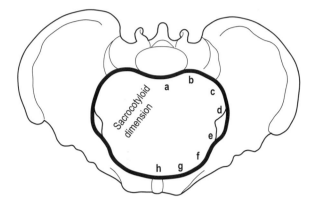

d. Iliopectineal line

_____. Sacral promontory

_____. Sacroiliac joint

_____. Superior ramus of the pubic border

_____. Sacral ala or wing

_____. Upper inner border of the symphysis pubis

e. Iliopectineal eminence

_____. Upper inner border of the pubic bone

Figure 1.5

Pelvic diameters

Contraction of any of the pelvic diameters can result in malposition or malpresentation of the presenting part of the fetus.

  Match and label

12. Fig. 1.6 provides a view of the pelvic brim showing diameters. Label the diameters of the pelvic brim by matching to the key provided.

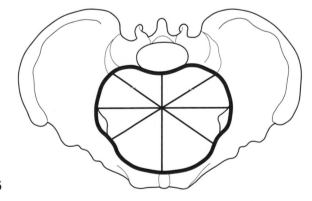

Transverse
Left oblique
Right oblique
Anteroposterior

Figure 1.6

Complete

13. Complete the following statements about pelvic brim diameter. Choose the correct key words taken from the following <u>extended</u> list of pelvis-related words.

Transverse diameter	Symphysis pubis	Sacral promontory
Conjugate diameter	Cavity	Ischial spines
Oblique diameter	Outlet	Iliac crest

  1. This diameter extends across the greatest width of the brim: _____.

  2. This diameter extends from the iliopectineal eminence of one side to the sacroiliac articulation of the

     opposite side: _____

  3. The anteroposterior diameter extends from the _____ _____ to

     the _____. The other term for this diameter is the

     _____ diameter.

 Complete

14. Complete Fig. 1.7 by inserting the correct measurement for each of the diameters (cm) of the pelvic brim, cavity and outlet in Fig. 1.7.

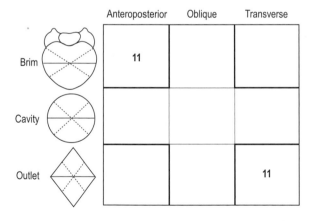

Figure 1.7

Conjugate diameters

Anatomical conjugate, obstetric conjugate and diagonal conjugate are three diameters that can be measured. Two diameters may be referred to as the 'true' conjugate. The midwife must be aware of this fact and be clear as to the conjugate measurement referred to in any given situation.

True/false

15. Consider the following statements and complete Table 1.5 by ticking to indicate if each statement is true or false.

Table 1.5

	Statement	True	False
a.	Pelvic planes are three-dimensional measurements at the brim, cavity and outlet of the pelvic canal		
b.	When standing upright, the pelvis is placed so that the anterior superior iliac spine and the front edge of the symphysis pubis are in the same vertical plane, perpendicular to the floor		
c.	The anatomical conjugate diameter is measured from the sacral promontory to the uppermost point of the symphysis pubis and averages 12 cm		
d	The anatomical conjugate is also referred to as the 'true' conjugate		
e	The diagonal (Internal) conjugate diameter is measured anteroposteriorly from the upper border of the symphysis to the sacral promontory		
f	The obstetrical conjugate diameter is measured from the sacral promontory to the posterior border of the upper surface of the symphysis pubis		
g.	The obstetrical conjugate diameter represents the shortest anteroposterior diameter through which the fetus must pass through		
h.	The obstetrical conjugate diameter measurement averages 12 to 13 cm		
i.	Each oblique diameter extends from the iliopectineal eminence of one side to the sacroiliac articulation of the opposite side. Measurement averages 12 cm		
j.	The obstetrical conjugate can be measured by examining fingers and a range of other techniques		

 Match and label

16. Fig. 1.8 represents the median section of the pelvis showing anteroposterior diameters. Label the following figure by matching the correct terms.

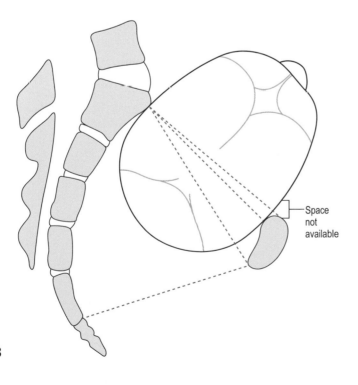

Obstetrical conjugate
Internal or diagonal conjugate
Obstetrical anterior of outlet
Anatomical conjugate (true)
Obstetrical anterior–posterior of outlet

Space not available

Figure 1.8

Asynclitism

 Complete

17. Carefully consider how the fetal head negotiates the pelvic brim and then complete the following section using the relevant key words from the extended subsequent list (some words may be used more than once).

Anterior	Sacral hollow	External	Parietal eminence
Flexion	Internal	Symphysis pubis	Lateral
Sacral promontory	Outlet	Posterior	Similar
Oblique	Opposite	Rotation	Anteroposterior
Ischial spines	Ischial tuberosity	Biparietal	Cavity
Posterior	Descent	Rotation	Bone

1. Engagement of the fetal head may necessitate _____ tilting, known as asynclitism, to

   allow the _____ diameter to pass the narrowest _____ diameter of

   the brim.

2. In anterior asynclitism, the _____ parietal bone moves down behind the

   _____ until the _____ enters the brim. The

   movement is then reversed and the fetal head tilts in the opposite direction until the _____

   parietal bone negotiates the _____ and the fetal head is engaged.

3. In posterior asynclitism, the movements of anterior asynclitism are reversed. The _____

   parietal bone negotiates the _____ before the _____ parietal

   bone moving down behind the _____. Once the pelvic brim has been negotiated,

   descent progresses normally accompanied by _____ and _____

   rotation.

Miscellaneous questions about the pelvis

 Complete

18. Consider the following statements and complete Table 1.6 to indicate all the correct statements.

Table 1.6

	Statement	Correct
a.	The sacroiliac joints are strong non-weight-bearing synovial joints	
b.	The sacrococcygeal joint permits the coccyx to be deflected forwards during the birth of the fetal head	
c.	The anterior superior iliac spine is the bony prominences felt at the back of the iliac crests	
d.	The concave posterior surface of the ilium is the iliac fossa	
e.	The lesser sciatic notch lies between the ischial spine and ischial tuberosity	
f.	The obstetrical outlet is of greater practical significance because it includes the narrow pelvic strait through which the fetus must pass	
g.	The obturator foramen is the space enclosed by the body of the pubic bone, the rami and the ileum	
h.	Sacrocotyloid dimension passes from the sacral promontory to the iliopectineal eminence on each side and measures 9 to 9.5 cm	
i.	A widening of 1–2 cm at the symphysis pubis during pregnancy above the normal gap of 7 to 8 cm is normal	
j.	The obstetrical outlet is the space between the narrow pelvic strait and the anatomical outlet	
k.	High assimilation pelvis occurs when the fifth lumbar vertebra is fused to the sacrum and the angle of inclination of the pelvic brim is increased	
l.	The sacrotuberous ligaments and sacrospinous ligaments pass between the sacrum and ischium	
m.	The narrow pelvic strait lies between the sacrococcygeal joint, the two ischial spines and the lower border of the symphysis pubis	
n.	The obstetrical outlet is the space between the narrow pelvic strait and the anatomical outlet	

 Multiple choice questions (MCQ)

19. Consider each of the following statements and circle the correct answer(s).

1. If the line joining the sacral promontory and the top of the symphysis pubis was extended, then the angle formed with the horizontal floor would be:

   a. 90 degrees

   b. 60 degrees

   c. 45 degrees

2. The cavity of the pelvic girdle is:

   a. heart-shaped

   b. funnel-shaped

   c. basin-shaped

3. The depth of the anterior wall and length of the posterior wall of the cavity are:

   a. 8 cm in depth and 12 cm in length

   b. 6 cm in depth and 14 cm in length

   c. 4 cm in depth and 12 cm in length

4. The sacrocotyloid dimension passes from the sacral promontory to the iliopectineal eminence on each side and measures:

   a. 9–9.5 cm

   b. 10–10.5 cm

   c. 11–11.5 cm

20. Consider the following statements.

   1. Choose the correct answer(s):

      a. The pelvis is said to be contracted if one of the diameters is smaller than normal by 2 cm or more.

      b. The anterior wall of the cavity is formed by the curve of the sacrum and is 12 cm in length.

      c. In the justo minor pelvis all pelvic diameters can be 1.25 cm smaller than average.

      d. All of the above.

      e. None of the above.

   2. Choose the correct answer(s):

      a. The ischial tuberosity is a bony prominence found on the ilium.

      b. The lateral walls of the outlet are mainly covered by the obturator internus muscles.

      c. The anatomical outlet is formed by the upper borders of each of the bones together with the sacrotuberous ligament.

      d. None of the above.

      e. All of the above.

   3. Choose the correct answer(s):

      a. The anatomical outlet is formed by the lower borders of each of the bones together with the sacrotuberous ligament.

      b. The ischial tuberosity is a bony prominence found on the ischium.

      c. The sacrocotyloid dimension is important with posterior positions of the occiput, when the parietal eminences of the fetal head may become caught.

      d. All of the above.

      e. None of the above.

   4. Choose the correct answer(s):

      a. In posterior positions of the occiput, it is the sacrocotyloid dimension that becomes important as the parietal eminences of the fetal head may become caught.

      b. In the standing position, the pelvis is placed such that the anterior superior iliac spine and the front edge of the symphysis pubis are in the same vertical plane.

      c. Pelvic planes are imaginary flat surfaces at the brim, cavity and outlet of the pelvic canal.

      d. None of the above.

      e. All of the above.

Pathophysiology: deformed pelves

21. Deformed pelves may occur for a variety of reasons, including developmental anomaly, dietary deficiency, injury or disease. Consider the following statements in Table 1.7 and tick the appropriate deformed pelvis or deformity the statement refers to.

Table 1.7

	Statement	Rachitic pelvis	Osteomalacic pelvis	Naegle's pelvis	Robert's pelvis	Spinal deformity
a.	This deformity results from the condition of rickets (malnutrition) in early childhood					
b.	This deformity is caused by an acquired deficiency of calcium (Ca++) (occurs in adulthood)					
c.	Failure in normal development results in this deformity/deformities					
d.	This deformity usually involves kyphosis or scoliosis					
e.	In this deformity, one sacral ala is missing, and the sacrum is fused to the ilium					
f.	In this pelvis, the weight of the body presses down onto softened pelvic bones					

Short answer

22. Identify and describe two features of the rachitic pelvis that differ from the gynaecoid pelvis. How may this impact on labour and birth outcome?

_____

_____

_____

THE PELVIC FLOOR

Functions of the pelvic floor

Soft tissues filling the outlet of the pelvis form the pelvic floor. The most important is the strong diaphragm of muscle slung like a hammock from the walls of the pelvis. The urethra, the vagina and the anal canal pass through this diaphragm of muscle.

Short answer

23. a.   Identify three important functions of the pelvic floor:

_____

_____

_____

b. Describe the influences the pelvic floor has during the childbirth process:

_____

_____

_____

Muscle layers

The two muscle layers of pelvic floor muscles are the superficial muscle layer (composed of five muscles, also termed the superficial perineal muscles) and the deep muscle layer (consists of four main pairs of muscles, collectively known as _Levator ani_).

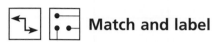 **Match and label**

24. Complete labelling of a range of figures to demonstrate your knowledge of the position of the muscles of the pelvic floor in relation to other pelvic structures.

   a) Fig. 1.9 shows the layers of the pelvic floor in relation to the uterus and vagina. Insert two labels to identify the positioning of the (i) superficial perineal muscles and (ii) levator ani.

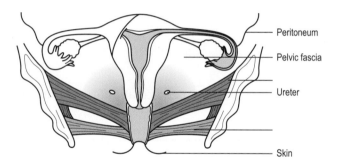

Figure 1.9

   b) Match and label the superficial perineal muscles in Fig. 1.10. An extended list of key words is provided for you to choose the three correct labels.

Ischiocavernosus	Bulbocavernosus (also named bulbospongiosus)	Iliococcygeal	Transverse perineal muscle
Pubococcygeus	Coccygeus	Puborectalis	

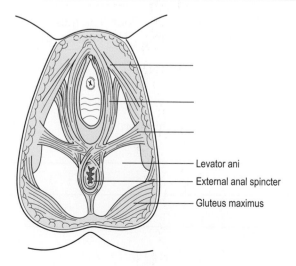

Figure 1.10

c) Match and label Fig. 1.11A,B, by identifying the deep pelvic floor muscles and structures of the pelvic floor. The two parts to the figure provide a superior view (A) and inferior view (B) of the muscles of the pelvic diaphragm. An exact list of labels is provided. Some labels are used in both views as indicated beside the labels listed.

Urethra × 2	Coccyx × 2	Coccyx × 2
Rectum	Pubococcygeus × 2	Sacral promontory
Iliococcygeus × 2	Puborectalis	Vagina x2

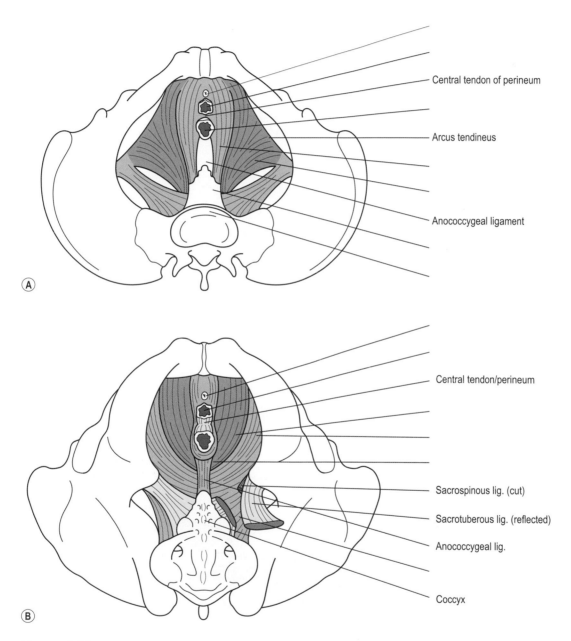

Central tendon of perineum

Arcus tendineus

Anococcygeal ligament

Ⓐ

Central tendon/perineum

Sacrospinous lig. (cut)

Sacrotuberous lig. (reflected)

Anococcygeal lig.

Coccyx

Ⓑ

Figure 1.11

d) Knowledge of the perineum and structures is crucial for midwifery practice. Fig. 1.12A,B focuses on the structures in the urogenital triangle. In Fig. 1.12B, the left bulbospongiosus (also known as bulbocavernosus) muscle has been removed to demonstrate the underlying tissues. Complete Figs 1.12A,B by selecting the correct terms from the subsequent list. Again, some labels are used in both views as indicated beside the labels listed.

Clitoris × 2	Bulbospongiosus (Bulbocavernosus) muscle	Pubococcygeus	Urethra × 2
Perineal body × 2	Superficial transverse perineal muscle	Vagina × 2	Anus
External anal sphincter × 2	Puborectalis	Bartholin's gland	Iliococcygeus
Ischiocavernosus muscle × 2	Vestibular bulb	External anal sphincter	Coccyx × 2

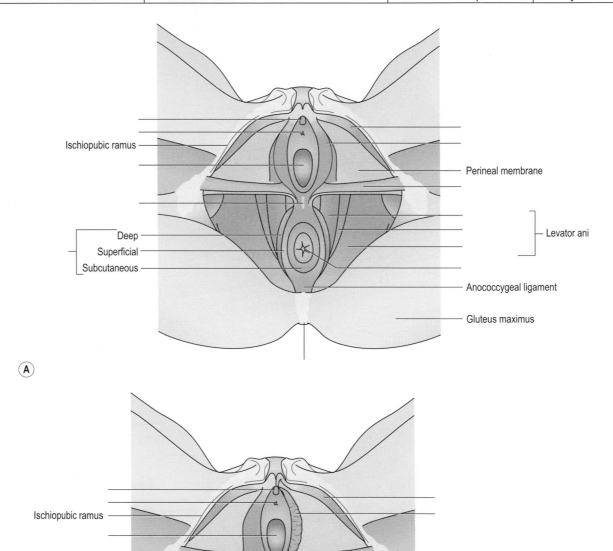

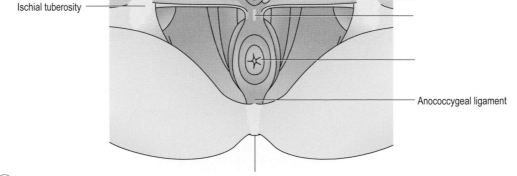

Figure 1.12

e) Fig. 1.13 presents (A) coronal section of the anorectum and (B) anal sphincter and levator ani. Complete this activity by matching and labelling this figure.

Terms
Levator ani
Perineal skin
Corrugator cutis ani
Deep muscles
Superficial muscles
Subcutaneous tissue
External anal sphincter-*(this term groups the structures involved)*

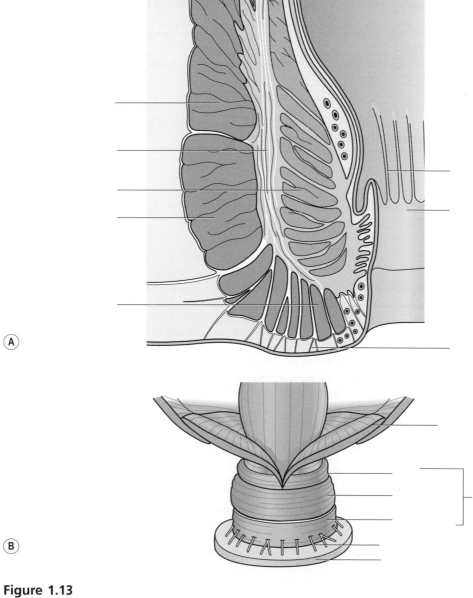

Ⓐ

Ⓑ

Figure 1.13

Complete

25. Carefully consider the descriptive statement presented in Table 1.8 about the superficial and deep muscles of the pelvic floor. Complete the table by identifying the correct statements.

Table 1.8

	Descriptive statement	Correct
a.	Iliococcygeus (deep muscle) converges with the pubococcygeus (deep muscles) where it inserts into the coccyx and lower sacrum	
b.	Bulbospongiosus (bulbocavernosus) superficial muscle arises in the centre of the perineum, with fibres passing on either side of the vaginal orifice and urethra	
c.	Pubococcygeus (deep muscle) passes around the rectum and continues to its insertion on the upper sacrum	
d.	Ischiococcygeus (deep muscle) originates from the ischial spine and adjacent sacroiliac fascia	
e.	The superficial transverse muscle is a narrow slip of muscle that arises from the inner and forepart of the ischial tuberosity and is inserted into the central tendinous part of the perineal body	
f.	Puborectalis (deep muscle) passes anteriorly, encircling the rectum becoming part of the anorectal ring	
g.	Iliococcygeus (deep muscle) forms a horizontal sheet that spans the opening in the posterior region of the pelvis and forms a shelf for pelvic organs to rest on	
h.	Pubococcygeus and puborectalis deep muscle pairs become interlaced to the point of becoming inseparable	
i.	Ischiococcygeus (deep muscle) originates from the coccyx and lower sacrum to the median portion of the sacrotuberous ligament	
j.	The ischiocavernosus superficial muscle is elongated, thinner in the middle than at either end, and is situated on the posterior boundary of the perineum	

Miscellaneous questions about the pelvic floor

True/false

26. Consider the following statements in Table 1.9 and choose if the statements are true or false by ticking the appropriate column. Correct any false statements identified.

Table 1.9

	Statement	True	False
a.	The pubococcygeus and the ischiocavernosus are collectively known as the *levatores ani*		
b.	The bulbocavernosus muscle is responsible for the erection of the clitoris and contraction of the vaginal walls		
c.	Pelvic fascia is tightly packed areolar tissue between and around muscle layers		
d.	The muscles of the levator ani differ from most other skeletal muscles in several ways. One example is that muscles maintain constant tone during functions, such as voiding and defaecation		
e.	The perineal body is the central point between the urogenital and the anal triangles of the perineum		
f.	The pelvic floor is a musculotendinous sheet that spans the pelvic outlet and consists entirely of the paired Levator ani muscles		
g.	Within the perineal body, there are interlacing muscle fibres from the bulbospongiosus (bulbocavernosus), superficial transverse perineal and external anal sphincter muscles		
h.	Another example of how the levator ani muscles differ from most other skeletal muscles is the inability to contract quickly at the time of acute stress (such as sneezing or coughing)		
i.	Levator ani muscles differ from other skeletal muscles in that they also have the ability to distend considerably during parturition and contract after birth to resume normal function		

Pathophysiology: pelvic floor complications

Loss of integrity and trauma to the soft tissues associated with childbearing can damage the pelvic floor. This may result in short-term and long-term reproductive anomalies and maternal morbidity issues.

Definitions

27. Define the terms and identify signs and symptoms:

Cystocele: _____

_____

Urethrocele: _____

_____

Uterovaginal Prolapse: _____

_____

Rectocele: _____

_____

Enterocele: _____

_____

Other definitions:

Dyspareunia: _____

Procidentia: _____

What is the typical treatment for pelvic floor prolapse? _____

_____

Short answers

28. The midwife can minimize the risk of prolapse. Use Box 1.1 to identify at least four possible actions by the midwife.

Box 1.1

1. _____.

    _____

2. _____.

    _____

3. _____.

    _____

4. _____

    _____

5. _____

    _____

6. _____

    _____

7. _____

2 The reproductive systems

The structure of the male and female reproductive systems is different. The common function is primarily to ensure reproduction and the passing of genetic material to children. Both systems produce gametes (sex cells), which fuse to form a potential human being. The female reproductive tract also has the significant responsibility of carrying, nurturing and producing the offspring of sexual reproduction. This chapter will test knowledge of the structures and some processes involved.

THE FEMALE REPRODUCTIVE SYSTEM

External structures of the female reproductive system

 Matching and labelling

1. Fig. 2.1 shows the external female genital organs. Label the structures by matching to the key word options provided.

Anus
Clitoris
External urethral orifice
Frenum
Fourchette
Hymen
Labium minus (or minora)
Labium majus (or majora)

Mons veneris
Opening of Bartholin's duct
Perineum
Prepuce
Vagina
Vestibule

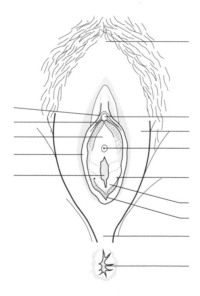

Figure 2.1

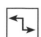 **Match and complete**

2. The vulva is the collective term for the external genitalia. Each structure of the external genitalia has a unique description. Complete the following activity in Table 2.1 by matching the name of the structure from the list to the correct description.

Mons pubis/ mons veneris	Vestibule	Skene ducts
Vaginal orifice	Hymen	Bartholin's glands
Labia majora	Labia minora	Prepuce
Urethral orifice	Clitoris	

Table 2.1

	Descriptive statement	Structure (vulva)
i.	This is a retractable piece of skin surrounding and protecting the clitoris	
ii.	These lie in the posterior part of the labia majora and secrete mucus lubricating the vaginal opening	
iii.	Anteriorly, these two small subcutaneous folds (lie between the labia majorus and enclose the clitoris)	
iv.	This is a small rudimentary sexual organ corresponding to the male penis	
v.	This area is enclosed by the labia minora in which the openings of the urethra and the vagina are situated	
vi.	This is a rounded pad of fatty tissue lying anterior to the pubic symphysis of the pubic bones (symphysis pubis). It is covered with hair from puberty	
vii.	This lies 2.5 cm posterior to the clitoris and immediately in front of the vaginal orifice	
viii.	These are two folds of fat and areolar tissue covered with skin and pubic hair on the outer surface and have a pink smooth inner surface	
ix.	These are two small blind-ended tubules 0.5 cm long running within the urethral wall	
x.	This is thin membrane that tears during sexual intercourse or during the birth of the first baby	
xi.	This structure occupies the posterior two-thirds of the vestibule. It is also known as the *introitus*	

Internal structures of the female reproductive system

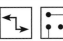 **Match, label and colour**

3. Fig. 2.2 displays a coronal section through the pelvis. Match and label the structures and tissues from the list provided. Optional—colour the structures as preferred.

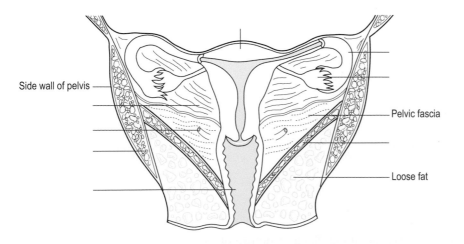

Label

Levator ani muscle
Ureter
Uterine tube
Vagina
Ovary
Uterus
Broad ligament
Obturator internus muscle

Side wall of pelvis

Pelvic fascia

Loose fat

Figure 2.2

4. Fig. 2.3 presents a lateral view of the female reproductive organs in the pelvis and their associated structures. Match and label the structures from the list provided. Optional—colour the structures as preferred.

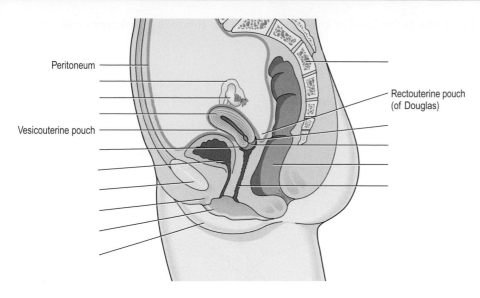

Peritoneum

Vesicouterine pouch

Rectouterine pouch
(of Douglas)

Label

| Uterine tube |
| Uterus |
| Anterior fornix |
| Pubic bone |
| Urinary bladder |
| Labium minorus (singular) |
| Clitoris |

| Vagina |
| Rectum |
| Sacrum |
| Posterior fornix of vagina |
| Cervix |
| Labium majorus (singular) |
| Ovary |

Figure 2.3

5. Fig. 2.4 shows the uterus and the left uterine tube and ovary. Label the following structures and colour as preferred.

Label key structures:

Ovary	Fimbriae	Fundus	Cornua
Uterine tube	Ampulla	Vagina	Uterine (fallopian) tube

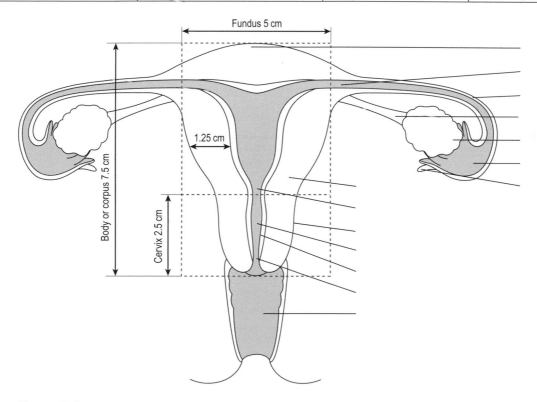

Fundus 5 cm

1.25 cm

Body or corpus 7.5 cm

Cervix 2.5 cm

Figure 2.4

Label the other areas/structures

External cervical os	*Cervix	Ovarian ligament	Myometrium	Cervical endometrium	Ovarian ligament
Isthmus	Internal cervical os	*Fundus	*Body or corpus		Cervical canal

*Measurement labels (arrows)

6. Fig. 2.5 shows the supports of the uterus at the level of the cervix. Label the following structures and colour if preferred.:

| Transverse cervical ligament |
| Rectum |
| Pubocervical ligament |
| Symphysis pubis |
| Uterine cervix |
| Uterosacral ligament |
| Bladder |

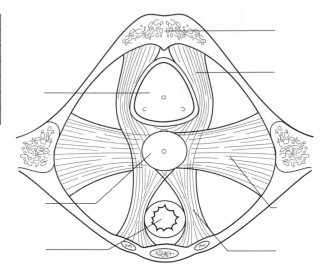

Figure 2.5

 True/false

7. It is essential for practitioners to have detailed knowledge of structures within the female reproductive system. Consider the following statements in Table 2.2 and then decide which structure is referred to by ticking the appropriate column.

Table 2.2

	Statement	True	False
a.	The mucous lining of the uterus is known as the *exometrium*		
b.	The nonpregnant uterus typically lies tilted posteriorly toward the sacrum		
c.	The ovaries are attached to the back of the broad ligament		
d.	The walls of the vagina are thrown into small folds known as *rugae*		
e.	The myometrium is composed of bundles of skeletal muscles		
f.	In labour, the cervix stretches because of the muscle fibres being embedded in collagen fibres		
g.	The endometrium forms a lining of ciliated epithelium (mucous membrane) on a base of connective tissue		
h.	The interstitial part of the uterine tube is the widest section		
i.	Lymphatic drainage of the uterus provides an effective defence against uterine infection		
j.	During the menstrual cycle, the basal layer of the uterine layers alters because of the influence of hormones		
k.	The perimetrium covers the anterior and posterior surfaces of the uterus		
l.	Myometrium fibres interlace to surround the blood vessels that pass to and from the endometrium		
m.	Bartholin's glands are connected to the vestibule		
n.	The folds of the labia minora are devoid of fat		
o.	The ovary is composed of a medulla and cortex		
p.	During pregnancy the isthmus of the uterus enlarges to form the lower uterine segment		

The uterus and uterine tubes

 Complete

8. The subsequent paragraph describes aspects of the uterus using correct and incorrect words. Cross out the incorrect words.

The uterus is a hollow **pear-/round**-shaped **muscular/visceral** organ, described as being a **thin/thick** organ and is located in the **true/false** pelvis between the **bladder/colon** and the **vagina/rectum**. The position of the uterus within the **true/false** pelvis is one of **ante-/retro**version and **ante-/retro**-flexion. **Ante-/retro**version means that the uterus leans forward and **ante-/retro**-flexion means that it bends forwards upon itself. When the woman is standing upright, the **anteverted/retroverted** uterus is in an almost **horizontal/lateral** position with the **cervix/fundus** resting on the bladder. The uterus has three layers: endometrium, perimetrium and myometrium. The **endometrium/perimetrium** is the **inner/middle** layer and the myometrium, the **middle/ outer** layer, is the **thinnest/thickest** of the three layers.

 Short questions

9. Enter the following measurements in Table 2.3.

Table 2.3

	Question	Numerical value
i.	**Vagina:**	
	a. Length of posterior wall	_____ cm
	b. Length of anterior wall	_____ cm
	c. Diameter	_____ cm
ii.	**Fallopian tubes:**	
	a. Length of each tube	_____ cm
	b. Lumen of the tube	_____ mm
	c. Isthmus	_____ cm
	d. Ampulla	_____ cm
iii.	**Nonpregnant uterus:**	
	a. Length	_____ cm
	b. Width	_____ cm
	c. Depth	_____ cm
	d. Weight	_____ g
	e. Thickness of each wall.	_____ cm
iv.	What is the pH value of the vagina fluid?	pH _____

Complete

10. Complete the short answers in Table 2.4.

Table 2.4

	Question	Short answer
a.	The labia minora are also known as:	
b.	The labia majora are also known as:	
c.	The upper end of the vagina is known as the:	
d.	Name the three layers of the vagina:	_____ _____ _____
e.	Name the four portions of the uterine tube:	_____ _____ _____ _____
f.	Name the cells within the lining of the uterine tube secreting glycogen to nourish the oocyte	_____
g.	The epithelial folds that line the uterine tubes are known as:	_____
h.	List three other terms used for the uterine tubes	_____ _____ _____
i.	Identify 3 missing words: pH value of vaginal fluid is created by (i) _____ bacilli acting on (ii) _____ to form (iii) _____acid.	

THE MALE REPRODUCTIVE SYSTEM

The male reproductive organs

 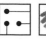 **Match, label and colour**

11. Fig. 2.6 shows the male reproductive organs. Some organs are partly visible and others are partly hidden within the body.

Label the following structures and colour if preferred.

| Urethra |
| Testis |
| Urinary bladder |
| Scrotum |
| Prostate gland |

| Ejaculatory duct |
| Seminal vesicle |
| |

| Penis |
| Spermatic cord and deferent duct |
| Prepuce |
| Glans penis |
| Deferent duct |
| Bulbourethral gland |
| |
| Epididymis |

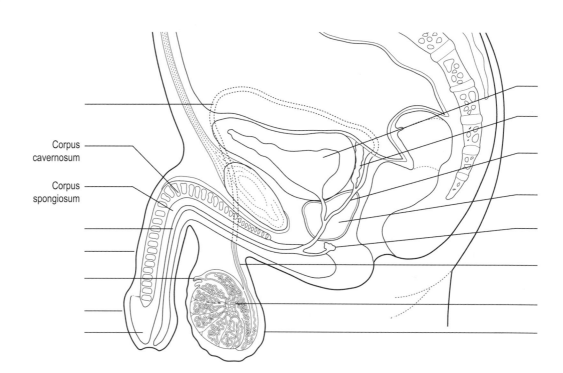

Corpus cavernosum

Corpus spongiosum

Figure 2.6

 True/false

12. Consider the following statements in Table 2.5. Select if they are true or false by ticking the appropriate column.

Table 2.5

	Statement	True	False
a.	Luteinizing hormone (LH) inhibits production of testosterone		
b.	The scrotum forms a pouch in which the testes are suspended outside the body, keeping them at a temperature higher than the rest of the body		
c.	The control of the male gonads is cyclical		
d.	Mature sperm are stored in the epididymis and the deferent duct until ejaculation		
e.	The testicular veins form a network around the testicular artery, known as the *pampiniform plexus* (tendril-like)		
f.	The testes are the body's main source of the male hormone testosterone		
g.	Spermatogenesis takes place in the epididymus		
h.	Normal spermatozoon move at a speed of 2–3 mm/min		
i.	Testes are components of the reproductive and endocrine systems		

13.

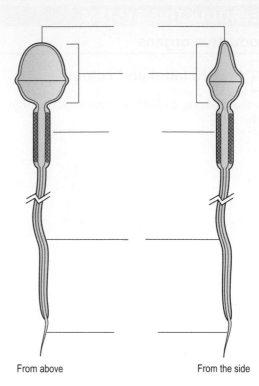

Figure 2.7

From above   From the side

 Multiple choice questions (MCQ)

14. Choose the correct response to the following questions about the male and female reproductive system. Other names used for uterine tubes include:

   a.   Isthmus tubes

   b.   Fallopian tubes

   c.   Salpinges

   e.   All of the above

   f.   b and c

15. The transverse cervical ligaments are sometimes known as:

   a.   Cardinal ligaments

   b.   Mackenrodt's ligaments

   c.   Round ligaments

   d.   All of the above

   e.   a and b

   f.   b and c

16. The isthmus of the uterine tube is:

   a.   The wider portion and is 5 cm long

   b.   The narrow portion and is 2.5 cm long

   c.   The funnel-shaped portion and is 5 cm long

   d.   None of the above

17. Which of the following statements are correct:

   a. The term 'Carunculae myrtiformes' refers to tags remaining once the hymen is torn during sexual intercourse or following the birth of the first baby.

   b. The prepuce is a nonretractable piece of skin surrounding and protecting the clitoris.

   c. The clitoris is a rudimentary sexual organ with the visible knob-like portion located near the anterior junction of the labia minora above the opening of the urethra and vagina.

   d. All of the above

   e. a and c

   f. b and c

18. Which of the following statements are correct:

   a. When the woman stands upright, the vaginal canal points in an upward-backward direction and forms an angle of approximately 45 degrees with the uterus.

   b. The uterovesical pouch lies between the bladder and uterus and is formed by the perimetrium draping over the anterior surface of the uterus reflecting onto the bladder.

   c. The ovary is supported from above by the ovarian ligament medially and the infundibulopelvic ligament laterally.

   d. All of the above

   e. b and c

19. Spermatogenesis takes place under the influence of:

   a. Follicle stimulating hormone (FSH) only

   b. Testosterone only

   c. Thyroxine

   d. Testosterone and FSH

20. The ideal temperature for the production of viable sperm is:

   a. 34.4°C

   b. 35.5°C

   c. 36.7°C

   d. 33.6°C

Pathophysiology

 MCQs

Choose the correct answer about pathophysiology in the female reproductive system.

21. Endometriosis is a condition where endometrial tissue is found outside the uterus. Symptoms include:

   a. Dysmenorrhoea

   b. Pelvic pain

   c. Hormonal disturbances

   d. Fatigue

   e. All of the above

22. Which of the following statements is true about polycystic ovarian syndrome (PCOS)?

    a.   It is the third most common cause of anovulatory infertility in the United Kingdom.

    b.   It is confirmed by the presence of hyperandrogenism, menstrual irregularities and polycystic ovaries.

    c.   Females with PCOS are less likely to be obese.

    d.   Insulin resistance is not a feature of the syndrome.

    e.   All of the above

 Correct/Incorrect

23. Table 2.6 provides descriptive statements about uterine malformations. Complete Table 2.6 by identifying the **correct** statements.

Table 2.6

	Descriptive statements	Correct
a.	In the general population, the prevalence of uterine malformation is estimated to be approximately 7%	
b.	The female genital tract is formed in late embryonic life when several pairs of ducts develop	
c.	Abnormal development of the Mullerian duct(s) during embryogenesis can lead to uterine abnormalities	
d.	A double uterus (duplication of body of uterus, cervix and vagina) will develop where there has been complete failure of fusion	
e.	Partial fusion will result in various degrees of duplication	
f.	One common malformation results when one Mullerian duct regresses and the result is a uterus with one horn termed—a unicornuate uterus	
g.	A single vagina with a double uterus will result from fusion of the upper end of the ducts only	
h.	A bicornuate is a result of complete fusion at the upper portion of the uterovaginal area	
i.	A problem for pregnancy occurs only when the tissue is insufficient to allow the uterus to enlarge for a full-term fetus lying longitudinally	
j.	In situations with one horn and a double uterus, the empty horn can cause obstruction in labour—resulting in a caesarean section	

3 The female urinary tract

The urinary system is an important excretory system that plays a vital role in maintaining homeostasis of water and electrolyte concentrations in the body. The urinary tract begins with the kidneys, and continues as a passage for urine in the ureters, bladder and urethra. Completing the activities will help you to understand how this occurs.

THE STRUCTURE AND FUNCTIONS OF THE KIDNEY

   Match, label and colour

1. The kidneys are a pair of bean-shaped excretory glands. Fig. 3.1 shows the longitudinal section of the kidney. Label the structures and tissues by matching to the options provided. Colour as preferred.

Label and colour

Pelvis of kidney
Renal vein
Renal artery
Ureter

Label

Cortex
Medulla
Medullary rays
Calyx

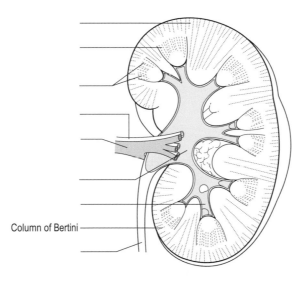

Column of Bertini

Figure 3.1

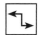 **Match**

2. The functions of the kidney can be summarized into categories of elimination, regulation and secretion. Draw a line to match the six broad functions of the kidneys.

Elimination of:	• pH of blood
Elimination of:	• Toxins
Regulation of:	• Hormones
Regulation of:	• Waste materials
Regulation of:	• Osmotic pressure of blood
Secretion of:	• Water content

The basic functional unit of the kidney

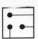 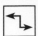 **Match, label and colour**

3. Fig. 3.2 shows a glomerular body. Match and label the structures from the list provided. Colour the structures if preferred.

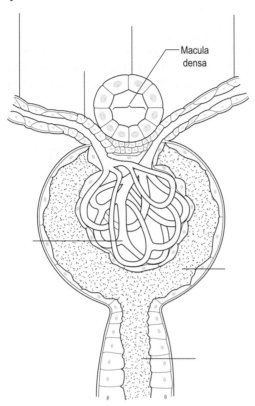

Afferent arteriole
Distal convoluted tubule
Efferent arteriole
Glomerulus
Glomerular capsule
Granular juxtaglomerular cells
Proximal convoluted tubule

Macula densa

Figure 3.2

4. Fig. 3.3 shows a nephron. Match and label the structures and tissues of the nephron from the list provided. Colour as preferred.

Label and colour

Afferent arteriole
Efferent arteriole
Branch of renal artery
Branch of renal vein

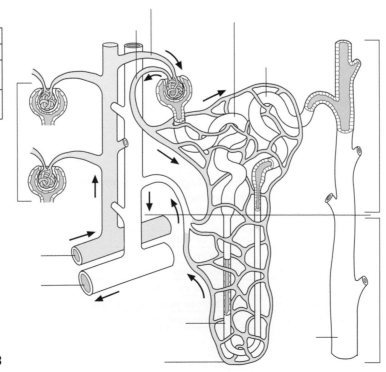

Label

Glomerular bodies
Distal convoluted tubule
Proximal convoluted tubule
Medulla
Cortex
Straight collecting tubule
Loop of Henle
Capillary

Figure 3.3

Complete

5. Complete the following activity about the production of urine by removing the incorrect words.

Three processes are involved in the production of urine: (i) **filtration/hydrolysis**; (ii) **nonselective absorption/ selective reabsorption**; and (iii) **secretion/absorption**.

In **filtration/hydrolysis**, fluid and solutes are forced through a **membrane/hilum** by **gravity/hydrostatic pressure**. Water and other small molecules pass through **easily/with difficulty**.

During **nonselective absorption/selective reabsorption**, removal of **two-thirds/one-fifth** of the filtrate takes place in the **proximal/distal** tubule. **Antidiuretic hormone (ADH)/Aldosterone** increases reabsorption of **sodium/calcium** and water. **ADH/Aldosterone** increases permeability of the tubules, **decreasing/increasing** water reabsorption.

Secretion/absorption is an important mechanism in clearing the blood of unwanted substances, for example, **drugs/sodium**.

 Multiple choice questions (MCQ)

6. The kidneys secrete several hormones. These include:

a. Cortisol and oxytocin

b. Erythropoietin, calcitriol and prostaglandins

c. Oestrogen and cortisol

d. Aldosterone, oxytocin and adrenaline

7. The glomerular filtration rate is:

a. The volume of urine produced per day

b. The systolic blood pressure within the glomerulus

c. The volume of plasma filtered through the glomeruli in 1 minute

d. The difference in plasma volume between the afferent arteriole and the efferent arteriole

8. In the healthy adult kidney there are:

a. 50,000 nephrons

b. 50,000 nephrons

c. 1 million nephrons

d. 5 million nephrons

e. 10 million nephrons

9. The main structures (renal artery, renal vein, nerves and lymphatics) enter and leave the kidney at the:

a. Medulla

b. Capsule

c. Hilum

d. Cortex

10. In the nephron, filtration takes place in the:
    a. Collecting duct
    b. Distal convoluted tubule
    c. Proximal convoluted tubule
    d. Loop of Henle
    e. Glomerulus

11. Which of the following statements is/are correct?
    a. The majority of nephrons are cortical nephrons (85%–90%) with short loops of Henle and their main function is to control plasma volume under normal circumstances.
    b. The juxtamedullary nephrons have longer loops of Henle extending into the medulla and facilitate reduced water retention when there is restricted water available.
    c. All of the above.
    d. None of the above.

12. Which options contain only normal constituents of filtrate?
    a. Water, salts and glucose
    b. Water, blood components and salts
    c. Blood corpuscles, platelets and plasma proteins
    d. Blood corpuscles, salts and glucose

13. Of the vast amount of fluid that passes out in the filtrate daily, how much of this fluid is reabsorbed?
    a. Less than 1%
    b. About 5%
    c. About 10%
    d. About 50%
    e. About 99%

14. ADH is produced by the:
    a. Cortex of the suprarenal gland
    b. Kidney
    c. Anterior pituitary gland
    d. Posterior pituitary gland
    e. Medulla of the suprarenal gland

15. Aldosterone is produced in the:
    a. Medulla of the suprarenal gland
    b. Anterior pituitary gland
    c. Posterior pituitary gland
    d. Kidney
    e. Cortex of the suprarenal gland

16. The reabsorption of sodium is primarily controlled by:

   a. ADH

   b. Aldosterone

   c. Calcitonin

   d. Adrenaline

   e. Aldosterone and antidiuretic hormone

Complete

17. Consider the following words relating to the constituents of glomerular filtrate (10 in total) and those remaining in the capillaries (5 in total). Complete Table 3.1.

Erythrocytes	Ketoacids	Plasma protein	Glucose
Water	Hormones (some)	Amino acids	Some drugs (large)
Platelets	Leucocytes	Nutrient salts	Some drugs (small)
Mineral salts	Uric acid	Creatinine	

Table 3.1

Constituents in glomerular filtrate	Constituents remaining in glomerular capillaries

The bladder, ureters and ligaments

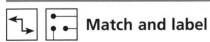 **Match and label**

18. Fig. 3.4 shows a section through the bladder. Label the structures from the list of options provided.

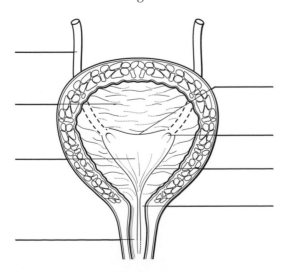

Bell's muscle
Internal urethral orifice
Interureteric bar
Rugae
Opening of the ureter
Trigone
Ureter
Urethra

Figure 3.4

Complete

19. Complete the following activity by inserting the missing word(s) and numerical values from the extended list provided:

pH	Low	High	hydrogen [H⁺]
1–14	7	7.4	6.8
Alkaline	Urine	Gastric juice	Electrolyte balance
Acidic	Blood	Osmosis	Saliva
Oxygen [O⁻]	Calcium [Ca⁺⁺]	Potassium [K⁺]	1–10

An important function of the renal system is _____. pH is a measure of

_____ ion concentration, and runs on a numerical scale of _____.

   More _____ ions result in an _____ solution demonstrated by a _____ pH

value. Less _____ ions result in an _____ solution, demonstrated by a

_____ pH value. A neutral pH value is _____. The typical pH of _____ is between 5 and 6,

compared with the pH of _____ which is 1 to 3.

Match

20. Table 3.2 provides the ligaments attached to the bladder. Using arrows, complete by correctly matching where each ligament extends from and where it is attached to.

Table 3.2

Name of ligament(s)	Extend(s) from:	Attached to:
Urachas	Bladder neck anteriorly	Symphysis pubis
Pubocervical (×2)	Bladder	Umbilicus
Lateral (×2)	Apex of bladder	Side walls of the pelvis

Correct/incorrect

21. Consider the following statements. Complete Table 3.3 by ticking the correct statements about the female urinary system.

Table 3.3

	Statement	Correct
a.	The kidneys only have an exocrine function	
b	During pregnancy, renal blood flow increases 60% by the end of the first trimester	
c.	Erythropoietin is a hormone secreted by the kidney, which stimulates the production of red blood cells	
d.	Glomerular filtration of fluids and solutes is largely a passive, non-selective process	
e.	Renal arterioles within the glomerular capillary bed are low-resistance vessels	
f	The anterior part of the bladder lies close to the symphysis pubis and is termed the *apex*	
g	The right kidney is longer, more slender and located slightly lower than the left kidney	
h	A low bacterial count of less than 100,000/mL is not significant to confirm a urinary tract infection	
i	The absence of ADH causes segments of the kidney's tubule system to become more permeable to water	
j	Certain substances, such as creatinine and toxins, are added directly to urine in the ascending arm of the loop of Henle	
k	The hormone renin is produced in the afferent arteriole and is secreted in response to a reduced blood supply and in response to low sodium levels	
l	During pregnancy, stasis of urine can result because of the relaxation influence progesterone has on the walls of the ureters	
m	In the days following birth, there is a rapid and sustained loss of sodium and a major diuresis occurs	
n	Glomerular filtration is reduced during pregnancy to compensate for the additional maternal and fetal metabolism	
o	The main changes of pregnancy are sodium retention and increased extracellular volume	

 Short answers

22. Complete Table 3.4 by providing short answers about the kidneys.

Table 3.4

A.	Name/identify the following about the kidney:	Answer
i.	The functional unit	
ii.	Cup surrounding the glomerulus	
iii.	Renal arteriole feeding the glomerulus	
iv.	Renal arteriole draining and removing blood from the glomerulus	
v.	The two distinct layers	
vi.	The intrinsic system whereby the kidneys can control its own blood supply over a wide range of arterial blood pressure	
vii.	Endocrine glands situated on the upper pole	
viii.	The hormone released from these glands into the blood when the body is stressed	
B	Identify the following measurements of the kidney:	
i.	Length	
ii.	Width	
iii.	Thickness	
iv.	Approximate weight	

23. Complete Table 3.5 by providing short answers about the bladder and urine.

Table 3.5

A	Name/identify the following about the bladder:	Answer
i.	The physiological movement propelling urine to facilitate the transport from the kidneys to the bladder for storage and elimination from the body	
ii.	Shape of the empty bladder	
iii.	Shape of the distending bladder	
iv.	The base of the bladder	
v.	Volume capacity (with range variation)	
B	Identify the characteristics of urine:	
i.	Specific gravity	
ii.	Average pH (range variation)	
iii.	% range of water content	
iv.	Average volume per day (normal circumstances)	

Pathophysiology

 True/false

24. Complete Table 3.6 by indicating which of the statements about renal agenesis are true or false.

Table 3.6

	Statement	True	False
i.	Renal agenesis is the congenital absence of only one kidney		
ii.	Non-pregnant adults with unilateral renal agenesis have a lower risk of developing hypertension		
iii.	The absence of fetal kidneys causes oligohydramnios		
iv.	Bilateral renal agenesis is a rare condition		
v.	The absence of fetal kidneys causes polyhydramnios		
vi.	Renal agenesis is the congenital absence of one or two kidneys		
vii.	Bilateral renal agenesis is a causative agent of Potter sequence (Potter syndrome)		
viii.	Adults with unilateral renal agenesis have a considerable higher risk of hypertension, which is more pronounced during pregnancy		

 Multiple choice questions (MCQ)

25. Which of the following statements accurately describes genital tract sepsis:

    a. Genital tract sepsis is a major cause of maternal morbidity and mortality.

    b. Genital tract sepsis arises from polymicrobial infections (e.g., streptococcal bacteria) which can lead to overwhelming septicaemia.

    c. Signs and symptoms include pyrexia, swinging pyrexia, hypothermia, tachycardia, tachypnoea, abdominal pain, diarrhoea and vomiting.

    d. All of the above

    e. a and b

26. Which of the following statements does not accurately describe urinary tract infection (UTI):

   a. *Escherichia coli* is the most common pathogenic bacteria involved in causing the UTI.

   b. On urinalysis, urine is opalescent, offensive and alkaline.

   c. Symptoms are similar to cystitis, including urinary frequency, dysuria and haematuria.

   d. Possible slight rise in maternal temperature.

   e. Pus and blood may be found on microscopic examination.

27. If UTI is inadequately treated and septicaemia results, then identify the possible outcomes:

   a. Acute renal failure

   b. Multiple organ failure

   c. Death

   d. All of the above

   e. a and b

28. Swelling of the kidney (or two kidneys) can result when urine fails to properly drain from the kidney to the bladder. This secondary condition is known as:

   a. Hydronephrosis

   b. Nephritis

   c. Acute pyelonephritis

   d. Chronic pyelonephritis

   e. UTI

 ## Short answers

29. Complete Table 3.7 by inserting short answers to address questions relating to pathophysiology of the urinary tract.

Table 3.7

	Questions	Answer
i.	What is the infection of the urinary tract called when there are no symptoms	
ii.	Name the investigation required to confirm diagnosis of UTI	
iii.	Name the condition if the infection is confined to the bladder	
iv.	Name the condition occurring if the infection ascends to the kidneys	
v.	In recurrent UTIs, identify one further investigation carried out to exclude underlying abnormality of the urinary tract	

4 Hormonal cycles: fertilization and early development

> The female hormonal cycles commence at puberty. This involves monthly physiological changes taking place in the ovaries and uterus and regulated by hormones produced by the hypothalamus, pituitary gland and ovaries. These cycles occur simultaneously and together are known as the *female reproductive cycle*. This chapter will help you to understand how this occurs and the processes involved.

Ovarian cycle

 Completion

1. The following paragraphs relate to the three phases of the ovarian cycle, which are all under the control of hormones. Cross out the incorrect options so that the phases involved in the ovarian cycle read correctly.

Phase one

In the **follicular/luteal** phase, low levels of ovarian hormones stimulate the **ovaries/hypothalamus** to produce **gonadotrophin releasing hormone (GnRH)/ovarian hormones**. This hormone causes the production of **oestrogen/follicle stimulating hormone (FSH)** and **luteinizing hormone (LH)/progesterone** by the **anterior/posterior** pituitary gland. Under the influence of this hormone, the Graafian follicle secretes **oestrogen/progesterone**, resulting in a surge in **LH/FSH**. The secretion of **LH/FSH** is inhibited when hormone levels reach a certain peak. Eventually, the largest and most dominant follicle secretes inhibin, which further suppresses **FSH/LH**, and this follicle prevails and becomes competent to ovulate. The time from growth and maturity of the Graafian follicles to ovulation is normally around **1/2** week(s), that is, day **5 to 14/10 to 21** of a 28-day cycle of events.

Phase two

Ovulation is stimulated by a sudden **surge/reduction** in **LH/progesterone** which matures the **oocyte/corpus luteum**. This surge occurs around day **2 to 4/12 to 13** of a 28-day cycle and lasts for **48 hours/72 hours**.

Phase three

In the final **follicular/luteal** phase, the **corpus luteum/corpus albicans** is formed by **proliferation/recession** of the residual ruptured follicle. This is a **yellow/white** irregular structure producing **oestrogen/LH** and **progesterone/FSH** for approximately **2/4** weeks. This develops the **endometrium/myometrium** of the **cervix/uterus**, which awaits the fertilized oocyte. The **corpus luteum/corpus albicans** continues its role, until the **placenta/endometrium** is adequately developed to take over this role. If fertilization does not occur, then the **corpus luteum/corpus albicans** degenerates and becomes the **corpus luteum/corpus albicans.** There is a decrease in **oestrogen and progesterone/FSH/LH hormones** and inhibin levels. These low hormone levels stimulate the **pituitary gland/hypothalamus** to produce **GnRH/FSH**. These rising hormone levels stimulate the **anterior/posterior** pituitary gland to produce **FSH/LH** and the cycle begins again.

Match, label and colour

2. Fig. 4.1 presents the cycle of a Graafian follicle in the ovary. Label Fig. 4.1 by matching from the options provided. Colour as preferred.

Developing corpus luteum	Fully developed corpus luteum	Ovarian ligament	Ovulation-released oocyte	Follicle reaching maturity
Uterine tube	Ruptured follicle	Large pre-ovulatory follicle	Developing follicles	Corpus albicans

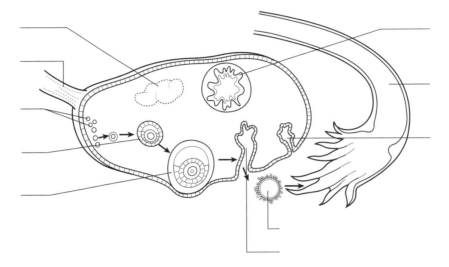

Figure 4.1

3. Fig. 4.2 shows a ripe Graafian follicle. Label Fig. 4.2 from the options provided.

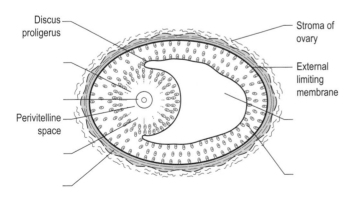

Figure 4.2

Granulosa cells
Oocyte
Zona pellucida
Theca
Follicular fluid
Corona radiata
Stroma of ovary; External limiting membrane; Discus proligerus; Perivitelline space

Female reproductive cycle and fertilization

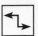 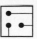 **Match, label and colour**

4. Fig. 4.3 details the female reproductive cycle during the menstrual cycle and early pregnancy. Carefully consider each section of this figure. Label the processes/structures involved by correctly matching the labels from the list provided. Colour as preferred.

1. Blastocyst	2. Embedded 'trophoblast'	3. Fertilization	4. Morula	5. Oocyte	6. Segmentation

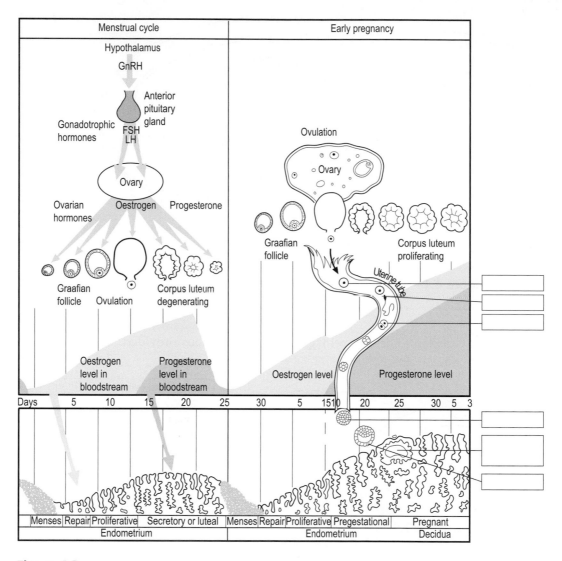

Figure 4.3

Completion

5. The menstrual cycle or endometrial cycle refers to the physiological changes that occur in the uterus in preparation to receive the fertilized oocyte. The cycle consists of three phases: menstrual, proliferative and secretory phases. Consider the following descriptive statements in Table 4.1 and tick the appropriate phase.

Table 4.1

	Statement	Menstrual phase	Proliferative phase	Secretory phase
a.	Eumenorrhoea occurs			
b.	This phase is simultaneous with ovulation			
c.	Physiologically, this is the terminal phase of the reproductive cycle			
d.	At the end of this phase, the endometrium consists of three layers			
e.	This phase is simultaneous with the beginning of the follicular phase of the ovarian cycle			
f.	In this phase, the fertilized oocyte implants itself within the endometrium			
g.	This phase follows the proliferative phase			
h.	In this phase, the spiral arteries of the endometrium go into spasm			
i.	In this phase, the functional layer of the endometrium thickens to approximately 3.5 mm thick			
j.	The blood supply to the area is increased			
k.	This phase is under the influence of progesterone and oestrogen secreted by the corpus luteum			
l.	In this phase, there is the formation of a new layer of endometrium			
m.	There is necrosis of the endometrium			
n.	This phase is under the control of oestradiol and other oestrogens secreted by the Graafian follicle			
o.	Some women experience dysmenorrhoea			
p.	Regeneration occurs			
q.	In this phase, a layer of cuboidal ciliated epithelium covers the functional layer			
r.	Glands produce nutritive secretions (such as glycogen)			
s.	In this phase, the functional layer, which contains tubular glands, is approximately 2.5 mm thick			

Fertilization

 Match and label

6. Fig. 4.4 shows a diagrammatic representation of the fusion of the oocyte and the spermatozoon (B–D are magnified). Label the figure A–D by correctly by matching to the options provided (some words may be used more than once).

Nucleus	Acrosomal vesicle	Corona radiata	Cell membrane
Release of enzyme	Zona pellucida	Plasma membrane	

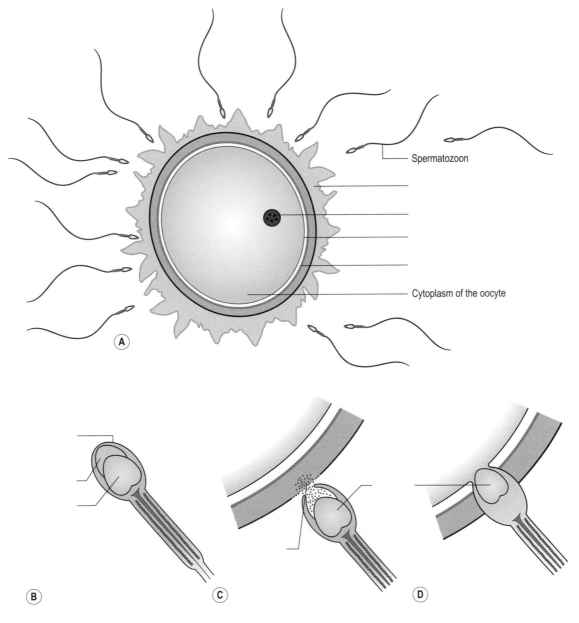

Figure 4.4

7. The following paragraph relates to the processes involved in fertilization. Cross out the incorrect word(s) so that the paragraph reads correctly.

Once inside the uterine tubes, the sperm undergo changes to the plasma membrane resulting in the removal of the glycoprotein coat. The **acrosomal/cortical** layer of the sperm becomes reactive with the release of the enzyme **hyaluronidase/hydrogenase.** This is known as the **acrosome/cortical** reaction. This reaction disperses the outermost layer of the oocyte called **corona radiata/zona pellucida,** allowing access to the **corona radiata/zona pellucida.** The first sperm that reaches the **zona pellucida/cortical layer** penetrates it with the aid of several enzymes. Upon penetration, **acrosomal/cortical** reaction occurs, which makes the **zona pellucida/cortical layer** impermeable to other sperm. The **plasma membranes/nuclei** of the oocyte and sperm fuse. The oocyte at this stage completes its **first/second** meiotic division and becomes **immature/mature.**

Development of the zygote

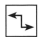

Match

8. Using arrows, match the term to the appropriate descriptive statement about the development of the zygote.

Haploid:
Blastocyst:

Diploid:
Morula:
Blastomeres:

a. The embryo now consists of 16–20 cells by the 3rd/4th day after fertilization.
b. Small cells produced by initial mitosis (cellular replication and division) of the zygote within 24 hours of fertilization.
c. Contains one of each pair of chromosomes (23 chromosomes, gamete).
d. A cell containing two sets of chromosomes 46 chromosomes, zygote).
e. This develops after cavitation, whereby the outermost cells secrete fluid into the morula resulting in a fluid filled cavity.

Short answers

9. Complete Table 4.2 by inserting brief answers to the list of questions related to fertilization and early development (zygote and embryo).

Table 4.2

	Question	Short answer
i.	In the development of the embryo, identify the layer forming the tissue that covers most of the body surfaces—the epidermis layer of the skin, hair, nails. It also forms the nervous system	
ii.	Each human cell has 46 chromosomes (23 pairs) with one pair of sex chromosomes. Name the term used for the remaining pairs	
iii.	In the development of the embryo, identify the layer forming the muscle, skeleton, connective tissue, blood vessels and blood, lymph cells, the urogenital glands and dermis of the skin	
iv.	In the healthy fertile male, identify the estimated number of sperm deposited in the vagina during intercourse	
v.	Estimate the number of sperm that will reach the oocyte following intercourse	
vi.	In the development of the embryo, identify the layer forming the epithelia lining of the respiratory, digestive, urinary systems and the glandular cells of organs, such as liver and pancreas	
vii.	In the development of the zygote, identify the cells giving rise to the cells of the embryo	

Development of the blastocyst

Completion

10. The following question relates to the blastocyst and development into the embryo. Complete the paragraph by inserting the correct words from the list provided. All words are used at least one, with some used more than once.

Decidua   Trophoblast   Uterus   Embryo
Placenta   Embryoblast   Amnion

In the first few days following fertilization, the zygote undergoes mitotic cellular replication and division as it journeys along the uterine tubes. The blastocyst, formed between days 3 and 5, enters the

_____. The blastocyst possesses an inner cell mass (or _____) and an outer

cell mass (or _____). Implantation of the _____ layer occurs into the

endometrium, and this layer is now known as the_____. The outer cell mass (or

_____) becomes the a) _____ and b) chorion, while the inner cell mass (or

_____) becomes the c) _____, d) _____ and e) umbilical cord.

True/False

11. Consider the following statements in Table 4.3 and indicate if they are true or false by ticking the appropriate column.

Table 4.3

	Statement	True	False
a.	Blastulation occurs around day 4 and refers to the process involved in the development of the morula to the blastocyst		
b.	Mittleschmerz is the term that refers to the varying degrees of abdominal pain experienced by women during ovulation		
c.	Under the influence of oestrogen the cervix secretes a flow of alkaline mucus that attracts the spermatozoa		
d.	The syncytiotrophoblast layer of the trophoblast cells or syncytium invade the decidua by forming villi		
e.	The oocyte moves along the uterine tube by the action of cilia and peristalsis		
f.	Implantation of the trophoblast layer into the endometrium is usually in the upper posterior wall of the uterus		
g.	Once inside the uterine tubes, the sperm undergo a process known as *decapacitation*		
h.	The syncytiotrophoblast cells produce human chorionic gonadotrophin (hCG) hormone		
i.	The preembryonic period is always a safe period in terms of early embryonic development		
j.	Hypoblast layer of the embryoblast give rise to extra-amniotic structures only, such as the yolk sac		
k.	Lacunae are spaces in the decidua that fill up with maternal blood		
l.	After birth, the only remains of the yolk sac is the vitelline duct at the base of the umbilical cord		

? Multiple choice questions (MCQs)

12. In the initiation of puberty, the following are thought to have a role:
   a. The interaction of leptin with GnRH
   b. The interaction of prolactin with GnRH and FSH
   c. The interaction of leptin, prolactin and FSH
   d. None of the above

13. The following is/are correct:
    a. Each sperm will carry only a Y chromosome
    b. Each sperm carries either an X or Y chromosome
    c. The oocyte always carries an X chromosome
    d. a and c
    e. b and c

14. The following is/are incorrect:
    a. Dizygotic twins (fraternal) are produced from two oocytes released independently (in the same time frame)
    b. Dizygotic twins (fraternal) are genetically different as they are fused with two different sperm
    c. Monozygotic twins are genetically identical.
    d. Monozygotic twins develop from two zygotes
    e. None of the above

15. The process of human fertilization normally takes approximately:
    a. 1 hour
    b. 24 hours
    c. 48 hours
    d. 4 hours

16. Human fertilization normally occurs in the:
    a. Ampulla of the uterine tube
    b. Fimbria of the uterine tube
    c. Fundus of the uterus
    d. Isthmus of the uterine tube

17. The embryoblast cells:
    a. Differentiate into epiblasts (closest to the trophoblast)
    b. Differentiate into hypoblasts (closest to the blastocyst cavity)
    c. Give rise to cells of the embryo
    d. All of the above

18. Following fertilization, the first appearance of the primitive streak is around:
    a. 2 days
    b. 5 days
    c. 10 days
    d. 15 days
    e. 20 days

19. Which of the following statements is/are correct:

    a. During embryological development, stem cells under predetermined genetic control become specialized.

    b. The zygote can give rise to a whole organism, known as a totipotent stem cell.

    c. Pluripont cells refer to stem cells, such as those in the inner cell mass, which can give rise to many different types of cells.

    d. Multipotent cells are specialization of pluripont cells giving rise to cells with more specific functions.

    e. All of the above.

Pathophysiology

The following are pathophysiology related questions.

 Correct/Incorrect

20. Consider each statement in Table 4.4. Identify the correct statements.

Table 4.4

	Statement	Correct
i.	Ectopic pregnancy or miscarriage can result from the inability for proper implantation	
ii.	Chromosomal defects and abnormalities in structure and in organ development can occur during the preembryonic period	
iii.	Stem cells taken from an embryo and transferred into another individual with no genetic match will not cause any rejection issues or problems	
iv.	Stem cells in adult organs have the potential to become any type of cell in a specific organ	
v.	Cytogenics is the study of chromosomes	
vi.	Translocation occurs when a chromosome fragment breaks off and is added to another chromosome	
vii.	An abnormal number of chromosomes present after fertilization is often caused by abnormal events during mitosis	
viii.	Down syndrome, one of the commonest chromosomal birth anomalies, has 47 chromosomes instead of 46 (termed trisomy 21)	

 Short answers

21. Complete Table 4.5 by inserting the answer to each question.

Table 4.5

	Question	Answer
i.	Identify one common chromosomal anomaly among sex chromosomes	
ii.	Provide an example of a recessively inherited autosomal condition	
iii.	Provide an example of a dominantly inherited autosomal condition	
iv.	Provide an example X-linked recessive disease	

5 The placenta

The fully developed placenta is a vital and complex organ serving as the interface between the mother and the developing fetus. Survival of the fetus depends upon the integrity and efficiency of the placenta, membranes and umbilical cord. This chapter will help you to understand the development, processes and function.

Early development of the placenta

 Label

1. Fig. 5.1 shows the chorionic villi. Match and label the structures and tissues from the list provided.

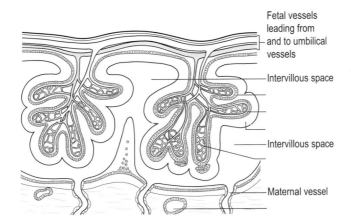

Fetal vessels leading from and to umbilical vessels

Intervillous space

Intervillous space

Maternal vessel

| Decidual gland |
| Cytotrophoblast |
| Fetal capillary |
| Syncytiotrophoblast |
| Mesoderm |

Figure 5.1

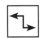 **Match, label and colour**

2. Fig. 5.2 shows the blood flow around the chorionic villi. Match and label the structures and tissues from the options provided. Colour as preferred.

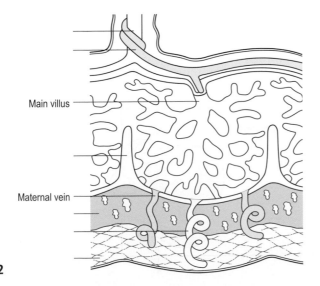

Main villus

Maternal vein

| Umbilical vein |
| Umbilical artery |
| Decidua |
| Septum |
| Maternal spiral artery |
| Uterine muscle |

Figure 5.2

Complete

3. Table 5.1 presents an overview of the sequence of events involved in the early development of the placenta. Complete the table by inserting the missing words from the list provided.

chorionic villi	trophoblasts	sinuses	chorion laeve
cytokines	blastocyst	decidua vera (× 2)	decidual basilis
decidua	blood spaces	decidua capsularis (× 2)	placenta

Table 5.1 Early development of the placenta

a.	By 10 days, the _____ is completely buried in the decidua. The _____ have a potent invasive capacity. The decidua secretes _____ and protease inhibitors that moderate this invasion.

↓

b.	From about 3 weeks after fertilization, proliferation of projections from the trophoblastic layer form the _____ This becomes more profuse in the _____ where there is a rich blood supply. This is known as the *chorion frondosum*, which will develop into the _____.

↓

c.	The portion of the decidua surrounding the blastocyst where it projects into the uterine cavity is known as the _____. The villi under this area degenerates (because of lack of nutrition) forming the _____ from where the chorionic membrane originates, The remaining decidua is known as the _____ (or parietalis).

↓

d.	As the uterus is filled with the enlarging fetus, the _____ thins and disappears and the chorion meets the _____ (or parietalis) on the opposite wall of the uterus.

↓

e.	The villi penetrate the _____ and erode the walls of the maternal blood vessels opening them up to form a lake of maternal blood in which they float. The opening blood vessels are known as _____ and the area surrounding the villi are called _____.

The mature placenta

 Complete

4. The placenta performs a variety of functions for the developing fetus. List the six key functions using the pneumonic SERPENT presented in Fig. 5.3.

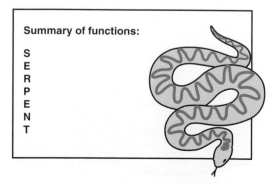

Summary of functions:

S
E
R
P
E
N
T

Figure 5.3

5. This question relates to placental circulation. Complete the subsequent paragraphs by removing the incorrect terms:

Maternal blood is discharged into the intervillous space by **25 to 50/80 to 100** spiral arteries within the decidua basilis after **2 to 4 weeks/10 to 12 weeks**. Blood flows **slowly/quickly** around the villi, eventually returning to the endometrial **veins/arteries** and the maternal circulation. There are about **50 mL/150 mL** of maternal blood in the intervillous spaces, which is exchanged **3 or 4/9 or 10** times per minute.

Fetal blood is **high/low** in oxygen. The fetal heart pumps the blood towards the placenta and along the umbilical **vein/arteries** and then transported along their branches to the **capillaries/arterioles** of the chorionic **villi/membrane**, where exchange of nutrients takes place between mother and fetus. After yielding **oxygen/carbon dioxide** and waste products and absorbing **carbon dioxide/oxygen** and nutrients, the blood is returned to the fetus via the umbilical **arteries/vein**.

 ## True/false

6. Consider the following statements in Table 5.2 and indicate if they are true or false by ticking the appropriate column.

Table 5.2

	Statement	True	False
a.	Between 12- and 22-weeks' gestation, the placenta weighs less than the fetus		
b.	Nitrogen is the main substance excreted from the placenta		
c.	The cytotrophoblast cells and the syncytiotrophoblast gradually degenerate as some of the fetal organs develop (an example is the liver)		
d.	The placenta cannot store iron and fat-soluble vitamins		
e.	Oxygen from the maternal haemoglobin passes directly into the fetal blood by simple diffusion		
f.	Fat-soluble vitamins (A, C, D and E) cross the placenta		
g.	Carbon dioxide passes into maternal blood by simple diffusion		
h.	Nutrients are actively transferred from maternal to fetal blood through the walls of the villi		
i.	The placenta provides only a limited barrier to infection		
j.	Amino acids are found at lower levels in the fetal blood than in maternal blood		

 ## Short answers

7. Complete the questions and short answers in Table 5.3.

Table 5.3

	Question	Answer
a.	Identify two types of villi:	_____ _____
b.	Identify one bacteria that can cross the placenta:	_____ _____
c.	Identify two viruses that can cross the placenta:	_____ _____
d.	List four key hormones produced by the placenta:	_____ _____ _____ _____

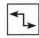

Match

8. Using arrows or lines, complete the following statements about nutritional function of the mature placenta by matching and connecting the correct terms from the list (a–e) provided.

1   Amino acids and glucose are required for
2   Calcium and phosphorus are required for
3   The placenta stores glucose in the form of
4   The placenta excretes carbon dioxide and also excretes
5   Iron is required for

a.   Blood formation
b.   Glycogen
c.   Bones and teeth
d.   Energy and growth
e.   Bilirubin

Placental membranes

Completion

9. The following words/phrases relate to either the amnion or the chorion membrane. Consider each and then complete Table 5.4 by matching them to the appropriate membrane.

Table 5.4

	Term	Chorion	Amnion
a.	Outer membrane		
b.	Inner membrane		
c.	Smooth		
d.	Tough		
e.	Thick		
f.	Translucent		
g.	Derived from the inner cell mass		
h.	Friable		
i.	Derived from the trophoblast		
j.	Opaque		
k.	Lines the surface of the placenta		
l.	Continues with the outer surface of the umbilical cord		
m.	Fibrous		
n.	Continuous with the edge of the placenta		

Amniotic fluid

Completion

10. Consider the main function of amniotic fluid in Table 5.5. Complete this table by appropriately matching each function to either 'during pregnancy' or 'in labour (intact membranes)'.

Table 5.5

During pregnancy	Function of amniotic fluid	In labour with intact membranes
	a. Has a small nutritional function	
	b. Maintains constant temperature for the fetus	
	c. Protects the placenta and umbilical cord from pressure during uterine contractions	
	d. Supports dilatation of the uterine os	
	e. Protects fetus from injury	
	f. Aids effacement of the cervix	
	g. Allows normal growth and free fetal movement	
	h. Equalizes pressure	

Correct/incorrect

11. Table 5.6 provides statements about the placenta and umbilical cord at term. Complete the activity by indicating if the statements are correct or incorrect.

Table 5.6

	Statements	Correct	Incorrect
a.	The maternal surface of the placenta is arranged into cotyledons (lobes) and is dark red in colour		
b.	It is approximately 35 cm in diameter		
c.	The fetal surface of the placenta has a shiny appearance		
d.	The thickness in the centre is approximately 2.5 cm		
e.	The fetal surface is covered by the chorion		
f.	The amnion can be peeled off the surface of the chorion to the umbilical cord		
g.	Normally the umbilical cord has two vessels only		
h.	The sulci separate the cotyledons (lobes)		
i.	Risks of a long cord include knotting and becoming wrapped around the fetal neck or body		
j.	The placenta weighs approximately one-fifth of the baby's weight		
k.	Wharton's jelly encloses and protects the umbilical blood vessels		
l.	The length of the umbilical cord is normally 50–60 cm with a diameter of 3–4 cm		
m.	There are two umbilical veins and one umbilical artery		

 Multiple choice questions (MCQ)

12. The placenta is completely formed and functioning in:

    a. 8 weeks after fertilization

    b. 10 weeks after fertilization

    c. 12 weeks after fertilization

    d. 14 weeks after fertilization

13. Antibodies in the form of immunoglobulin G (IgG) transferred to the placenta offer the baby passive immunity for the first:

    a. 1 month

    b. 2 months

    c. 3 months

    d. 6 months

14. Maternal and fetal blood is separated by:

    a. Two layers of tissues

    b. Three layers of tissues

    c. Four layers of tissues

    d. Six layers of tissues

15. Amniotic fluid is thought to be:

    a. Exuded from maternal vessels in the deciduas

    b. Exuded from fetal vessels in the placenta

    c. Secreted by the amnion

    d. All of the above

16. The water in amniotic fluid is exchanged approximately:

    a. Hourly

    b. 3-hourly

    c. 6-hourly

    d. Daily

17. The volume of amniotic fluid is greatest at approximately:

    a. 36 weeks' gestation

    b. 38 weeks' gestation

    c. 40 weeks' gestation

    d. None of the above

18. A hydatidiform mole will produce excessive amounts of which placental protein hormone:

    a. Oestrogen

    b. Human placental lactogen (hPL)

    c. Human chorionic gonadotrophin (hCG)

    d. Schwangerschaftsprotein

19. Which of the following **is** not secreted by the maternal part of the placenta and the decidua.

    a. Prolactin

    b. Estradiol

    c. Relaxin

    d. Prostaglandins

20. Which of the following is not considered a cause of polyhydramnios:

    a. Multiple pregnancy

    b. Fetal renal anomalies

    c. Maternal diabetes mellitus

    d. Rhesus isoimmunization

Anatomical variations of placenta and cord

 Short answers

21. The following Figs 5.4 to 5.6 relate to anatomical variations of the placenta and cord. Name and describe the type of variation and identify any associated risks:

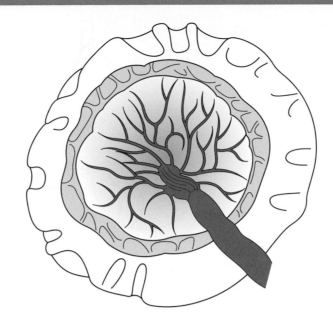

Figure 5.4

A. Type of placenta: 5.4: _____

Description: _____

_____

_____

Risk factors: _____

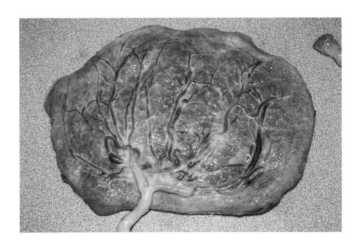

Figure 5.5

B. Type of placenta: 5.5: _____

Description: _____

_____

Risk factors: _____

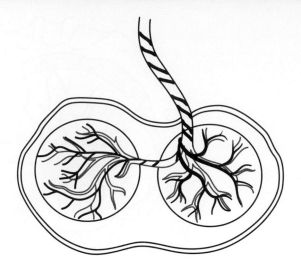

Figure 5.6

C. Type of placenta: 5.6: _____

Description: _____

_____

Risk factors: _____

6 The fetus

This chapter focuses on fetal growth and development, the fetal circulation and fetal skull. Knowledge of fetal development is essential to understand the situation for both preterm and term babies born. The following activities will help you to assess your knowledge in these areas.

FETAL DEVELOPMENT

Development of the embryo

 Complete

1. Embryological development is complex and occurs from week 2 to 8 after fertilization followed by fetal development, until birth of the baby. The statements in Table 6.1 relate to embryological or fetal development up to 20 weeks' gestation. Complete Table 6.1 by ticking the appropriate gestational age range for each statement.

Table 6.1

Embryological and fetal development	Weeks of gestation				
	0–4	4–8	8–12	12–16	16–20
a. Rapid weight gain					
b. Meconium present in gut					
c. Swallowing begins					
d. External genitalia distinguishes gender					
e. 'Quickening'—mother feels fetal movements					
f. Limb buds form					
g. Primitive streak appears					
h. Nasal septum and palate fuse					
i. Early movements					
j. Urine passed					
k. Vernix caseosa appears					
l. Lanugo appears					
m. Fetal heart heard on auscultation					
n. Gender determined					

Development of the fetus

2. The statements in Table 6.2 relate to fetal development from 20 weeks' gestation until birth of the baby. Complete Table 6.2 by ticking the appropriate gestational age range for each statement.

Table 6.2

Fetal development	Weeks of gestation				
	20–24	24–28	28–32	32–36	36–birth
a. Weight gain 25 g/day					
b. Respiratory movements					
c. Lanugo disappears from body					
d. Responds to sound					
e. Skull formed but soft and pliable					
f. Head hair lengthens					
g. Begins to store fat and iron					
h. Plantar creases visible					
i. Increased fat makes body more rounded					
j. Eyelids open					
k. Skin red and wrinkled					
l. Testes descend into scrotum					
m. Surfactant secreted in the lungs					

Fetal circulation

The placenta is the source of oxygenation, nutrition and excretion of waste products of metabolism for the fetus. In addition, several temporary structures enable the fetal circulation to occur. Sound knowledge of the structures and processes involved in the fetal circulation and adaptation to extrauterine life is essential for midwives.

Match and label

3. Fig. 6.1 presents a diagram of the fetal circulation. Match and label the structures as listed subsequently. In addition, two different shading formats indicate oxygenated blood flow and deoxygenated blood flow. Please identify which shade correlates to each on the figure.

Label

Superior vena cava
Aorta (descending aorta)
Umbilical vein
Inferior vena cava
Pulmonary artery
Pulmonary veins
Umbilical arteries
Umbilicus
Left lung
Liver
Right lung
Portal vein
Renal vein
Renal artery
Temporary structures:
• Foramen ovale
• Ductus venosus
• Ductus arteriosus
• Hypogastric arteries

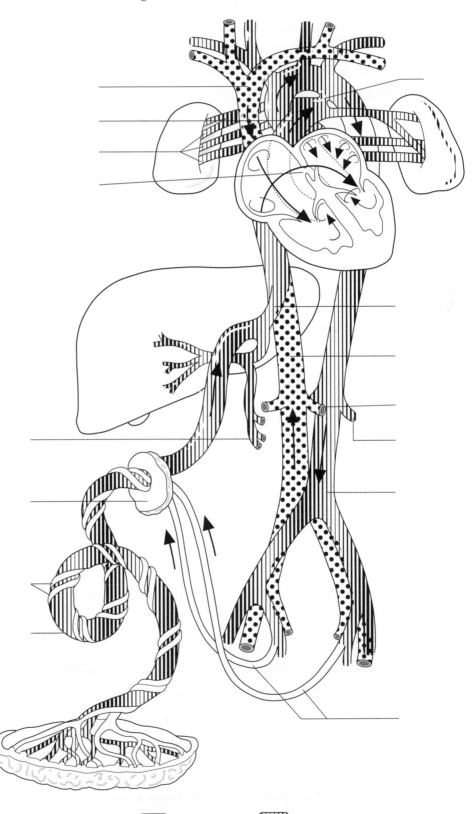

Figure 6.1

Complete

4. Complete Table 6.3 by inserting the missing terms relating to the temporary structures in the fetal circulation (refer to Fig. 6.1).

Table 6.3

Temporary structures	
a.	The _____ connects the umbilical vein to the inferior vena cava
b.	The _____ leads from the bifurcation of the pulmonary artery to the descending aorta
c.	The _____ . _____ is an opening between the right and left atria
d.	The _____ . _____ branch off from the internal iliac arteries and become the umbilical arteries when they enter the umbilical cord

5. Table 6.4 presents the sequence of events relating to the blood flowing in the fetal circulation. Complete the table by removing the incorrect word(s).

Table 6.4

a. Oxygenated blood from the placenta travels **to/from** the fetus in the **umbilical vein/umbilical arteries**. The **umbilical vein/ umbilical arteries divide(s)** into two branches: one that supplies the **portal vein/inferior vena cava** in the liver, the other the **ductus venosus/ductus arteriosus** joining the **inferior/superior** vena cava.

b. Most of the oxygenated blood that enters the **right/left** atrium passes across the foramen ovale to the **right/left** atrium and from here into the **left/right** ventricle, and then to the **aorta/pulmonary artery**. The head and **upper/lower** extremities receive about half of the blood supply via the coronary and carotid arteries, and subclavian arteries, respectively. The remainder of blood travels in the **descending aorta/inferior vena cava**, mixing with **oxygenated/deoxygenated** blood from the **right/left** ventricle.

c. **Oxygenated/deoxygenated** blood collected from the upper parts of the body returns to the **right/left** atrium in the **inferior/superior** vena cava. Blood that has entered the **right/left** atrium from the inferior and superior vena cava passes into the **left/right** ventricle. A small amount of blood travels to the lungs in the **pulmonary artery/pulmonary veins** for lung development.

d. Most blood passes through the **ductus venosus/arteriosus** into the **ascending/descending** aorta. **Deoxygenated/ oxygenated** blood travels back to the placenta via the **internal/external** iliac arteries leading into the hypogastric **arteries/ veins**, which lead into the umbilical **vein/arteries**.

 Short answers

6. Table 6.5 relates to the adaptation to extrauterine life. Complete the following statements by inserting the missing terms:

Table 6.5

	Statement	Answer
a.	The ductus venosus becomes the _____	
b.	The umbilical vein becomes the _____	
c.	The ductus arteriosus becomes the _____	
d.	The foramen ovale becomes the _____	
e.	The hypogastic arteries are known as the _____	
	except for the first few centimetres which remain open as the:_____	
	_____	

Multiple choice questions (MCQ)

The following MCQs relate to the embryo/fetal growth and development, fetal circulation and adaptation to extrauterine life.

7. Fetal erythrocytes have a life span of:

    a. 60 days   b. 90 days   c. 120 days   d. 150 days

8. Surfactant:

    a. Is a lipoprotein that reduces surface tension

    b. Is produced by type II alveolar cells

    c. Assists gaseous exchange

    d. All of the above

9. What is the approximate circulating blood volume of the neonate at birth?

    a. 65–75 mL/kg

    b. 75–85 mL/kg

    c. 85–90 mL/kg

    d. 90–95 mL/kg

10. The neural tube is derived from the:

    a. Ectoderm

    b. Endoderm

    c. Mesoderm

    d. None of the above

11. Fetal haemoglobin (HbF):

    a. Has greater affinity for oxygen than adult haemoglobin (HbA)

    b. Has greater concentrations (18–20 g/dL at term) than adult haemoglobin (HbA)

    c. Is found in the erythrocytes produced by the yolk sac and liver

    d. All of the above

12. In developed countries, the average birth weight is around:

    a. 2400 g

    b. 3000 g

    c. 3400 g

    d. 3800 g

13. What percentage of oxygenated blood is directed through the pulmonary artery to the lung tissue in fetal life?

    a. 10%

    b. 20%

    c. 30%

    d. 40%

Pathophysiology

 Correct/Incorrect

14. Table 6.6 provides statements related to pathological changes in fetal development. Complete the table by indicating if the statements are correct or incorrect.

Table 6.6

	Statement	Correct	Incorrect
a.	In the classification of conjoined twins, OMPHALOPAGUS indicates they are joined at the anterior abdominal wall		
b.	Twin-twin transfusion syndrome **only** occurs in monoamniotic twin pregnancies		
c.	A single uterine artery is always indicative or renal abnormalities and requires investigation		
d.	Asymmetric fetal growth retardation is when fetal weight is reduced out of proportion to length and head circumference		
e.	During a fetomaternal haemorrhage (FMH), 0.5 mL to 5 mL of fetal blood enters the maternal circulation		
f.	Severe maternal protein calorie malnutrition has no impact on fetal growth and development		

FETAL SKULL

Structures of the fetal skull

 Complete

15. The skull is divided into the vault, the base and the face. Complete Table 6.7 by providing short answers to the related activities/questions.

Table 6.7

	Activity	Response
a.	The face is composed of firmly united small bones. How many bones are present?	
b.	The bones are described as being:	
c.	Identify the main structures the base of the skull protects:	
d.	List three key ossification centres on the skull:	i.
		ii.
		iii.
e.	The vault is dome-shaped and situated above an imaginary line drawn between two landmarks. Identify the landmarks.	i.
		ii.
f.	What does ossification relate to?	
g.	Define the terms suture and fontanelle:	
	Suture:	
	Fontanelle:	

16. Table 6.8 provides information on the three bones of the vault. Complete the table by providing the missing information.

Table 6.8

	Name the main bone(s) of the vault	Brief description of position	Ossification centre
a.		Form the forehead and sinciput	
b.		Lie on either side of the skull	
c.		Lies at the back of the head	

17. Table 6.9 provides information about the sutures. Complete the table by inserting the name of the suture to match the description.

Table 6.9

	Name of suture	Describe position of each suture
a.		Separates the frontal bones from the parietal bones, passing from one temple to the other
b.		Runs between the two halves of the frontal bone
c.		Separates the occipital bone from the two parietal bones
d.		Lies between the two parietal bones

18. Table 6.10 relates to the two fontanelles. Complete the table by providing the correct responses.

Table 6.10

	Activity	Answer
i)	**Posterior fontanelle**	
a.	What is the alternative name?	
b.	Describe the size and shape	
c.	Describe the position of this fontanelle and identify sutures involved	
d.	When does it close?	
ii)	**Anterior fontanelle**	
a.	What is the alternative name?	
b.	Describe the size and shape	
c.	Describe the position of this fontanelle and identify sutures involved	
d.	When does it close?	

 ## Label and colour

19. Fig. 6.2 shows the division of the skull. Label the three main divisions—face, vault and base. Colour as preferred.

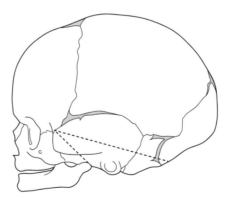

Figure 6.2

The skull is further separated into regions with important landmarks. During vaginal examinations, the landmarks provide useful information in relation to the position of the fetal head.

Match, label and colour

20. Fig. 6.3 presents a view of the fetal head from above with the head partially flexed. Label the figure from the list provided. Colour as preferred.

Label and colour

Frontal eminence or boss
Occipital protuberance
Parietal eminence

Label

Anterior fontanelle
Occipital bone
Posterior fontanelle
Frontal bone
Parietal bone

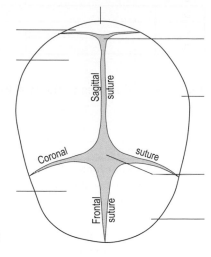

Figure 6.3

 Complete

21. Table 6.11 relates to the regions of the fetal head. Complete the table by inserting the missing information from the list provided.

Occipital protruberance   Orbital ridges   Parietal eminences
Glabella   Foramen magnum   Mentum
Neck   Coronal suture

Table 6.11

	Name of region	Position boundaries
a.	Forehead/sinciput	This region extends from the anterior fontanelle and the _____ to the orbital ridges.
b.	Face	The face extends from the _____ and the root of the nose to the junction of the chin or _____ (landmark) and the _____. The point between the eyebrows is known as the _____ (landmark).
c.	Occiput	This region lies between the _____ and posterior fontanelle. The part below the _____ (landmark) is known as suboccipital region.
d.	Vertex	This region is bounded by the posterior fontanelle, the _____ and the anterior fontanelle.

Landmarks of the fetal skull

 Label

22. Fig. 6.4 shows the fetal skull regions and landmarks. Label the following structures:

Anterior fontanelle
Mentum
Posterior fontanelle
Frontal bone
Occipital protuberance
Suboccipital region
Glabella
Parietal eminence

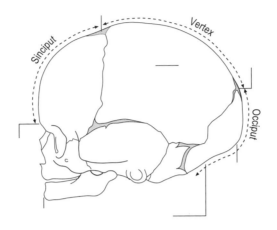

Temporal bone
Frontal bone
Parietal bone
Lambdoidal suture
Coronal suture

Figure 6.4

Knowledge of the diameters of the skull and diameters of the pelvis is essential for midwives to determine the relationship between the fetal head and maternal pelvis during labour.

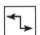 **Match**

23. Table 6.12a,b relate to the six longitudinal diameters of the fetal skull. Using lines, complete Table 6.12a by appropriately matching the diameter to the correct areas measured for each diameter. Using lines, complete Table 6.12b by matching the diameter to the correct length (cm).

Table 6.12a

Name of diameter	Areas the diameter is measured between:
Suboccipitofrontal (SOF) 10	i. From the point of the chin to the highest point on the vertex
Occipitofrontal (OF) 11.5	ii. From the point where the chin joins the neck to the centre of the anterior fontanelle
Suboccipitobregmatic (SOB) 9.5	iii. From below the occipital protuberance to the centre of the frontal suture
Submentovertical (SMV) 11.5	iv. From the occipital protuberance to the glabella
Submentobregmatic (SMB) 9.5	v. From the point where the chin joins the neck to the highest point on the vertex
Mentovertical (MV) 13.5	vi. From below the occipital protuberance to the centre of the anterior fontanelle

Table 6.12b

Diameter	Length (cm)
MV, Mentovertical	• 11.5
SOB, Suboccipitobregmatic	• 10
SMV, Submentovertical	• 9.5
SOF, Suboccipitofrontal	• 13.5
OF, Occipitofrontal	• 11.5
SMB, Submentobregmatic	• 9.5

Short answers

24. Complete the short answers to the activities related to landmarks and fetal diameters in Table 6.13. It is important to have knowledge of the diameters of the fetal trunk for delivery of the shoulders and breech births.

Table 6.13

	Activity	Answer
a.	Identify the alternative name for the anterior fontanelle	
b.	**Bisacromial diameter:**	
	Identify the length	
	This diameter is measured as the distance between which areas of the fetus?	
c.	**Bitrochanteric diameter:**	
	Identify the length	
	This diameter is measured as the distance between which areas of the fetus?	
	Identify the presenting diameter in breech presentation	

 ## Label

25. Fig. 6.5 shows the transverse diameters of the fetal skull. Label the biparietal diameter and bitemporal diameter and include each measurement (cm).

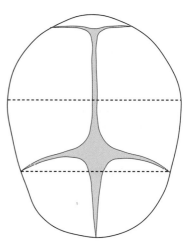

Figure 6.5

 ## Completion

26. The presenting diameters of the fetal head (a longitudinal diameter and transverse diameter) are those that are at right angles to the curve of Carus. The presenting diameters determine the presentation of the fetal head. Table 6.14 provides an activity about the three presentations of the fetal head. Complete the table by correcting the paragraphs by crossing out the incorrect diameters and numerical values.

Table 6.14

a.	**Vertex presentation:** When the head is well flexed the **suboccipitobregmatic diameter (9.5 cm)/submentobregmatic (9.5 cm)** and the biparietal diameter (**9.5 cm/10 cm**) present. The **suboccipitofrontal (10 cm)/suboccipitobregmatic (9.5 cm)** diameter distends the vaginal orifice. When the head is deflexed, the presenting diameters are the occipitofrontal (**10.0 cm/11.5 cm**) and the **biparietal (9.5 cm)/bitemporal (8.2 cm)**. This often arises when the occiput is in a **posterior/anterior** position. If this remains, then the occipitofrontal diameter (**10.5 cm/11.5 cm**) distends the vaginal orifice and the biparietal (9.5 cm). This often arises when the occiput is in a posterior position. If this remains, then the occipitofrontal diameter (11.5 cm) distends the vaginal orifice.
b.	**Face presentation:** When the head is completely **flexed/extended**, the presenting diameters are the **submentobregmatic (9.5 cm)/suboccipitobregmatic (10.5 cm)** and the **biparietal (9.5 cm)/bitemporal (8.2 cm)**. The submentovertical diameter (**10.5 cm/11.5 cm**) will distend the vaginal orifice.
c.	**Brow presentation:** This occurs when the head is **partially/fully** extended and the **mentovertical (13.5 cm)/submentovertical (11.5 cm)** diameter and **biparietal (9.5 cm)/bitemporal (8.2 cm)** present. Vaginal birth is unlikely.

Moulding of the fetal skull

 Short answers

27. Complete the following questions:

a Define the term moulding:

b Why does this happen?

Internal structures of the fetal skull

 Label

28. Fig. 6.6 shows a coronal section through the fetal head to show intracranial membranes and venous sinuses. Label the structures and tissues using the list provided:

Arachnoid mater
Lateral sinus
Pons Varolii
Cerebrum
Medulla oblongata
Sagittal suture
Cerebellum
Parietal bone
Superior sagittal sinus
Falx cerebri
Periosteum
Tentorium cerebelli
Inferior sagittal sinus
Pia mater
Two layers of dura mater

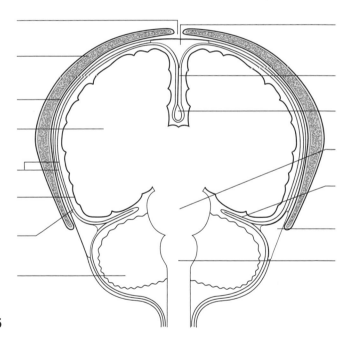

Figure 6.6

29. Fig. 6.7 shows intracranial membranes and venous sinuses. Label the structures and tissues using the list provided:

Confluence of sinuses
Inferior sagittal sinus
Superior sagittal sinus
Falx cerebri
Lateral sinus
Tentorium cerebelli
Great cerebral vein
Straight sinus
To internal jugular vein

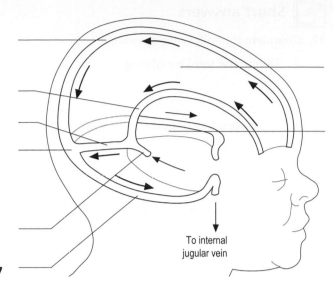

To internal jugular vein

Figure 6.7

 Multiple choice questions (MCQ)

30. The bitrochanteric diameter is the presenting diameter in:

    a. Brow presentation

    b. Face presentation

    c. Breech presentation

    d. Vertex presentation

31. The articulation of the clavicles on the sternum may reduce the diameter slightly in the:

    a. Mentovertical diameter

    b. Bitemporal diameter

    c. Bisacromial diameter

    d. Bitrochanteric diameter

32. A tear in the tentorium cerebella may result in:

    a. Bleeding from the great cerebral vein

    b. Bleeding from the arachnoid mater

    c. Bleeding from the lateral sinuses

    d. None of the above

33. Craniosynostosis describes a condition whereby the sutures on the skull are

    a. Irregularly positioned

    b. Abnormally wide

    c. Closed or fused prematurely

    d. None of the above

34. Which term correctly identifies a condition whereby a significant portion of brain, skull and scalp is absent?

    a. Holoprosencephaly

    b. Anencephaly

    c. Lissencephaly

    d. Brachycephaly

35. Which of the following is a serious birth injury commonly associated in births assisted by vacuum extraction?

    a. Subaponeurotic haemorrhage

    b. Intraparenchymal haemorrhage

    c. Porencephalic cysts

    d. Intracranial haemorrhage

7 Anatomy and physiology: body systems revision

This chapter focuses on the anatomy and physiology of body systems, including the haematological, cardiovascular, respiratory, gastrointestinal, central nervous and endocrine systems. The reproductive and renal systems are in previous chapters. It is important for midwives to have knowledge about these systems in the nonpregnant individual to fully understand and appreciate the dramatic and profound changes occurring in body systems during pregnancy.

Haematological—physiology of blood

 Match

1. Complete Table 7.1 by drawing a line between the terms in column A with the correct role or function in column B.

Table 7.1

A	B
Haemopoiesis	• Oxygen and carbon dioxide transport function
Erythrocytes	• Represents the percentage of total blood volume occupied with erythrocytes
Leucocytes	• Has a function in haemostasis
Thrombocytes	• Has a function in osmotic distribution of fluid between compartments
Pluripotent stem cell	• Blood cell formation
Haematocrit	• Blood plasma without fibrinogen and other clotting factors
Serum	• All blood cells descend from this bone marrow cell
Electrolytes	• Defence against microorganism function

 Complete

2. Complete Table 7.2 by inserting the correct numerical values from the numerical list provided.

55	120	6–8	5–6
7.35–7.45	4–5	>99	45

Table 7.2

	Component	Numerical value
i.	pH of blood	
ii.	Volume of blood in an adult woman	litres
iii.	The % of the content of cells in blood	%
iv.	The % blood comprises of body weight	%
v.	Lifespan of an erythrocyte	days
vi.	The % of cellular content of blood consisting of erythrocytes	%
vii.	Volume of blood in an adult man	litres
viii.	The % of plasma content in blood	%

Correct/incorrect

3. Complete Table 7.3 by ticking only the correct statements.

Table 7.3

	Statement	Correct
i.	The formation of erythrocytes is called *erythropoiesis*	
ii.	In the western world, about 85% of people are rhesus positive (Rh⁺) and have the Rh agglutinogen on their red cells	
iii.	Under normal circumstances, platelets stick to each other and to the endothelial lining of blood vessels	
iv.	The production of platelets is called *thrombopoiesis* and occurs in the bone marrow	
v.	Unnecessary blood clots are removed by fibrinolysis to prevent occlusion of blood vessels	
vi.	Heparin is a synthetic anticoagulant	
vii.	Folate is a vitamin found in leafy green vegetables, such as spinach	
viii.	Prolonged boiling during cooking does not destroy folic acid	

Cardiovascular

 Label

4. The diagram in Fig. 7.1 represents the interior of the heart. Label the structures and chambers from the list provided.

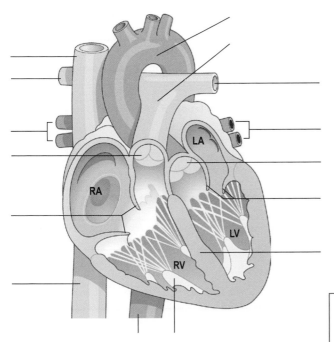

Inferior vena cava
Septum
Pulmonary artery
Right pulmonary artery
Pulmonary valve
Aortic valve
Right arterioventricular valve
Left arterioventricular valve
Superior vena cava
Aorta
Left pulmonary veins
Papillary muscle with chordae tendinae
Right pulmonary veins
Arch of aorta
Left pulmonary artery

RA – Right atrium
LA – Left atrium
RV – Right ventricle
LV – Left ventricle

Figure 7.1

5. The diagram in Fig. 7.2 shows the structures involved in the conducting system of the heart. Label the structures and vessels from the list provided.

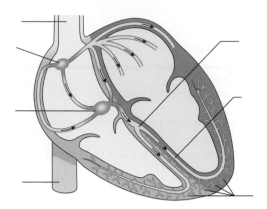

Network of purkinje fibres
Sino atrial node (SA)
Left atrioventricular bundle branch
Atrioventricular bundle
Superior vena cava
Inferior vena cava
Atrioventricular node (AV)

Figure 7.2

 True/false

6. Consider the following statements in Table 7.4 and complete the table by ticking if they are true or false statements.

Table 7.4

	Statement	True	False
a.	The Bainbridge reflex occurs when the atrial walls are stretched (because of increased blood volume or increased venous return); this then causes the heart rate to increase by 10%–15%		
b.	Parasympathetic stimulation on the heart increases the heart rate and increases the strength of cardiac contraction		
c.	Sympathetic stimulation of blood vessels causes most vessels to constrict. There is dilation of arteries supplying the brain and skeletal muscles		
d.	Chemoreceptors, situated in the arch of the aorta and in the carotid bodies, respond to a fall in blood oxygen and increase in blood acidity		
e.	Osmosis is the movement of water down a concentration gradient across a semi-permeable membrane		
f.	Baroreceptors provide a short-term feedback mechanism responding to changes and activity levels		
g.	Diffusion is always the movement of substances along a concentration gradient from low concentration to high concentrations		

Respiration

 Label

7. Fig. 7.3 presents the structures involved in the respiratory system. Label the structures from the list provided.

Diaphragm
Nostril
Intercostal muscles
Tongue
Second rib
Alveolus
Clavicle
Alveolar sac
Teeth
Respiratory bronchioles
Alveolar duct
Mediastinum
Nasal cavity

Laryngopharynx
Visceral pleura
Parietal pleura
Trachea
Bronchi
Larynx
Respiratory bronchioles
Oral cavity
Bronchioles
Intrapleural 'space'

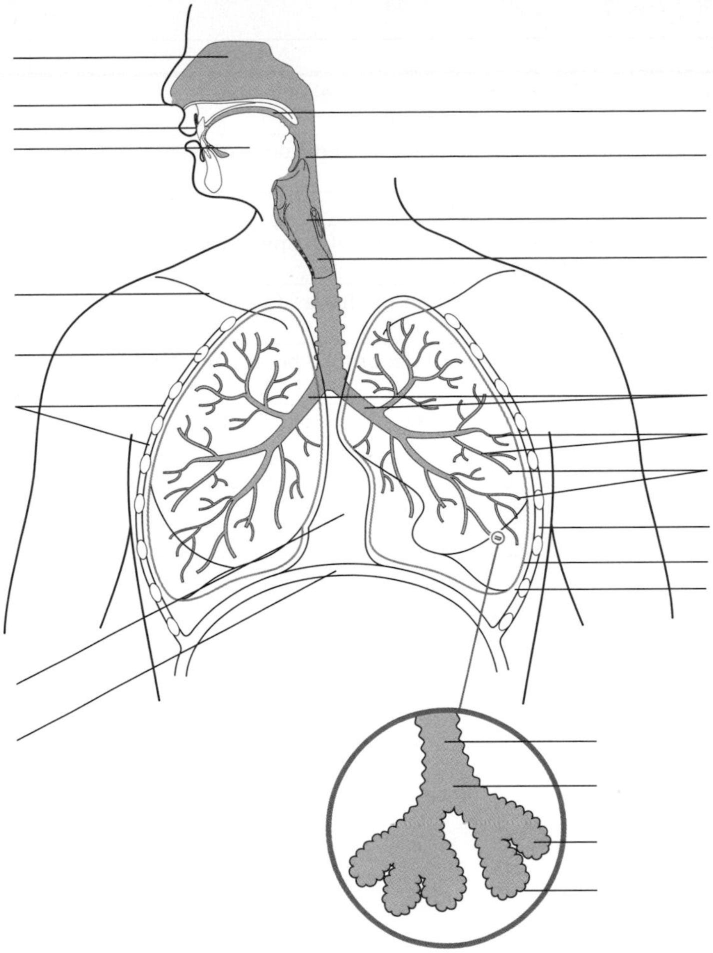

Figure 7.3

 Match

8. Complete Table 7.5 by drawing a line to connect the terms in column A with the correct respiratory description of ventilation in column B.

Table 7.5

A	B
Residual volume (RV)	Volume of air entering and leaving the lungs during a single breath
Tidal volume (TV)	Total volume of air exchanged with the atmosphere in 1 minute
Functional residual capacity (FRC)	Amount of air remaining in the lungs after normal expiration
Total lung capacity (TLC)	Volume of air remaining in the lungs at the end of maximal active expiration
Minute volume (pulmonary ventilation)	Amount of air in the lungs at the end of a maximum inspiration

 Short answers

9. Complete Table 7.6 by providing short answers to a range of physiologically related revision questions.

Table 7.6

	Questions	Answer
a.	What term is used to describe reduction in the blood vessel diameter as a result of increasing contraction of the circular muscle fibres?	
b.	What term is used to describe the amount of blood ejected from each ventricle with each heartbeat?	
c.	What term is used to describe the thickness of blood?	
d.	What term is used to describe increase in the blood vessel diameter caused by relaxation of the circular muscle fibres?	
e.	What is the term used for the 'pressure' describing the force of water pushing against the cell membrane?	
f.	What blood group is referred to as the universal donor type because it is compatible with any blood type?	
g.	What term is used to describe for the normal state of contraction in the smooth muscle of blood vessels?	
h.	What blood group is referred to as the universal recipient type because a person with this blood type can receive blood from any blood type?	
i.	What are the four cardinal signs of inflammation? List:	

Gastrointestinal tract and accessory organs

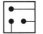 **Label**

10. Fig. 7.4 presents the structures involved in the gastrointestinal tract. Label the structures from the list provided.

Label

Nasal cavity
Laryngopharynx
Appendix
Soft palate
Gall bladder
Parotid salivary gland
Caecum
Liver
Anal canal

Label

Bile duct
Ascending colon
Fundus of stomach
Tail of pancreas
Diaphragm
Tongue
Submaxillary salivary gland
Cardia of stomach
Teeth
Duodenum
Sublingual salivary gland
Transverse colon
Rectum
Oesophagus
Position of pyloric sphincter
Small intestine (jejunum and ileum)
Descending colon

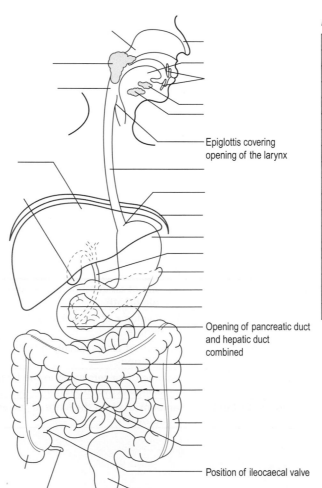

Epiglottis covering opening of the larynx

Opening of pancreatic duct and hepatic duct combined

Position of ileocaecal valve

Figure 7.4

Correct/incorrect

11. Table 7.7 provides statements related to the gastrointestinal tract and digestion. Complete the table by ticking the correct statements.

Table 7.7

	Statement	Correct
a.	Taste is aided by the sense of smell, which sends impulses to the brain via the olfactory nerve	
b.	The mucosal layer of the stomach has fold called *rugae*, which allows distension. The stomach is j-shaped when empty	
c.	Bile, produced in the gall bladder is stored in the liver	
d.	The vagus nerve is the source of sympathetic nerve supply to the oesophagus, stomach, pancreas and intestine	
e.	Fat-soluble vitamins include A, D, E and K	
f.	Iron is actively absorbed in the upper part of the small intestine	
g.	Peristalsis moves the faeces toward the rectum	
h.	The liver plays a major role in controlling plasma cholesterol	

 Short answers

12. Complete Table 7.8 by inserting the correct answers to the questions detailed.

Table 7.8

	Question	Answer
a.	What is the normal range of blood glucose levels in a healthy individual?	
b.	**What physiological process occurs when:**	
	(i) Glucose is converted to glycogen under the influence of insulin?	
	(ii) Blood glucose levels fall and liver glycogen is broken down to release glucose?	
	(iii) Glycogen levels in the liver are depleted and the liver manufactures glucose from amino acids and glycerol?	
c.	What is the process called that takes place in the mitochondria of cells where glucose is oxidized to form energy?	

Central nervous system

 Complete

13. Fig. 7.5 presents the structures of a whole nerve fibre. Label the structures from the list provided.

Label

Myelin sheath
Axon hillock
Axon
Dendrites covered with dendrite spines
Cell body
Cellular sheath
Axon terminals
Nodes of Ranvier
Synaptic knobs
Collateral branch
Nucleus

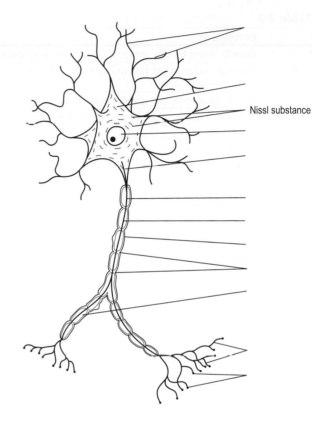

Nissl substance

Figure 7.5

14. Fig. 7.6 illustrates the component structures involved in a reflex arc. Label the structures from the list provided.

Label

Receptor
Motor efferent nerve
Effector organ, for example, muscle or gland
Sensory afferent fibre
Central nervous system (CNS): brain or spinal cord
Cell body or sensory neuron
Synapse x 2
Interneuron

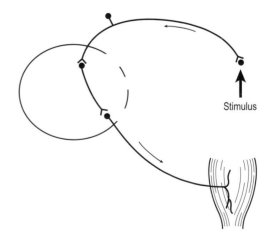

Stimulus

Figure 7.6

15. Fig. 7.7 presents the position of the endocrine glands in the body. Label the endocrine main glands/organs and the tissue/glands with secondary endocrine function from the list provided.

Label main endocrine glands/organs

| Adrenal gland (right) |
| Pineal body |
| Testes (males) |
| Pituitary gland |
| Thyroid gland |
| Pancreatic islets (of Langerhans) |
| Ovaries (female) |
| Parathyroid glands (behind thyroid) |

Label tissues and glands (secondary endocrine function)

| Kidneys |
| Thymus gland |
| Heart |
| Stomach |

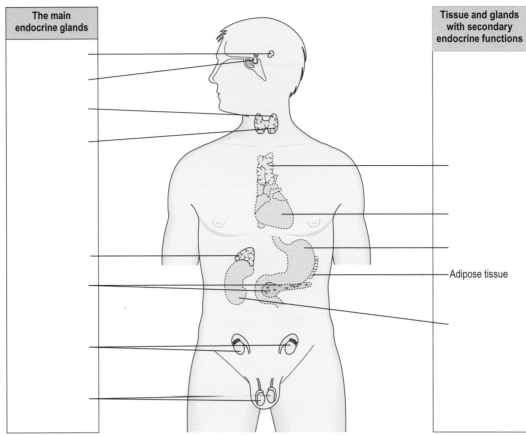

Figure 7.7

 Match

16. Table 7.9 lists endocrine glands and hormones. Complete the table by drawing line/s to connect the hormone to the correct endocrine gland.

Table 7.9

Endocrine gland	Hormone
Pineal body:	• Antidiuretic hormone (ADH)
	• Prolactin (PRL)
	• Follicle stimulating hormone (FSH)
Pituitary (posterior):	• Thyroxine
	• Adrenocorticotrophic hormone (ACTH)
	• Growth hormone (GH)
Pituitary (anterior):	• Thyroid stimulating hormone (TSH)
	• Melatonin
	• Luteinizing hormone (LH)
Thyroid:	• Oxytocin
	• Triiodothyronine

True/false

17. Complete Table 7.10 by indicating if the range of physiologically related statements are true or false.

Table 7.10

		Statements	True	False
a.		Oedema is the accumulation of fluid within the interstitial space		
b.		Potassium (K+), the main cation in intracellular fluid (ICF), is necessary for normal neuromuscular functioning		
c.		Immunoglobulin (Ig)G antibodies provide active immunity to the fetus		
d.		Fever is an elevation of the body temperature in response to chemicals called *pyrogens* (e.g., interleukins)		
e.		Interferons (IFNs) limit the spread of viral infections		
f.		Aldosterone is produced by the cortical cells of the adrenal gland with release mediated by renin production by the kidney		
g.		Antibodies are also called *immunoglobulins* and are a group of glycoproteins present in blood and tissue fluids		
h.		The spleen is the smallest lymphoid tissue in the body		
i.		The thymus gland (bilobed gland), found in the mediastinum of thorax, is more active during adulthood		
j.		Clotting proteins form a fibrin mesh limiting the spread of harmful agents and acting as scaffolding for tissue repair		
k.		Potassium is toxic, especially to the heart muscle		

8 Changes and adaptation in pregnancy

The anatomical and physiological adaptations throughout pregnancy affect almost every body system. Variations in the timing and intensity of changes between systems are designed to support fetal growth and development through each stage of pregnancy and prepare the woman for childbirth. Midwives need to appreciate the anatomical and physiological adaptations to pregnancy to appropriately manage pregnancy and childbirth and recognize abnormal findings. Therefore, it is fundamental for them to have knowledge of the anatomy and physiology of the body systems and the changes that occur during pregnancy. The activities in this chapter will assess your knowledge of changes and adaptations during each stage of pregnancy.

Signs of pregnancy

 Complete

1. Signs and symptoms of pregnancy are often enough for a woman to suspect pregnancy. Diagnosis usually confirms probable signs and positive signs. Complete Table 8.1a–c by drawing a line to connect the signs or activities in column A with the correct timing of the occurrence in column B

Table 8.1a

	A. Possible (presumptive) signs	B. Time of occurrence (weeks)
a.	Early breast changes (primigravidae)	• 16–20
b.	Amenorrhoea	• 3–4+
c.	Nausea and vomiting	• 6–12
d.	Bladder irritability	• 4
e.	Quickening	• 4–14

Table 8.1b

	A. Probable signs	B. Time of occurrence
a.	Changes in skin pigmentation	• 9–10 days
b.	Uterine souffle	• 8+ weeks
c.	Ballottement of fetus	• 8+ weeks
d.	Braxton Hicks contractions	• 6–12 weeks
e.	Blueing (or purpling) of vagina	• 14 days
f.	Softened isthmus	• 16 weeks
g.	Timing when the hCG hormone is present in urine	• 12–16 weeks
h.	Timing when the hCG hormone is present in blood	• 8+ weeks
i.	Pulsation in fornices	• 16–28 weeks

Table 8.1c

	A. Positive signs	B. Time of occurrence (weeks)
a.	Fetal heart sounds by doppler	• 20+ weeks
b.	Gestational sac visible by abdominal ultrasound	• 24+ weeks
c.	Fetal movements palpable	• 5.5 weeks
d.	Gestational sac visible by transvaginal ultrasound	• ≥22 weeks
e.	Fetal parts palpated	• 11–12 weeks
f.	Fetal heart sounds by fetal stethoscope	• 4–5 weeks

Complete

Midwives need to keep an open mind when women report possible/probable signs and symptoms of pregnancy. These signs and symptoms may result from other conditions. Differential diagnosis always needs to be considered.

2. Table 8.2 presents a list of possible alternative conditions, which may result in possible or probable signs of pregnancy. A list of these signs of pregnancy is provided for you to match to each condition. Complete Table 8.2 by inserting the correct sign or symptom of pregnancy each condition produces. Some signs from the list are used more than once.

Early breast changes (nulliparous woman)

Nausea and vomiting
Presence of hCG in blood

Presence of human chorionic gonadotropin (hCG) in urine
Pulsation of fornices
Amenorrhoea

Bladder irritability

Quickening

Table 8.2

	Differential diagnosis	Possible sign of pregnancy
a.	Urinary tract infection (UTI)	
b.	Pyrexial illness	
c.	Emotional stress	
d.	Gastrointestinal (GI) disorders	
e.	Intestinal movement, wind	
f.	Hydatidiform mole	
g.	Pelvic tumour	
h.	Pelvic congestion	
i.	Hormonal imbalance	
j.	Tumours	
k.	Choriocarcinoma	
l.	Cerebral irritation	
m.	Illness	
n.	Contraceptive pill	

The uterus during pregnancy

The uterus plays an essential role in pregnancy by expanding to accommodate the growing fetus and providing support and protection for the fetus, placenta and amniotic fluid. Complete the following activities related to the uterus, vagina and cervix.

True/false

3. Table 8.3 provides statements about the uterus. Complete the table by deciding if each statement is true of false.

Table 8.3

	Statement	True	False
a.	The perimetrium is a draped over the uterus, uterine tubes and is continuous laterally with the broad ligaments		
b.	In the first 12 weeks of pregnancy, uterine growth is partly because of hyperplasia and mainly because of hypertrophy		
c.	The perimetrium is a thick layer of peritoneum composed of connective tissue (collagen and elastin fibres)		
d.	The myometrium, the muscular wall of the uterus, is composed mainly of bundles of smooth myometrial cells (myocytes) embedded in a supporting extracellular matrix (ECM)		
e.	There is little change in the size of the myometrial thickness of the uterine body across pregnancy in spite of the increased volume		
f.	With ascent from the pelvis, the uterus usually undergoes dextrorotation, with tilting to the right because of the rectosigmoid on the left side of the pelvis		
g.	Progesterone withdrawal is responsible for the awakening of the quiescent uterus throughout pregnancy		
h.	The ECM is composed of tension-bearing proteins, including elastin, fibronectin and collagen		
i.	The junctional zone is a separate and distinct functional unit within the uterus lying between the myometrium and deciduas		
j.	Relaxin produced by the decidua plays a part in myometrial quiescence		
k.	The decidua in the cervix and isthmus is more developed than in the corpus		
l.	During normal pregnancy, the uterus weighs approximately 1100 g at term		
m.	Between 38 and 40 weeks, the increase in myometrial tone results in smoothing and shortening of the upper uterine segment		

Match

4. Table 8.4 provides a list of uterine changes in column A and a list of numerical weeks of gestation in column B. Draw a line to accurately match and connect the two columns.

Table 8.4

	A. Uterine changes	B. Weeks' gestation
a.	The isthmus has fully developed into the lower uterine segment by week:	30
b.	The uterus is usually palpable just above the symphysis pubis by the end of week:	20
c.	The enlarging uterus displaces the intestines laterally and superiorly by around week:	12
d.	The uterus is the size of a grapefruit by week:	38
e.	The fundus reaches the tip of the xyphoid cartilage by week:	10
f.	Uterine souffle is detected from week:	36
g.	The physiological retraction ring develops at the junction between lower and upper segments by week:	20
h.	The uterus changes from pear shaped to ovoid shaped by week:	15
i.	The initial softening phase of the cervix begins at conception and continues until approx:	32

Changes in the cervix

Complete and short answers

5. Table 8.5 provides descriptive statements about signs and sounds unique to pregnancy. Complete the table by matching and inserting the correct term from the list provided. Some terms are used more than once.

Osiander's sign   Hegar's (or Goodnell's) sign   Chadwick's (or Jacquemeir's) sign
Funic souffle   Uterine souffle   Placental souffle

Table 8.5

	Descriptive statement	Sign or sound
a.	This refers to violet or dark purplish discolouration and congestion of the vulvar and vaginal mucous membranes.	
b.	This refers to the soft blowing sound made by blood passing through the dilated uterine vessels	
c.	This refers to the stronger and harder vaginal pulsations in the lateral fornices caused by the increased blood supply and enlarged uterine artery. It occurs from 8+ weeks	
d.	This sign is caused by increased vascularity and is first detected between the fourth and eighth week of pregnancy	
e.	This refers to the muffled 'ocean-like' sound of blood coursing through the placenta	
f.	This sound is synchronous with the maternal pulse	
g.	This sound is synchronous with the fetal heart	
h.	This sign refers to the softening of the lower parts of the isthmus felt in contrast to a firm cervix (about 6–8 weeks) on bimanual pelvic examination	
i.	This sound is heard distinctly at the lower portion of the uterus	
j.	This sound is a muffled swooshing sound produced by the pulsation of blood as it is propelled through the arteries of in the umbilical cord	

 ## Complete

6. This activity involves completing the physiological processes involved in 'ripening' of the cervix. Complete the activity by removing the incorrect word so the paragraphs read correctly.

   a. Cervical ripening is a more **slower/accelerated** phase occurring in the **middle/final** weeks of pregnancy. The process of cervical ripening involves **inflammatory/stroma** cells but is probably dependent upon **endogenously/exogenously** produced **prostaglandins/oestrogen**.

   b. Collagen is **reduced/increased** and the cervix becomes **thin/thick.** The rearrangement and degradation of **collagen/elastin** fibres creates an **increase/decrease** in the space between them, **shortens/lengthens** them and **increases/decreases** acidic solubility, along with **increased/reduced** capacity to **retain/lose** water.

   c. The cervix changes to a **soft/firm** and **distensible/rigid** structure with **reduced/increased** resistance to effacement and dilatation.

  ## Complete and short answers

7. Table 8.6 presents a range of activities and questions. An extended list of possible responses is provided. Complete the table by inserting the 10 correct terms/responses from this extended list of options.

Oedema	Doderlein's bacillus	Lower uterine segment	Oestrogen
pH 5.5–8.5	Progesterone	hCG	pH 3.5–6
Antibacterial plug	Upper uterine segment	Leucorrhoea	Vascularity
Effacement	Braxton-Hicks	Candida albicans	Engagement
Lightening	Funnelling	Dextrorotation	Isthmus

Table 8.6

	Activity	Answer
i.	Name the dominant flora in the vagina	
ii.	Identify the thick, white vaginal discharge produced because of high levels of hCG hormone	
iii.	Insert the normal pH range of the vagina during pregnancy	
iv.	Identify the development in the cervix as a result of the endocervical mucosal cells producing copious amounts of tenacious fluid	
v.	Identify the term used to refer to descent of the fetal head into the pelvic brim	
vi.	Identify this uterine segment: 'the middle layer of the myometrium forms 8-shaped fibres around the blood vessels to control postpartum haemorrhage (living ligatures)'	
vii.	Identify the hormone with a relaxing effect that blocks the myometrial response to oxytocin	
viii.	Identify the term used to describe shortening of the cervical canal form about 2 cm (length) to a circular orifice with paper-thin edges	
ix.	Identify the two factors that because of their increase cause the cervix (following conception) to become softer and cyanosed	
x.	Identify this uterine segment: 'the peritoneum is loosely attached, the decidua is poorly developed and the membranes are loosely attached'	

? Multiple choice questions (MCQ)

8. In the first 12 weeks of pregnancy, the smooth muscle cells in length from nonpregnant levels by up to:
   a. 5-fold (50–250 µm)
   b. 10-fold (50–500 µm)
   c. 15-fold (50–750 µm)
   d. 20-fold (50–1000 µm)

9. During pregnancy, the weight of the uterus increases:
   a. 5-fold
   b. 10-fold
   c. 15-fold
   d. 10–20-fold

10. Comparison between the uterus and fruit has become a fairly reliable way to measure uterine size in early pregnancy. The uterus would feel like an unripe pear at:
    a. 5 weeks' gestation
    b. 8 weeks' gestation
    c. 10 weeks' gestation
    d. 12 weeks' gestation

11. The fundus of the uterus becomes dome-shaped in the first half of pregnancy. Indicate the weeks of gestation this occurs.
    a. 6–10 weeks
    b. 8–12 weeks
    c. 12–16 weeks
    d. 16–20 weeks

12. Which of the following statements relates to Doderlein's bacillus (*Lactobacillus acidophilus*):
    a. This is a normal commensal of the vagina
    b. It metabolizes glycogen to lactic acid
    c. It leads to increased vaginal acidity
    d. All of the above
    e. b and c

13. In preparation for the distension that occurs in labour, the vaginal walls undergo the following changes:
    a. Mucosa thickens, connective tissue loosens and smooth muscle cells hypertrophy
    b. Mucosa thins, connective tissue loosens and smooth muscle cells hypertrophy
    c. Mucosa thickens, connective tissue and smooth muscle cells remain unchanged
    d. None of the above

14. The forceful, synchronous contractions of labour are caused by:
    a. The rise in gap junction density
    b. The increase in progesterone resistance
    c. Excitation of myocytes
    d. All of the above
    e. a and c

15. Which of the following statement is incorrect about the increasing uterine size:
    a. The bladder is displaced as the uterus comes into contact with the anterior abdominal wall
    b. There is increased tension exerted on the broad and round ligaments
    c. The diaphragm is raised by about 4 cm
    d. The transverse diameter of the thoracic cavity increases

Changes in the main body systems

Pregnancy is associated with profound and predominantly reversible changes in maternal haemodynamics and cardiac function.

Complete

16. All components of the cardiovascular system (CVS) undergo a degree of adaptation during pregnancy. Box 8.1 focuses on the CVS. Column **B** provides an extended list of changes. Complete this activity by identifying only the correct changes and drawing a line to connect directly with the **A**. CVS (heart, blood and blood pressure [BP]).

Box 8.1

A. CVS (heart, blood and blood pressure [BP])	**B** Cardiac output (CO): increases by 35%–50% CO: minimal change only CO: increases by 15%–25% Heart: no change in size, displaced: backwards and to the right Heart increases in size and displaced upward and to the left Heart rate: decreases 10–20 beats per minute (mainly first trimester) Heart rate: increases 10–20 beats per minute (mainly first trimester) Heart rate: increases 30 beats per minute in pregnancy Systemic and pulmonary vessels: no change Veins: vasodilation and impeded venous return in lower extremities Systemic and pulmonary vessels: dramatic vasodilation to increase blood flow Systemic and pulmonary vessels: vasodilation to increase blood flow (third trimester only) Systemic blood pressure: minimal change/no reduction Systemic blood pressure: dramatic increase Diastolic blood pressure: increase, returning to normal by term Diastolic blood pressure: decrease, returning to normal by term Pulmonary and systemic vascular resistance: decrease Pulmonary and vascular resistance: increase Capillaries: increased permeability Capillaries: decreased permeability

17. There are important haematological and biochemical blood changes occurring during pregnancy. An extended list of changes are provided in column **B/C** in Box 8.2. Complete this activity by identifying only the correct changes that occur during pregnancy. Draw a line to connect the correct changes in B/C directly with **A**.

Box 8.2

A. HAEMATOLOGICAL SYSTEM: BLOOD COMPONENTS	**B. HAEMATOLOGY:** Total body water: increase Total body water: no change Plasma volume: marked increase 45%–50% Plasma volume: slight increase Red cell mass increases 18% Red cell: slight reduction Platelets: slight decrease Platelets: no change Total blood volume: slight increase 5%–10% Total blood volume increases 30%–45% White cell count: reduces White cell count: normal levels **C. BIOCHEMISTRY:** Potassium–unchanged Potassium increases Creatinine levels: lower in mid pregnancy (rises toward term) Creatinine levels: no change Urea levels: higher Urea levels: lower

Correct/incorrect

18. Table 8.7 provides a list of statements. Complete the table by identifying the correct statements.

Table 8.7

	Statement	Correct
a.	The changes in cardiac output in early pregnancy are mainly caused by an increase in heart rate	
b.	The secretion of atrial natriuretic peptide (ANP) is not increased during pregnancy because the ANP-volume is reset during pregnancy	
c.	During pregnancy, there is an increased capacity for clot formation	
d.	Haemoglobin (Hb) level below 105 g/L at 28 weeks' gestation does not require investigation	
e.	Haemodilution occurs in pregnancy because of an increase in plasma volume resulting in the 'apparent anaemia' found in pregnancy	
f.	Creatinine levels are higher in mid pregnancy but lower toward term	
g.	Coagulation factors VII, VIII and X increase during pregnancy	
h.	While total haemoglobin increases the mean haemoglobin concentration falls	
i.	The majority of increased iron requirements occur in the first trimester	
j.	Reduced total serum protein content is always a sign of pathology	

 Short answers

19. Using your knowledge of supine hypotension, complete Table 8.8 by inserting short answers.

Table 8.8

	Supine hypotension	Answer
a.	Name the two major vessels compressed by the enlarging uterus	
b.	List three signs the woman may report	
c.	List two symptoms the midwife may find	
d.	What physiological reasons would lead the woman to losing consciousness?	
e.	What physiological reasons may cause fetal compromise?	

 Complete

20. Table 8.9 provides a summary of changes in the respiratory system. Choose the direction of change by ticking the appropriate column.

Table 8.9

Direction	Oxygen (O_2) consumption	Metabolic rate	Minute volume	Tidal volume	Functional residual capacity	Arterial O_2 tension (PaO_2)	Arterial CO_2 tension ($PaCO_2$)	Arterial pH
Increase	x	x	x	x		x		x
Decrease					x		x	

True/false

21. Table 8.10 provides statements relating to aspects of pregnancy. Complete the table by indicating if the statements are true or false.

Table 8.10

	Statement	True	False
a.	The anterior pituitary gland decreases in size during pregnancy		
b.	The opioid active form of β endorphin produced by the pituitary may play a major role in raising the maternal threshold for pain and discomfort in the latter stages of pregnancy		
c.	Glycosuria provides substrates for bacterial growth and can cause asymptomatic bacteruria		
d.	The renin-angiotensin-aldosterone system is important in fluid and electrolyte homeostasis and maintaining blood pressure		
e.	The gall bladder enlarges with slower emptying because of reduced mobility leading to bile stasis and increased concentrated bile salts (predisposing to physiological cholestasis and pruritis)		
f.	Pregnancy always results in dental caries leading to tooth decay		
g.	The fetus draws the calcium required from the maternal skeleton		
h.	Maternal calcium absorption doubles by 36 weeks to support maternal and fetal bone mineralisation		
i.	Accelerated starvation refers to a pregnancy induced switch in fuels from glucose to lipids with ketonaemia rapidly appearing		

Complete

22. Complete this activity about the ureters during pregnancy by crossing out the incorrect words.

   a. Dilatation of the ureters is rarely present **below/above** the pelvic brim. Dilation is possibly caused by compression by the enlarging uterus and **ovarian plexus/enlarged kidneys**.

   b. The early onset of ureteral dilatation suggests that smooth muscle relaxation, caused by **oestrogen/progesterone**, possibly plays an additional role.

   c. Dilatation of the ureters is more marked on the **right/left** side, because of the cushioning effect of the **ascending/sigmoid** colon on the **right/left** and because of the uterine tendency to **flexion/dextrorotation**.

Match and connect

23. Table 8.11 relates to the distribution of weight gain during pregnancy. Column A provides maternal weight gain and column B provides fetal-related weight gain. Draw a line to correctly match and connect the maternal and fetal weight gains.

Table 8.11

Distribution of total weight gain in pregnancy (total 12.5 kg)			
A. Maternal gain (64%) (7.7 kg)		**B. Fetal-related gain (36%) (4.8 kg)**	
Uterus:	• 1.2 kg	Fetus:	• 0.7 kg
Breasts:	• 0.4 kg	Placenta:	• 0.8 kg
Fat:	• 1.2 kg	Amniotic fluid:	• 3.3 kg
Blood:	• 0.9 kg		
Extracellular fluid:	• 4.0 kg		

Complete

24. Consider the following paragraph about insulin levels and remove the incorrect words.

   a. In late pregnancy, although basal insulin levels are **elevated/reduced** maternal blood glucose levels are similar to nonpregnant levels and do not **increase/reduce** as rapidly as usual even with **higher/lower** circulating levels of insulin. This diabetogenic state protects the fetus, even if the mother is fasting by keeping glucose in the blood and thus available for placental transfer.

   b. Normal glucose ranges during pregnancy are **3.4 to 5.5 mmol/L/5.2 to 7.9 mmol/L**. After a meal, however, the pregnant woman's levels of glucose and insulin are **lower/higher** than those of nonpregnant women and **glycogen/glucagon** is suppressed resulting in **hyper-/hypo**-insulinaemia, **hyper-/hypo**-glycaemia and insulin resistance.

 Short answers

25. Table 8.12 provides a range of activities. Using your own knowledge, complete the activities by inserting the correct answer.

Table 8.12

	Activity	Answer
a.	Identify the following hormones:	
(i)	The hormone mainly responsible for relaxing all smooth muscle and leading to many minor disorders. It has a sedative effect on uterine muscle contractibility	
(ii)	The hormone termed the 'growth stimulator'. It causes hypertrophy and hyperplasia of uterine muscle, as well as development of breasts	
(iii)	The hormone with a major role in the changes, remodelling collagen fibres and softening pelvic joints and ligaments in preparation for birth	
(iv)	The hormone with a key role in the regulation of body fat and energy expenditure. It is a peptide hormone secreted by the placenta and adipose tissue	
b.	Name two joints that may contribute to the alteration in maternal posture leading to the characteristic 'waddling gait' and back pain of pregnancy	
c.	Identify the benign vascular lesion of the skin and mucosa in the mouth developing from gingivitis (minor trauma/inflammation in the presence of bacterial plaque)	
d.	Name the term used to refer to excessive salivation in pregnancy	
e.	Identify the term used to refer to persistent craving and compulsive consumption of unusual substances	
f.	What is the term used for the 'mask of pregnancy'?	
g.	List three other skin changes or conditions occurring in pregnancy	

Changes in the breasts

 Complete

It is fundamental for midwives to have a clear understanding of the changes in the breast to appropriately advise and reassure women of normal changes expected at each stage of pregnancy.

Match

26. Column A and column C of Table 8.13 are mixed up. Consider each breast change listed and then correctly match and connect by drawing a line between the correct timing of the change and the correct reason or influence for the change.

Table 8.13

A. Time	B. Breast changes	C. Reason/influence
Late pregnancy:	Prickling, tingling sensation, particularly around the nipple	Oestrogen
16 weeks:	Development of duct system	Prolactin/oestrogen
8–12 weeks:	Development of lobular formation	Hypertrophy of the alveoli. Human Placental Lactogen (hPL) and oestrogen
3–4 weeks:	Increase in size, painful, tense and nodular, delicate, bluish surface, veins become visible just beneath skin	Progesterone
6–8 weeks:	Montgomery tubercles become more prominent on the areola. Glands secrete sebum to keep nipple soft	Prolactin/progesterone
From early pregnancy:	The pigmented area around the nipple (primary areola) darkens and may become more erectile	Hypertrophy of the glands. Human Placental Lactogen (hPL) and oestrogen
	Colostrum can be expressed/the secondary areola develops with further extension of the pigmented area (often mottled in appearance)	Increased blood supply
	Colostrum may leak from the breast/the nipple becomes more prominent and mobile	Increased melanin activity

Multiple choice questions (MCQ)

27. Which of the following statements about clotting in pregnancy are correct:

   a. Clotting time is reduced from 12 minutes to 8 minutes.

   b. Peripheral oedema in the lower limbs in the third trimester is a feature of normal pregnancy.

   c. The haematocrit is lower.

   d. All of the above

   e. a and c

28. Which of the following statements about respiratory function in pregnancy are correct:
    a. Changes in the respiratory function result in a state of compensated respiratory acidosis.
    b. Hyperventilation of pregnancy causes a 15% to 20% decrease in maternal carbon dioxide partial pressure (PaCO2) in late pregnancy.
    c. Expansion of the rib cage causes tidal volume to increase by 30% to 40%, gradually rising from 8 weeks until term.
    d. a and c
    e. b and c

29. By the 16th week of pregnancy, renal blood flow has increased by as much as:
    a. 10%–25%
    b. 25%–50%
    c. 50%–65%
    d. 70%–80%

30. Blood flow in the lower limbs is slowed in late pregnancy by:
    a. The enlarging uterus compressing the iliac veins
    b. The enlarging uterus compressing the inferior vena cava
    c. The hydrodynamic effects of the decreased venous return from the uterus
    d. a and b

31. Normal oxygen consumption at rest is:
    a. 80 mL/min
    b. 100 mL/min
    c. 150 mL/min
    d. 250 mL/min

32. Hyperventilation during pregnancy may lead to mild:
    a. Metabolic alkalosis
    b. Respiratory acidosis
    c. Metabolic acidosis
    d. Respiratory alkalosis

33. During pregnancy, renin and aldosterone activity are both:
    a. Increased by oestrogens, progesterone and prostaglandins, leading to increased fluid and electrolyte retention
    b. Increased by oestrogens, progesterone and prostaglandins, leading to decreased fluid and electrolyte retention
    c. Increased by oestrogens, progesterone and prostaglandins, with no influence on fluid and electrolyte retention
    d. None of the above

34. Renin release is stimulated by:
    a. Higher blood pressure
    b. Oestrogens
    c. Relaxin
    d. Decreased levels of plasma and urinary prostaglandins

35. By 36 weeks' gestation, the fetus accumulates the following amount of maternal calcium per day:

    a. 50–100 g

    b. 100–200 g

    c. 250–350 g

    d. 350–400 g

36. The percentage of women experiencing nausea and vomiting during pregnancy is:

    a. 40%–50%

    b. 50%–60%

    c. 60%–70%

    d. 70%–85%

9 Antenatal care and problems in pregnancy

Antenatal care refers to the care of pregnant women from the time pregnancy is confirmed, until the beginning of labour. This chapter will assess your knowledge of aspects relating to assessment and progress in pregnancy, including routine and specialized investigations. Activities will also focus on abnormalities and problems experienced during pregnancy.

ASSESSMENTS DURING PREGNANCY

First antenatal assessment

 Complete

1. Estimated date of birth (EDB) is normally calculated using the method known as *Naegele's rule* (i.e., 9 calendar months and 7 days from the first day of the last menstrual period, LMP). Assumptions are made when using this method for EDB. Table 9.1 provides a list of statements relating to assumptions when using Naegele's rule for EDB and related factors. Identify the correct statements.

Table 9.1

	Statement	Correct
a.	Conception occurred 14 days after the first day of the LMP (only if woman has a 30-day cycle)	
b.	Conception occurred 14 days after the first day of the LMP (only if woman has a 35-day cycle)	
c.	Conception occurred 14 days after the first day of the LMP (only if woman has a 28-day cycle)	
d.	Regular record of regularity and length of time between periods	
e.	Regular record of menstrual loss	
f.	The last period of bleeding was true menstruation	
g.	The last period of bleeding was of shorter and lighter duration than normal	
h.	Breakthrough bleeding and anovulation can be affected by the contraceptive pill, thus impacting the accuracy of the LMP as defined as the last day of menstrual period	
	Based on Naegele's rule, the duration of pregnancy is:	
i.	- 280 days	
j.	- 270 days	
k.	- 280 days	
l.	- 290 days	

Complete the following activities relating to the first antenatal assessment:

2. Body mass index (BMI) is the weight in kg divided by the height in m². Using your own knowledge, complete Table 9.2 by identifying the BMI (cut-off or range) for the following BMI classifications:

Table 9.2

BMI classifications	Underweight	Normal/Healthy	Overweight	Obese	Very obese
kg/m² (cut-off or range)					

Antenatal tests

 Short answers

Maternal assessment of health and well-being in pregnancy usually commences at the antenatal booking visit when the midwife conducts a series of routine antenatal tests. Antenatal assessment of the fetus is now a mainstream aspect of care involving both routine and more specialized screening and diagnostic tests for fetal anomaly.

3. Table 9.3 presents a list of activities/questions related to the routine antenatal tests conducted by the midwife at booking visit. Complete the table by providing short answers or lists.

Table 9.3

	Activity/Questions	Answer
a.	What needs to breakdown in the body to result in ketones?	
b.	List three reasons for ketonuria:	
c.	Untreated asymptomatic bacteriuria can lead to key medical and obstetrical conditions. Name the medical condition and the possible obstetrical outcome.	
d.	Urinalysis performed at all antenatal visits excludes proteinuria. Which serious pregnancy-related condition can this be a symptom of?	
	Antenatal: blood and screening tests:	
e.	List the routine blood tests normally investigated:	
f.	List the other screening tests normally investigated:	
g.	List the infections not currently recommended as being routinely screened for antenatally:	

True/false

4. Table 9.4 provides statements relating to screening and diagnostic tests conducted during pregnancy. Complete the table by deciding if the statements are true or false.

Table 9.4

	Statement	True	False
a.	A diagnosis of Down syndrome can be accurately made using chorionic villus sampling (CVS) or amniocentesis		
b.	'False negative rate' from screening tests is the proportion of affected pregnancies that would not be identified as high risk		
c.	CVS can be performed from 11 weeks of pregnancy		
d.	CVS is mainly carried out by the transcervical (TC) route		
e.	On ultrasound scan in early pregnancy, the femur is a reliable indicator of gestational age		
f.	After 13+ weeks of pregnancy, gestational age is primarily assessed using the head circumference (HC)		
g.	Amniocentesis can be performed after 15 weeks of pregnancy		
h.	Alphafetoprotein (AFP) is used as a biochemical marker for neural tube defects		
i	On ultrasound, a fetal sac can be seen from 5 weeks' gestation and a small embryo from 9 weeks' gestation		
j.	Atrial atresia has a clear appearance on ultrasound		
k.	Fetuses with excessive growth (macrosomia) are associated with maternal diabetes mellitus		
l.	In fetal blood sampling, blood can be sampled from the umbilical cord or the intrahepatic umbilical vein		
m	Raised AFP levels can be predictive of intrauterine growth restriction and preeclampsia		
n	Nuchal translucency (NT) of >3.5 mm is considered to be the threshold definition of an increased NT above which the risk of other (nonchromosomal) abnormalities increases		
o	The combined test comprises measurement of the crown-rump length (CRL) and nuchal transparency (NT) space and maternal blood for serum markers of pregnancy-associated plasma proteins A (PAPP-A) and human chorionic gonadotropin (hCG) levels		

Terminology and facts relating to assessment of pregnancy

It is essential that the midwife has detailed knowledge of the terminology and definitions related to assessment of pregnancy. The following activities will test this knowledge.

 Complete

5. Box 9.1 presents information about terminology and descriptions relating to the fetus in utero. Draw a line to accurately match and connect the terminology in column A with the correct description in column B.

Box 9.1

A	B
Attitude:	• Vertex, brow and shoulder are all cephalic presentations
	• Refers to the name of the part of the presentation used when referring to fetal position
Lie:	• This refers to the uterus when it is tilted to one side (usually left side)
	• Refers to the name of the part of the fetal head identifying the attitude
Presentation:	• Refers to the relationship of the fetal head and limbs to the trunk
	• Vertex, face and brow are all cephalic presentations
Position:	• Refers to the relationship between the denominator of the presentation and the 10 points on the pelvis
	• Refers to the relationship between the denominator of the presentation and the six key points on the pelvic brim
	• Refers to the part of the fetus lying at the pelvic brim or in the lower pole of the uterus
Denominator:	• Refers to the relationship between the long axis of the fetus and long axis of the uterus
	• Refers to the part of the fetus lying at the in the upper pole of the uterus

Fundal height

 Complete

6. Complete Fig. 9.1 by drawing a curved line to represent the height of the fundus at the following weeks of gestation: 12, 16, 24, 30, 36, 40 weeks.

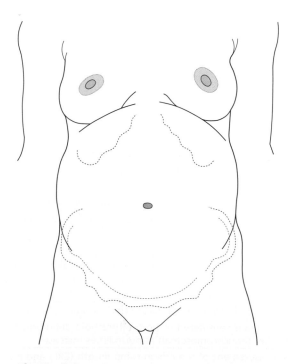

Figure 9.1

Presentations

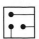 **Label**

7. Fig. 9.2 shows five presentations (over six illustrations). Label the presentations.

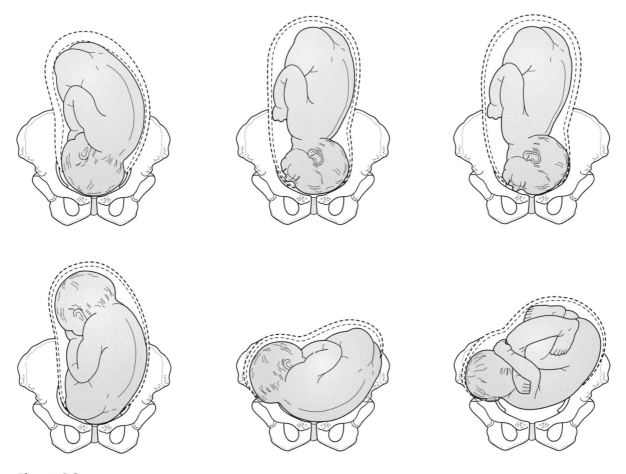

Figure 9.2

8. Fig. 9.3 shows four varieties of cephalic or head presentations. Label the figures.

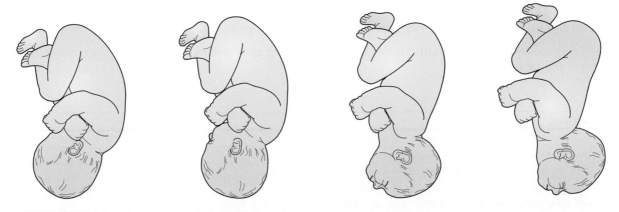

Figure 9.3

9. Fig. 9.4 illustrates six positions of vertex presentations. Identify each of the presentations.

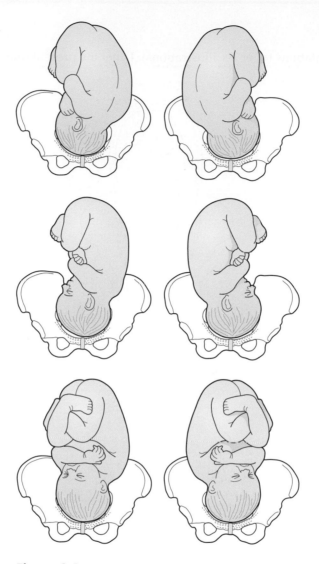

Figure 9.4

Engagement

 Short answers

Engagement has occurred when the key presenting diameter has passed through the brim of the pelvis.

10. Table 9.5 presents activities relating to 'engagement'. Using your own knowledge, provide answers to complete the table.

Table 9.5

	Activity	Answer
a.	Identify the key diameter relating to engagement:	
b.	Identify when engagement is likely to occur in a first time pregnancy:	
c.	Identify the engaging diameter (cm) in a cephalic presentation	
d.	Identify the engaging diameter (cm) in a breech presentation	
e.	List pregnancy-related factors that cause of nonengagement of the head:	
f.	List other factors that cause of nonengagement of the head:	

11. Table 9.6 presents activities relating to the fetal lie, attitude and denominator of presentation. Using your own knowledge, complete the table by inserting the correct response.

Table 9.6

	Activity	Response
a.	List the three types of lie of the fetus:	
b.	Identify the preferred attitude of the fetus:	
	Identify the denominator in the:	
c.	• face presentation:	
d.	• breech presentation:	
e.	• vertex presentation:	
f.	List three key indicators of fetal well-being:	

Vertex positions

 Match

12. Complete Table 9.7 by drawing a line between the descriptions of the relationship of landmarks to the points on the pelvic brim in column A with the correct vertex position in column B.

Table 9.7

Description of the occiput in relation to the six points of the pelvis	
A	B
a. Occiput points to symphysis pubis; sagittal suture is in anteroposterior diameter of the pelvis:	• Direct occipitoposterior (DOP)
b. Occiput points to left iliopectineal eminence; sagittal suture is in right oblique diameter of the pelvis:	• Left occipitolateral (LOL)
c. Occiput points to right iliopectineal line midway between the iliopectineal eminence and sacroiliac joint; sagittal suture is in transverse diameter of the pelvis:	• Direct occipitoanterior (DOA)
d. Occiput points to right iliopectineal eminence; sagittal suture is in left oblique diameter of the pelvis:	• Left occipitoposterior (LOP)
e. Occiput points to sacrum; sagittal suture is in anteroposterior diameter of the pelvis:	• Right occipitoposterior (ROP)
f. The occiput points to the left sacroiliac joint; sagittal suture is in the left oblique diameter of the pelvis:	• Right occipitoanterior (ROA)
g. Occiput points to left iliopectineal line midway between iliopectineal eminence and sacroiliac joint; sagittal suture is in transverse diameter of the pelvis:	• Left occipitoanterior (LOA)
h. Occiput points to right sacroiliac joint; sagittal suture is in right oblique diameter of the pelvis:	• Right occipitolateral (ROL)

Label

13. Label the six vertex positions shown in Fig. 9.5. Insert the relative frequency of each position.

ROP:	%	ROA:	%	ROL:	%
LOP:	%	LOA:	%	LOL	%

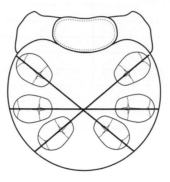

Figure 9.5

Multiple choice questions (MCQ)

14. Identify the correct statement/s:

   a. The detailed fetal anomaly scan screens for anomalies that may benefit from intrauterine therapy.

   b. One of the purposes of the first trimester pregnancy scan is to detect gross fetal abnormalities, such as anencephaly.

   c. The detailed fetal anomaly scan can reveal echogenic bowel in cases of cystic fibrosis and fetal infection.

   d. All of the above

   e. a and c only

15. Examples of diagnostic tests include:

   a. Amniocentesis

   b. Ultrasound scan

   c. Chorionic villus sampling

   d. All of the above

16. The estimated incidence of pregnant women in UK carrying group B Streptococcus (GBS) is:

   a. <10%

   b. 15%

   c. 20%

   d. 25%

17. Increased nuchal translucency is associated with:
   a. Structural disorders
   b. Genetic disorders
   c. Chromosomal disorders
   d. All of the above
   e. b and c

18. Detailed fetal anomaly screening ultrasound scan is usually performed between:
   a. 10–12 weeks' gestation
   b. 14–16 weeks' gestation
   c. 18–20 weeks' gestation
   d. 22–24 weeks' gestation

19. Gestational age is accurately assessed by crown-rump length (CRL):
   a. Before 13 weeks' gestation
   b. In early second trimester
   c. In mid pregnancy
   d. In late pregnancy

PROBLEMS IN EARLY PREGNANCY

Problems in pregnancy relate to mildly irritating to life-threatening conditions and situations. Regular antenatal assessment often helps to prevent many complications and the associated problems, contribute to timely diagnosis and facilitate the relationship between the midwife and woman.

 Short answers

20. Table 9.8 includes activities relating to pregnancy-related causes of abdominal pain. Complete the activities by providing the correct answers.

Table 9.8

	Activity	Answer
In relation to abdominal pain in pregnancy:		
a.	List four incidental and more common pathological causes	
b.	List four other miscellaneous causes:	
c.	Identify one physiological pregnancy-related cause that can become pathological	

Match

21. The activities in Box 9.2 relate to the other causes resulting in abdominal pain during pregnancy (i.e., other than pregnancy-related causes). Identify your knowledge of their classification into physiological causes or pathological causes by drawing a line to correctly match and connect column A (classification) and column B (causes).

Box 9.2

A	B
Causes of abdominal pain in pregnancy	
Physiological:	• Heartburn • Ectopic pregnancy • Soreness from vomiting • Chorioamnionitis • Round ligament pain • Preterm labour • Hyperemesis gravidarum (straining) • Braxton hicks contractions • Uterine/ovarian tumours • Spontaneous uterine rupture
Pathological:	• Constipation • Spontaneous miscarriage • Abdominal pregnancy • Placental abruption • Pressure from growing fetus (vigorous/malpresenting)

  Complete and match

22. Table 9.9 provides descriptive statements relating to definitions and terminology associated with bleeding in early pregnancy. Using your own knowledge, draw a line to match and connect the statement to the condition/problem.

Table 9.9

	Descriptive statement	Condition
a.	Three or more successive pregnancy losses before the age of viability:	Spontaneous miscarriage
b.	Any pregnancy when the fertilized ovum implants outside the uterine cavity:	Criminal termination of pregnancy
c.	Small amount of vaginal bleeding occurring as blastocyst implants into endometrium 5–7 days after fertilization:	Incomplete miscarriage
d.	Overarching term relating to termination of the products of conception before 24 weeks' gestation:	Cervical ectropion (cervical erosion)
e.	Termination of pregnancy is induced under the terms of legal act/s:	Missed or silent miscarriage
f.	Terminology of pregnancy conducted out with the terms of legal act/s:	Ectopic
g.	Abdominal pain persists, bleeding increases, cervix opens with the products of conception entering vagina:	Cervical polyps
h.	Identifiable fetal parts are seen on ultrasound but there is no fetal heart:	Threatened miscarriage
i.	Occurs when all products of conception are spontaneously passed from uterus:	Induced/therapeutic termination of pregnancy
j.	Vaginal bleeding occurs with or without abdominal pain - pregnancy continues:	Implantation bleeding
k.	Occurs when some of the products of conception remains in the uterus:	Recurrent miscarriage
l.	This change in the cervix is a physical response occurring due hormonal changes in pregnancy:	Inevitable miscarriage
m.	Small, vascular pedunculated growths on the cervix:	Complete miscarriage

Early pregnancy loss

 Short answers

23. An estimated 10% to 20% of clinically recognized pregnancies will end in miscarriage often with no definite known cause. Table 9.10 provides related activities. Provide the correct response to complete the activities.

Table 9.10

	Activity	Answer
a.	Identify one fetal cause	
b.	Identify one maternal cause	
c.	Identify two structural causes of miscarriage	
d.	Name four pathophysiological causes of miscarriage	
e.	Infection in genital tract may occur in the process of miscarriage: List three clinical findings present	
f.	List four manifestations or complications of overwhelming infection	
g.	Name two common organisms invading the uterine cavity	

Ectopic pregnancy

 Label

24. Fig. 9.6 shows the site of implantation of ectopic pregnancy. Label the sites.

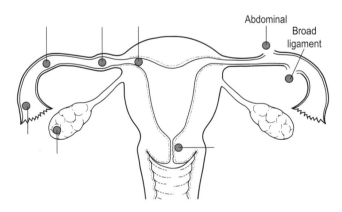

Figure 9.6

Complete

25. Tables 9.11A,B relate to ectopic pregnancy. Table A relates to the classical pattern of symptoms of ectopic pregnancy and Table B relates to the clinical findings. Complete both tables by ticking the correct responses.

Table 9.11A

Classical pattern of symptoms:	Tick
Amenorrhoea	
Vaginal bleeding	
Lower abdominal pain of sudden onset starting locally usually on one side	
Abdominal pain spreads wider as blood loss extends into the peritoneal cavity	
High abdominal pain becoming generalized as blood loss extends into the uterine cavity	
Subdiaphragmatic irritation by blood with no effect on breathing and no referred pain	
Subdiaphragmatic irritation by blood produces referred shoulder tip pain and discomfort on breathing	
No episodes of syncope	
May be episodes of syncope	

Table 9.11B

Clinical findings	Tick
Hypotension	
Normotensive	
Hypertension	
Tachycardia	
Bradycardia	
Abdominal distension	
Guarding of abdomen with rebound tenderness	
No guarding of abdomen	
On pelvic examination the cervix is: Closed and acutely tender when moved	
Closed with no discomfort when moved	
Open and acutely tender when moved	

Trophoblastic disease

Complete

26. Box 9.3 relates to gestational trophoblastic disease (GTD). Complete the paragraphs to read correctly by scoring out the incorrect words or phrases and inserting the missing words.

Box 9.3

a. In molar pregnancy, the development of the placenta is **normal/abnormal** resulting in complete or incomplete hydatidiform mole with **a viable fetus/no viable fetus**. The grape-like appearance of the mole is caused by **over-proliferation/under-proliferation** of the **chorionic villi/endometrial cells**. The condition becomes apparent in **first trimester/second trimester/third trimester** and most commonly presents with **bleeding/abdominal pain**. The four associated conditions characterizing the condition include: _____. _____, _____, and _____.

b. Initially, it is usually diagnosed as a **threatened miscarriage/appendicitis**. The uterus is **larger/smaller** than dates in about half of the cases. If the mole remains in situ, diagnosis is confirmed by ultrasound examination revealing a **'snowstorm'/striated** appearance and continuing raised **hCG levels/prolactin levels**. Treatment is by **conservative monitoring/evacuation of the uterus**. Another associated disorder arising if the mole does not spontaneously miscarry is a variation of the disease progressing to **choriocarcinoma/uterine fibroids**.

Miscellaneous activities related to problems in early pregnancy

 True/false

27. Table 9.12 provides a range of statements. Complete the table by deciding if the statements are true or false.

Table 9.12

	Statement	True	False
a.	Ectopic pregnancy is the least common cause of direct maternal death in early pregnancy		
b.	Cervical excitation refers to the tenderness of the cervix when moved		
c.	A transvaginal ultrasound of the lower abdomen confirms the site of the ectopic pregnancy		
d.	Gestational trophoblastic disease (GTD) is always benign		
e.	Symptoms of pain, bleeding and amenorrhoea may be absent in the subacute phase of ectopic pregnancy		
f.	The retroverted uterus is where the long axis of the uterus and the axis of the vagina is ≤90 degrees		
g.	Hyperemesis gravidarum is the severest form of nausea and vomiting leading to weight loss and dehydration.		
h.	Clinical features of dehydration include both bradycardia and loss of skin turgor		
i.	Prolonged vomiting can be associated with other life-threatening complications, including hyponatraemia, confusion and seizures (if untreated can lead to respiratory arrest)		

PROBLEMS IN LATE PREGNANCY

Bleeding in late pregnancy

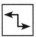 **Match**

28. Table 9.13 relates to definitions related to bleeding in late pregnancy. Column A provides a list of conditions and column B provides descriptive statements. Complete the table by drawing a line to correctly match and connect the condition and statement.

Table 9.13

A. Condition	B. Descriptive statement
Antepartum haemorrhage:	• Blood is retained behind the placenta where it is forced back into the myometrium
Placenta abruption:	• At least two-thirds of placenta has detached with ≥2000 mL blood loss from circulation
Placenta praevia:	• Bleeding from the genital tract after the 24th week of pregnancy and before the onset of labour
Concealed haemorrhage:	• Blood escapes from the placental site, separates the membranes from the uterine wall and drains through the vagina
Couvelaire uterus (uterine apoplexy):	• Premature separation of a normally situated placenta occurring after the 24th week of pregnancy
Revealed haemorrhage:	• The placenta is partially or wholly implanted in the lower uterine segment
Acute emergency obstetric haemorrhage:	• In haemorrhage, seepage of blood outside the normal vascular channels can cause marked damage (uterus observed as bruised, oedematous enlarged at operation)

Classification of placenta praevia

 Complete

29. Table 9.14 provides a list of statements related to the classification of placenta praevia. Complete the table by ticking the appropriate column each statement applies to.

Table 9.14

	Statement	Type 1	Type 2	Type 3	Type 4
a.	Fetal hypoxia is more likely to be present than maternal shock				
b.	The placenta is located over the internal os but not centrally				
c.	This is also described as being a marginal placenta praevia				
d.	The placenta is located centrally over the internal os				
e.	Blood loss is usually moderate, although the conditions of the mother and fetus may vary				
f.	Torrential haemorrhage is likely				
g.	Majority of the placenta is in the upper segment				
h.	Vaginal birth is not appropriate because the placenta precedes the fetus				
i.	Caesarean section is essential to save the lives of mother and baby				
j.	Placenta is partially located in the lower segment near the internal os				
k.	Blood loss is usually mild and the mother and fetus remain in good condition				
l.	Vaginal birth is possible				
m.	Vaginal birth is possible, particularly if the placenta is anterior				
n.	Bleeding is likely to be severe particularly when the lower segment stretches and the cervix begins to efface and dilate in late pregnancy				

True/false

30. Table 9.15 provides a range of statements. Complete the table by indicating if these statements are true or false.

Table 9.15

	Statement	True	False
a.	HELLP (haemolysis, elevated liver enzymes, low platelets) syndrome is a pregnancy-specific cause of jaundice in pregnancy		
b.	In placenta praevia, bleeding is always fresh (bright red) and painless		
c.	In placental abruption, blood retained behind the placenta may be forced into the myometrium		
d.	In a completely concealed abruption with no vaginal bleeding, the woman will have all the signs and symptoms of hypovolaemic shock		
e.	Placenta accreta is a complication in over 50% of women with placenta praevia		
f.	Pituitary necrosis is also known as *Sheehan's syndrome*. This is a serious complication of haemorrhage		
g.	Uterine apoplexy is another term for placenta praevia (stage 4)		
h.	On no account must any vaginal or rectal examination be performed to assess a woman with an antepartum haemorrhage		

Blood clotting

 Complete

31. Box 9.4 provides the normal stages involved in normal clotting. Remove the incorrect words to correct the paragraphs.

Box 9.4

> Normal blood clotting occurs in three main stages:
> (1) When tissues are damaged and **erythrocytes/platelets** break down, **thromboplastin/thrombin** is released;
> (2) In the presence of **potassium/calcium** ions, **thromboplastin/thrombin** leads to the conversion of **fibrin/prothrombin** into **fibrinogen/thrombin**;
> (3) **Thrombin/fibrinogen** is a proteolytic (protein-splitting) enzyme that converts **thrombin/fibrinogen** into fibrin. **Fibrin/fibrinogen** forms a network of long-sticky strands that entrap blood cells to form a clot. The coagulated material contracts and exudes a serum which is **erythrocytes/plasma** depleted of **fibrin/clotting factors**. The coagulation mechanism is normally held at bay by the presence of **vitamin K/heparin** which is produced in the liver. **Fibrinolysis/fibrinogenolysis** is the breakdown of fibrin and occurs in response to the presence of clotted blood. Coagulation will continue unless **fibrinolysis/fibrinogenolysis** takes place.

Complications: bleeding in pregnancy

Bleeding in pregnancy can result in a range of short-term and long-lasting complications. Prompt recognition and action by the midwife can reverse these complications. One life-threatening condition is disseminating intravascular coagulation (DIC). Bleeding can result in inappropriate coagulation leading to consumption of clotting factors. As a result, clotting fails and triggers widespread clotting with the formation of microthrombin throughout the circulation.

 Short answers

32. Table 9.16 provides activities related to placental abruption and bleeding in late pregnancy. Complete the table by providing correct responses.

Table 9.16

	Activity	Responses
a.	List four causes:	
b.	List the initial symptoms for moderate and severe blood loss:	
c.	Findings on abdominal examination:	
d.	In a severe antepartum haemorrhage resulting in an acute obstetric emergency, which two body systems may feature impaired function?	
e.	Identify four obstetric situations/events that may trigger DIC:	

Hepatic disorders and jaundice in pregnancy

 True/false

33. Table 9.17 provides statements related to hepatic disorders and jaundice in pregnancy. Consider the statements and tick the appropriate column to indicate if the statement is true or false.

Table 9.17

	Statement	True	False
a.	Obstetric cholestasis of pregnancy begins in the second trimester		
b.	If there is no active management, there are increased risks associated with obstetric cholestasis (an idiopathic condition)		
c.	Acute fatty liver of pregnancy is a rare and serious condition to mother and fetus if a diagnosis is not made or correct treatment given		
d.	Pregnancy appears to increase the risk of gallstone formation		
e.	Hepatitis A occurs as an acute infection spread mainly by ingesting water contaminated with faecal matter		
f.	In hepatitis B, the risk of liver damage is considered to be greater in the fetus than the mother through transplacental passage of the virus and particularly through blood and body fluids at birth		
g.	Hepatitis C virus is easier to acquire than hepatitis B and carries a lower risk of chronic liver disease		
h.	Generalized pruritus may be a symptom of hepatic related conditions and women should always be referred to a medical practitioner		
i.	Pregnancy increases the risk of women developing acute cholecystitis		

Miscellaneous related problems

  Complete and match

34. Box 9.5 provides statements about hydramnios and preterm prelabour rupture of the membranes (PPROM). Draw a line to match and connect the correct statements in columns A and B.

Box 9.5

	A	B
a.	Normal amniotic fluid increases in amount until 38 weeks is:	• 1 litre
b.	PPROM occurs before:	• Severe fetal abnormality
		• Cord prolapse
c.	Acute hydramnios usually occurs in pregnancy around:	• 800 mL
d.	Two main factors frequently associated with acute hydramnios include:	• 20 weeks' gestation
e.	Chronic hydramnios has a gradual onset usually starting at:	• 300–500 mL
f.	Two risks associated with PPROM include:	• 30 weeks' gestation
		• 37 completed weeks
g.	Normal amniotic fluid at term is:	• Monozygotic twins
h.	Amniotic fluid volume at term in oligohydramnios is:	• Antepartum haemorrhage

Multiple choice questions (MCQ)

35. The following relate to the pelvic girdle during pregnancy:

    a. Activity of pregnancy hormones causes pelvic joint ligaments to relax

    b. The main pregnancy hormone responsible for relaxation of ligaments is placental hormone hCG

    c. Excessive relaxation results in movement of pelvic bones when walking causing pain or discomfort termed pelvic girdle pain (formerly symphysis pubis dysfunction)

    d. All of the above

    e. b and c

    f. a and c

36. Which of the following statements about placental abruption is correct?

    a. Occurs in 5% of all pregnancies

    b. Always involves vaginal bleeding

    c. Partial separation of the placenta causes bleeding from the maternal venous sinuses in the placental bed

    d. Is not associated with a reduction in uterine size

    e. All of the above

37. Disseminating intravascular coagulation (DIC) results in situations involving intrauterine fetal death retained in utero for longer than 3 weeks because of the dead fetal tissue releasing:

    a. Thromboplastin

    b. Thrombin

    c. Fibrin

    d. Heparin

    e. None of the above

38. Pemphigoid gestationis (herpes gestationis) is a:

    a. Condition related to herpes virus

    b. Disease not specific to pregnancy

    c. Condition initiated by a maternal autoimmune response to paternal antigens

    d. Skin disorder only affecting the face

    e. All of the above

39. The most common two causes of cancer during pregnancy are:

    a. Cervix and ovary

    b. Breast and leukaemia

    c. Melanoma and colorectum

    d. Leukaemia and lymphoma

10 Conditions in pregnancy

The physiological changes during pregnancy have a dramatic and profound impact on many of the body systems. These can become further complicated by conditions and disorders experienced during pregnancy or by preexisting conditions. This chapter combines a range of topics including conditions and disorders of significance to midwifery practice. The range includes medical conditions and disorders impacting body systems in pregnancy, sexually transmitted infections of the reproductive tract and multiple births. The activities will assess your knowledge of physiology and pathophysiology related aspects to these topic areas.

Cardiac, haematological and hypertensive disorders in pregnancy

Many congenital heart diseases (CHD) should have been surgically corrected in childhood resulting in more women with CHD achieving pregnancy. In addition, women may experience acquired heart disease in pregnancy.

 Match

1. Table 10.1 provides a range of cardiac disorders with descriptions. Draw a line to match and connect the condition (column A) with the accurate description/s (column B).

Table 10.1

A	B
Common CHD in pregnancy:	• A large left-right shunt of blood is apparent through patent ventricular septal defect (VSD), atrial septal defect (ASD) and patent ductus arteriosus (PDA). Pregnancy is not advised.
	• ASD
	• The condition affects the musculoskeletal system, cardiovascular system (CVS) and eyes
Eisenmenger's syndrome:	• Aortic stenosis
	• Autosomal-dominant (chromosome 15) disorder of connective tissue.
	• VSD
Marfan syndrome:	• This condition causes inflammation and scarring of the heart valves resulting in valve stenosis with or without regurgitation
	• PDA
	• Teratology of Fallot
Rheumatic heart disease:	• May result in aortic dilatation and rupture late in pregnancy/labour
	• Pulmonary stenosis

Completion

2. Table 10.2 provides statements related to cardiac disease in pregnancy. Complete the table by indicating the correct statements.

Table 10.2

	Statement	Correct
a.	The most dangerous cardiac lesions are those that involve pulmonary hypertension	
b.	The three sensitive periods of CVS stress (most critical and life-threatening) are 28–32 weeks of pregnancy, labour and 12–24 hours after birth	
c.	Symptoms of the physiological changes in pregnancy can mimic signs and symptoms of cardiac disease	
d.	The hypercoagulable state in pregnancy decreases the risk of thromboembolic disease in women with arrhythmias, mitral valve stenosis or mechanical valve replacements	
e.	Epidural anaesthesia may be of benefit in labour as it causes peripheral vasodilation and decreases venous return (alleviates pulmonary congestion)	
f.	In active third stage, ergometrine is contraindicated as it can cause vasoconstriction and hypertension	
g.	Cardiac output in labour is not affected by the position of the woman	

Haematological disorders

Short answers

3. Table 10.3 provides a range of questions/activities related to anaemia. Provide short answers to complete the table.

Table 10.3

	Question/activity	Answer
a.	What is the defined level of anaemia in pregnancy (WHO)?	
b.	Identify two physiological reasons for iron deficiency:	
c.	Identify one pregnancy-related reason for iron deficiency:	
d.	Iron deficiency interferes with body functions, identify two of these functions:	
e.	Folic acid is part of which vitamin complex?	
f.	What is folic acid necessary for in pregnancy?	
g.	Name the anaemia that is an abnormality of erythroblasts in bone marrow:	
h.	Name the collective term used for the group of inherited conditions with abnormalities of haemoglobins	

Match

4. Table 10.4 provides risk factors for venous thromboembolism. Draw a line to accurately match and connect the three factors identified in column A with the correct risk factor in column B.

Table 10.4

A	B
	• Systemic infection
Preexisting factors:	• Preeclampsia
	• Previous venous thromboembolism (VTE)/family history of VTE
	• Dehydration/hyperemesis gravidarum
Obstetric factors:	• Age >35 years
	• Ovarian hyperstimulation syndrome
	• Prolonged labour
	• Obesity, BMI >30 kg/m²
Transient factors:	• Varicose veins
	• Immobility, travel >4 hours
	• Parity >3
	• Smoking

True/false

5. Table 10.5 provides a range of statements. Complete the table by deciding if the statements are true or false.

Table 10.5

	Statement	True	False
a.	Pregnant woman has a 10-fold increased risk of developing venous thromboembolism (VTE) compared with a nonpregnant woman.		
b.	Gradient compression (TED) stockings provide a pressure gradient mimicking the pumping action of the deep leg vein calf muscle.		
c.	A thrombus is a blood clot formed within a blood vessel.		
d.	Virchow's triad outlines predisposing factors for thrombus formation.		
e.	Postpartum, the risk of a woman developing VTE increases to a 25-fold risk.		
f.	Disseminated intravascular coagulation (DIC) is a common minor clotting disorder.		
g.	Pulmonary embolism occurs when a deep vein thrombosis (DVT) detaches (embolus) and becomes mobile.		

Hypertensive disorders

 Match

6. Table 10.6 presents the main categories of hypertension and related factors during pregnancy (column A) and descriptive statements (column B). Draw a line to match and connect the statement/s in column B with the correct category in column A.

Table 10.6

A. Category	B. Detailed description
	• Hypertension present at booking or <20 weeks, or on antihypertensive medication when referred (primary or secondary aetiology).
Mild hypertension:	• Hypertension developed as a result of an underlying physiological condition or pathology.
Moderate hypertension:	• Development of preeclampsia with preexisting hypertension and/or preexisting proteinuria.
Severe hypertension:	• Condition is unrelated to other cerebral pathological conditions.
Chronic hypertension:	• Neurological condition associated with preeclampsia manifesting with onset of seizures (pregnancy/postpartum).
New, gestational or pregnancy-induced hypertension:	• Diagnosed on the basis of new hypertension with significant proteinuria ≥20 weeks
New proteinuria:	• A multi-system disorder affecting the placenta, kidney, brain and other organs.
Preeclampsia:	• Diastolic BP 90–99 mmHg, systolic BP 140–149 mmHg.
Eclampsia:	• New hypertension presenting after 20 weeks without significant proteinuria.
Superimposed preeclampsia:	• Proteinuria defined as 1+ (≥300 mg/L) on dipstick, a protein-creatinine ratio of ≥30 mg/mmol on random sample, or urine proteinuria excretion ≥300 mg/24 hours.
Secondary hypertension:	• Diastolic BP 100–109 mmHg, systolic BP 150–159 mmHg.
	• Diastolic BP ≥110 mmHg, systolic BP ≥160 mmHg.

True/false

7. Table 10.7 provides statements related to hypertensive disorders of pregnancy. Complete the table by identifying if the statements are true or false.

Table 10.7

	Statement	True	False
a.	Increased haemoglobin levels and haematocrit suggest the onset of preeclampsia		
b.	The placenta is not the primary cause of preeclampsia		
c.	The coagulation cascade is activated because of disruption of the vascular endothelium and vasoconstriction		
d.	Thrombocytopenia results from the consumption of platelets		
e.	Where there is a large placental mass, hypertensive disorders are more likely to occur		
f.	Renal damage is reflected in increased creatinine clearance, and reduced serum creatinine and uric acid levels		
g.	In the kidneys, hypertension leads to vasospasm of the afferent arterioles resulting in decreased renal function		
h.	In a severe case of oedema in the liver cells, swelling causes lower abdominal pain and can lead to intracapsular haemorrhages		
i.	In hypertensive encephalopathy, the autoregulation of cerebral blood flow is disrupted resulting in vasospasm, cerebral oedema and blood clot formation		
j.	Women with preeclampsia are hypovolaemic		
k.	Preeclampsia is associated with thrombocytopenia (low platelets), prolonged clotting times and increased serum creatinine (>90 mm/L)		

HELLP syndrome

  ## Complete and short answers

8. Table 10.8 provides two sets activities relating to HELPP syndrome. Complete activities a and b by removing the incorrect words or numerical values for these paragraphs to read correctly. Insert the answers to the questions provided.

Table 10.8

	HELLP syndrome
a.	HELLP syndrome is **a multisystem/bi-system** disorder occurring either on its own or in association with **gestational diabetes/preeclampsia**. Of all cases, **70%/40%** will present in the antenatal period and **30%/60%** postpartum. Antenatally, the disorder typically manifests itself between **20 and 26 weeks/32 and 34 weeks'** gestation and typical onset postpartum is within **48/96** hours of birth.
b	The disorder involves activation of the **renin-angiotensin-aldosterone/coagulation** system. This causes increased deposits of protein **fibrin/thrombin** throughout the body resulting in fragmentation of **erythrocytes/platelets**. **Fibrin/thrombin** deposits on blood vessel walls initiate clumping of **erythrocytes/platelets** resulting in blood clots and lowering of the **erythrocyte/platelet** count. Deposits **increase/decrease** the diameter of blood vessels, **lowering/raising** the blood pressure and **increasing/reducing** blood flow to organs. The **kidneys/liver are/is** especially affected.
c.	What does the acronym HELLP stand for?
d.	What are the presenting symptoms? (Identify three symptoms)
e.	What are **serious** maternal complications? (Identify four)

Eclampsia

9. Table 10.9 provides activities related to eclampsia and impending eclampsia. Using your own knowledge of the condition, complete the table by scoring out the incorrect words and inserting the visual disturbances.

Table 10.9

Sign or symptom	Statement
Eclampsia	This is a **neurological/endocrine** condition associated with **convulsions and coma/respiratory distress** that cannot be attributed to other conditions, such as **epilepsy/asthma**. Eclampsia can develop from **late pregnancy and immediately following birth/20 weeks' gestation until 6 weeks' postpartum.**
Blood pressure	There is a sharp **rise/fall** in BP.
Headache	Described as being **severe/dull** and **intermittent/persistent**. It is usually located in the **frontal/occipital** region. This is caused by **cerebral vasospasm/dehydration**.
Level of consciousness	The woman is typically **awake/drowsy** and **alert/confused**. This is caused by **cerebral vasospasm/dehydration**.
Visual	Visual disturbances are caused by **cerebral vasospasm/dehydration**. The main two disturbances include: _____
Urinary output	Urinary output is **diminished/increased**. Proteinuria may increase/decrease. This woman is in **hepatic/renal** failure.
Abdominal pain	There is **liver/pulmonary** oedema. This causes the woman to complain of **upper/lower** abdominal pain. The woman may also have **nausea and vomiting/ pyrexia.**

DIABETES MELLITUS

The rising incidence of diabetes mellitus across the lifespan is now a global public health issue. This endocrine disorder interferes with the metabolism of glucose. It is chronic and progressive and if untreated, can result in a range of physical and health-related complications.

 Complete

10. Table 10.10 provides a range of activities related to diabetes mellitus. Complete the table by removing incorrect words and by providing a response to the activities/questions.

Table 10.10

Classification	Statement
Type 1 diabetes (IDDM)	Insulin dependent diabetes mellitus (IDDM) - Occurs when **alpha/beta** cells in the Islets of Langerhans located in the **gall bladder/pancreas** are destroyed, stopping the production of **insulin/glycagon**.
Type 2 diabetes (NIDDM)	Noninsulin dependent diabetes mellitus (NIDDM) - Results from a **surge/defect** in the action of **insulin/glucagon**. Three main factors increase the risk of developing diabetes 2. Identify these factors: _____ _____
Gestational diabetes (GDM)	GDM is defined as **glucose intolerance/carbohydrate intolerance** resulting in **hypoglycaemia/ hyperglycaemia** of variable severity. Onset or first recognition occurs during **adolescence/ pregnancy**.

	Activity/question	Answer
a.	What are the two key characteristics of this disorder?	
b.	Identify the three classic signs and symptoms:	
c.	Identify four long-term effects:	

Physiological values

11. Table 10.11 provides physiological values for haematological and blood plasma glucose values (based on the World Health Organization [WHO] and the National Institute for Clinical Excellence [NICE] recommendations). Complete the table by inserting the correct values from the list of numerical values provided.

12 g/dL	<7 g/dL	>25.0 mmol/L	4–7 mmol/L
120 days	17 days	5.3 mmol/L	150–400 × 10⁹/L
6.4 mmol/L	<2.2 mmol/L	7.8 mmol/L	3–5 mmol/L
11 g/dL	5–7 mmol/L		

Table 10.11

	Haematological-related values	Blood plasma glucose (metabolic) values
a.	Hb levels (woman): Non pregnant: _____g/dL Pregnant: _____ g/dL Severe anaemia: _____ g/dL	Normal nonpregnant range: _____ mmol/L Nonpregnant with diagnosed DM: Normal fasting range: _____ mmol/L Range before meals: _____ mmol/L
b.	Normal lifespan: Healthy erythrocytes: _____ days Sickle cells (fragile_____ days	Pregnant with DM: Fasting: _____ mmol/L 1 hour after meals: _____ mmol/L 2 hours after meals: _____ mmol/L
c.	Platelet range:	Hypoglycaemia:
d.		Severe hyperglycaemia: _____ mmol/L

Risks of diabetes on pregnancy

Diabetes in pregnancy is associated with risks to the woman and the developing fetus. This results in a significant increase in fetal and maternal morbidity. Midwives need to have knowledge of these risks, so they are vigilant in their observations and assessment.

 Short answers

12. Table 10.12 provides factors related to diabetes in pregnancy and the impact on the fetus. Using your own knowledge, provide short answers to complete the activities.

Table 10.12

	Activities/question	Answer
a.	List three risk factors for GDM assessed at booking visit:	
b.	Identify the test carried out for GDM in women with risk factors:	
c.	Identify the term used for breakdown of fatty acids:	
d.	List three complications for the pregnancy (woman with preexisting DM):	
e.	List two increased risks to the fetal development during pregnancy:	
f.	List two possible fetal complications at birth:	
g.	List two long-term maternal complications:	

Complete

13. Table 10.13 provides statements relating to diabetes mellitus. Complete the table by indicating the correct statements.

Table 10.13

	Statement	Correct
a.	The Coxsackie virus B4 causing childhood infection may be implicated in the onset of type 1 diabetes	
b.	Type 2 DM (NIDDM) results from increased insulin resistance because of the decreased number of cellular insulin receptors	
c.	GDM is diagnosed if the woman has either fasting blood glucose level of ≥5.6 mmol/L OR a 2-hour plasma glucose level of ≥7.8 mmol/L	
d.	Women with GDM are not at risk of developing GDM in a future pregnancy or developing NIDDM in later life	
e.	In later pregnancy, placental hormones (e.g. oestrogen and human placental lactogen) cause progressive insulin resistance which decreases insulin efficiency	
f.	No interventions are offered to women with GDM as it does not impact of the health of pregnancy, mother or baby	
g.	Women with DM are more at risk from infection	

Miscellaneous medical conditions during pregnancy

 Multiple choice questions (MCQ)

14. In relation to asthma, which of the following statements is incorrect:

a. It is an inflammatory disease with hyper-responsiveness of the airways.

b. It is characterized by constriction of the smooth muscles of the bronchioles, mucosal oedema and hypersecretion of mucous.

c. The work of breathing is increased and excessive negative intrapleural pressure can cause increase in the demands of the right ventricle.

d. There is a rise in pulmonary arterial pressure and a decrease in arterial systolic pressure and pulse pressure.

e. None of the above

15. In relation to pathophysiology, which of the following statements relating to asthma is incorrect:

a. Respiratory rate is not changed by pregnancy; however, the effects of progesterone does increase hyperventilation by term.

b. Women with asthma are not at any increased risks in pregnancy.

c. Expiratory and residual volumes may be decreased because of the effect of the gravid uterus on the diaphragm.

d. Bronchoconstriction occurs after exposure to an allergen, and this causes immunoglobin E (IgE) antigen to bind to mast cell surface receptors.

e. A small number of women in pregnancy may develop status asthmaticus, which is recurrent asthmatic episodes, leading to partial or complete obstruction of airways.

16. Which of the following statements relating to the pathophysiology of the following condition is/are correct:

    a. Tuberculosis (TB) is an infectious bacterial disease transmitted from person to person via droplets from the throat and lungs of people with active respiratory disease.

    b. The bacillus responsible for TB can lie dormant (latent TB) inside macrophages with a small percentage becoming active some years later.

    c. In the treatment of TB during pregnancy, streptomycin is contraindicated because of the incidence of hearing loss in neonates exposed in utero.

    d. All of the above

    e. b and c only

17. Which of the following statements is/are incorrect:

    a. A rare serious complication of hyperemesis gravidarum is Wernicke's encephalopathy.

    b. Acute kidney injury (AKI) usually results from a severe deficit in cortical renal blood flow leading to ischaemia in the kidneys.

    c. If the pregnant woman suffers from acute pyelonephritis, then bradycardia and hypertension may indicate the development of endototoxic shock.

    d. Pregnant women with chronic renal failure experience pathophysiological oedema caused by loss of protein in the urine and electrolyte imbalance because of low urine output from the kidneys.

    e. All of the above

    f. None of the above

18. Which of the following statements is/are correct:

    a. The typical signs of appendicitis may not be present because of the growing uterus gradually displacing the appendix.

    b. Ileostomy or colostomy (for previous urinary or alimentary diversion) should not affect the course of pregnancy, with approximately 75% of women progressing to a normal vaginal birth.

    c. Ultrasound scan cannot be used to diagnose appendicitis.

    d. All of the above

    e. a and b

    f. b and c

19. Which of the following statements relating to epilepsy is/are incorrect:

    a. Epilepsy is a curable condition.

    b. Pathophysiology of seizures involves the abnormal discharge of electricity spreading throughout the brain and resulting in a tonic phase followed by a clonic phase.

    c. The tonic phase involves generalized muscle contraction and increased muscle tone with the clonic phase interrupting the seizure discharge and leading to intermittent contract/relax pattern of muscle action.

    d. All of the above.

    e. None of the above

True/false

20. Table 10.14 provides a range of statements relating to medical conditions during pregnancy. Complete the table by indicating if the statements are true or false.

Table 10.14

	Statement	True	False
a.	Tea and coffee have no effect of the absorption of iron in the woman's diet		
b.	Biochemical thyrotoxicosis may occur in women who develop hyperemesis gravidarum because of the similarity between thyrotropin (TSH) and human chorionic gonadotropin (hCG)		
c.	The onset of primary TB is often insidious and the symptoms nonspecific		
d.	Thyroid crisis (thyroid storm) is rare and characterized by extreme hypermetabolic state. This medical emergency can occur in labour (women with hyperthyroidism) because of stressful delivery or infection		
e.	Hashimoto's disease is the underactivity of the thyroid gland		
f.	Some normal pregnancy features mimic Cushing's syndrome which is excessive levels of corticosteroids		
g.	Alcohol may interfere with the utilization of folic acid		
h.	Severe hyperthyroidism is not associated with infertility		
i.	Untreated hypothyroidism is often associated with infertility as thyrotropin-releasing hormone (TRH) stimulation induces hyperprolactinaemia which prevents ovulation		
j.	Women who suffer from spherocytosis may have had a splenectomy.		
k.	Many autoimmune diseases are more prevalent in women between puberty and the menopause		
l	Grave's disease is the most common cause of hyperthyroidism in pregnancy		

SEXUALLY TRANSMITTED INFECTIONS

 Match

21. Table 10.15 provides a range of genital, bacterial and viral infections of the reproductive tract (column B). Draw a line between the sexual infection (column B) to correctly match and connect with the correct mode of transmission (column A). Some conditions may be transmitted via multiple routes.

Table 10.15

A	B
	• Vulvovaginal candidiasis
Transmitted sexually:	• Human cytomegalovirus (CMV)
	• Hepatitis B virus (HBV)
	• Herpes simplex virus (HSV). Type 1 HSV-1
	• Trichomiasis
Not transmitted sexually:	• Group B streptococcus (GBS)
	• Chlamydia
	• Herpes simplex virus (HSV) I. Type 2 HSV-2
	• Genital warts
	• Gonorrhoea
Close sexual contact (increased sexual activity):	• HIV - Human immunodeficiency virus
	• Syphilis
	• Bacterial vaginosis (BV)
	• Hepatitis B virus (HBV)

Correct/incorrect

22. Table 10.16 provides a list of statements related to sexual-related infections. Complete the table by identifying the correct statements.

Table 10.16

	Statement	Correct
i.	Trichomoniasis is one of the most common sexually transmitted infections. A classic frothy yellow-green discharge occurs in 10%–30% of women	
ii.	Bacterial vaginosis (BV) is the most common cause of vaginal discharge. Associated with sexual activity, the infection often co-exists with other sexually transmitted infections	
iii	Factors predisposing to vulvovaginal candidiasis include: changes to vaginal flora (e.g. antibiotics, spermacides), poor diabetic control, pregnancy and immunosuppressant disease	
iv.	Gonorrhoea may cause systemic disease and arthritis	
v.	Syphilis is an acute and chronic infection that can be transmitted transplacentally to the fetus from 9th week of gestation onwards	
vi.	Group B streptococcus (GBS) is the leading cause of serious neonatal infection in the UK	
vii.	Hepatitis B virus (HBV) belongs to a family of deoxyribonucleic acid (DNA) viruses that cause infection of the liver.	
viii.	Human papillomavirus (HPV) does not cause genital warts	
ix.	Syphilis has an early noninfective stage and a late infective stage	

MULTIPLE PREGNANCIES

The term 'multiple pregnancy' describes the development of more than one fetus in utero at the same time. The following activities relate to twin pregnancies.

Match

23. Complete Table 10.17 by drawing a line to match and correct the type of twin (column A) with the correct statement in column B.

Table 10.17

A	B
	• Binovular twins
	• Same or different sex
	• Identical twins
Monozygotic twins (MZ):	• Two oocytes fertilized by two spermatozoa
	• Develop from the fusion of one oocyte and one spermatozoon
Dizygotic twins (DZ):	• Have the same genes, blood group and physical features
	• Fraternal twins
	• Uniovular twins
	• Always the same sex

Short answers

24. Table 10.18 presents a list of activities and questions relating to twin pregnancy. Complete the table by providing the correct answer/s.

Table 10.18

	Activity/question	Answer
a.	Name the term when twins are conceived from sperm of different men (> 1 partner during menstrual cycle):	
b.	Name the term used for twins conceived as a result of two coital acts in different menstrual cycles	
c.	Name the term used to determine whether twins are monozygotic or dizygotic	
d.	Which method usually confirms diagnosis of multiple birth pregnancy:	
e.	List two maternal complications of twin pregnancy during pregnancy:	
f.	List two fetal complications of twin pregnancy:	
g.	List one obstetric complications during pregnancy:	
h.	List one serious complication occurring in labour:	

True/false

25. Table 10.19 provides a range of statements about twin pregnancy. Complete the table by indicating if each statement is true or false.

Table 10.19

	Statement	True	False
a.	Both monozygotic and dizygotic twins can have separate placentae, two chorions and two amnions		
b.	Twin babies with a single outer membrane (chorion), they must be monochorionic and monozygotic		
c.	At birth dichorionic twins have a greater weight variation than monochorionic twins		
d.	In both monozygotic and dizygotic twins, the type of placenta produced is determined immediately at conception		
e.	Both monozygotic and dizygotic twins can have fused placentae, two chorions and two amnions		
f.	Only monozygotic twins can have a single placenta, one chorion and two amnions		
g.	Monochorionic twin pregnancies have a 3–5 times higher risk of perinatal mortality and morbidity than dichorionic twin pregnancies		
h.	'Lambda sign' relates to the tongue of placental tissue between the two chorions seen on ultrasound scan		
i.	DNA testing to compare each baby is the most accurate method of determining zygosity		

Multiple choice questions (MCQ)

26. The incidence of twin births in the United Kingdom is:
    a. 1 in 33 births
    b. 1 in 45 births
    c. 1 in 63 births
    d. 1 in 88 births

27. With monozygotic twins, the type of placenta produced is determined by the time the fertilized oocyte splits. The most common is:
    a. 0–3 days: dichorionic diamniotic placenta (DCDA)
    b. 4–8 days: monochorionic diamniotic placenta (MCDA)
    c. 8–12 days: monochorionic monoamniotic placenta (MCMA)
    d. 12–13 days

28. There is a familial history of:
    a. Dizygotic twins on the male side
    b. Dizygotic twins on the female side
    c. Both monozygotic and dizygotic twins
    d. Monozygotic twins on the female side
    e. Monozygotic twins on the male side

29. In relation to polyhydramnios which of the following statements is correct:
    a. Polyhydramnios is associated with fetal abnormalities
    b. Polyhydramnios is associated with twin to twin transfusion syndrome (TTTS)
    c. Acute polyhydramnios may occur in pregnancy as early as 16 weeks' gestation
    d. All of the above
    e. None of the above

11 Labour: first and second stages

The aetiology of labour is complex and not yet fully understood. What is known is that the transition from pregnancy to labour and birth is a sequence of events that often begins gradually. This chapter focuses on the physiology of first stage and second stage of labour. The range of activities will test your knowledge of terminology and the physiological and physical developments related to the onset, first and second stages of labour.

ONSET OF LABOUR

 True/false

1. Table 11.1 provides a range of evidence-based statements relating to physiological and other factors associated with the onset of labour in uncomplicated pregnancies. Complete the table by indicating if the statements are true or false.

Table 11.1

	Statements	True	False
a.	Normal labour occurs between 39 and 42 weeks (259–294 days) gestation.		
b.	Uterine quiescence is maintained during pregnancy by high levels of circulating progesterone.		
c.	Maternal oxytocin plays a major part in the initiation of labour.		
d.	Timing of onset may be related to fetal brain activity via adrenocorticotrophic hormone (ACTH) and the fetal pituitary-adrenal axis.		
e.	Cortisol secreted by the fetal adrenal cortex acts on the placental enzymes to convert progesterone to oestrogen.		
f.	Levels of oestrogen increase the sensitivity of the uterus to prostaglandins and oxytocin produced by maternal tissues and the fetoplacental unit.		
g.	A reduction in progesterone levels results in uterine contractions which are powerful enough to expel the fetus.		
h.	The hormone, dehydroepiandrosterone sulphate (DHEAS), is the major precursor of placental oestradiol and estrone synthesis. This hormone may be implicated in fetal control of the onset of labour.		
i.	Oestrogen stimulates uterine contractions and cervical dilatation.		
j.	Prostaglandin release in labour probably involves oxytocin release.		
k.	Evidence indicates that the hormone oestradiol brings about the changes in the collagen content of the cervix for labour.		
l.	Cortisol levels in umbilical cord blood after birth are difficult to assess. However, the increase in cortisol levels found is now thought to be caused by the stress of labour rather than being responsible for the onset of labour.		
m.	The chorion is the only membrane involved in the production of prostaglandins.		
n.	The decidua is a major source of prostaglandins during labour.		

Maternal physiological adaptation in labour

Labour influences maternal physiological changes. It is important that the midwife has knowledge of the physiological changes in relation to the extent, direction and timing of the changes, and recognizes the changes and why these occur.

Completion

2. Table 11.2 provides a range of statements relating to maternal physiological changes in labour. Remove the incorrect words/numerical values so that each statement reads correctly.

Table 11.2

	Statements
a.	First stage is associated with a progressive **rise/fall** in cardiac output as each contraction **adds/removes** 300–500 mL of blood **to/from** the circulating volume.
b.	Cardiac output **rises/falls** in first stage **10%–15% above/10%–15% below** pregnancy values and **50% above/50% below** pregnancy levels, during second stage.
c.	Within **1 h/4 h** of birth, cardiac parameters **fall/increase** to prelabour levels and may take up to **6–8 weeks/12 weeks** to return to prepregnancy levels.
d.	Haemoglobin levels tend to **increase/decrease** slightly in labour because of the haemoconcentration from muscular activity and dehydration.
e.	Erythropoiesis (formation of red blood cells [RBCs]) and white blood cell (WBC) count **increase/decrease** caused by the stress of labour and postpartum.
f.	A transitory **increase/decrease** in the activity of the coagulation system occurs during labour and **immediately/within 4 hours** following placental separation.
g.	Clot formation in the torn blood vessels on placental separation needs to be **maximized/minimized** and blood loss from haemorrhage **maximized/minimized**.
h.	A **decrease/increase** in fibrinolytic activity enhances clot formation at the placental site.
i.	Placental site is **rapidly/gradually** covered by a fibrin mesh utilizing **5%–10%/20%–30%** of circulating **prothrombin/fibrinogen**.
j.	Too frequent occurrence of contractions results in the **decrease/increase** in the oxygenation of the myometrium resulting in **metabolic acidosis/metabolic alkalosis**.
k.	Strong frequent uterine contractions **increase/decrease** in Pco_2 (because of the change to anaerobic metabolism) leading to a **fall/rise** in pH and causing **maternal acidosis/metabolic alkalosis**.
l.	During labour, pain cause the respiratory rate to **increase/decrease** and tidal volume to **increase/decrease**.
m.	Maternal hyperventilation leads to **respiratory alkalosis/respiratory acidosis**.
n.	During labour, the **increase/decrease** found in maternal and fetal renin-angiotensin may be important for **reducing/increasing** uteroplacental blood flow following birth.

 Multiple Choice Questions (MCQ)

3. Identify the correct statement/s about the physiological effects during labour:

   a. Uterine contractions cause profound changes in the cardiovascular system.

   b. There is further magnification of the hypercoagulable state present in pregnancy.

   c. Cardiovascular changes are limited by epidural analgesia, supine hypotension and by the alleviation of pain and anxiety.

   d. Epidural analgesia appears to prevent progressive increases in cardiac output.

   e. Supine hypotension lowers cardiac output and decreases stroke volume.

   f. Supine hypotension causes a compensatory increase in heart rate.

4. Identify the incorrect statement/s related to blood pressure (BP) changes **in labour**:

   a. Pain, anxiety and apprehension do not influence systolic and diastolic BP.

   b. During the first stage, blood pressure may rise by 5 mmHg and may rise even higher in second stage.

   c. Blood pressure begins to rise 5 seconds before the contraction begin and returns to normal after the contraction has ended.

   d. Diastolic pressure can rise by 25 mmHg in first stage and up to 55 mmHg in second stage.

   e. There is only a small change in the peripheral vascular resistance.

5. Identify the incorrect physiological event/s occurring in the presence of strong frequent uterine contractions:
    a.   Ischaemia and tissue hypoxia
    b.   Ischaemia does not cause pain
    c.   During active stage involving pushing, the partial pressure of carbon dioxide (PCO_2) may rise
    d.   During active stage involving pushing, fetal PCO_2 will rise if the mother is acidotic
    e.   Increased fetal PCO_2 will lead to fetal acidosis and distress

6. Hyperventilation can be caused by:
    a.   Pain and anxiety
    b.   Drugs
    c.   Breath-holding
    d.   Panic and excessive use of breathing exercises

7. Hyperventilation will result in:
    a.   Rise in PCO_2
    b.   Fall in PCO_2
    c.   Tingling of maternal fingers and toes
    d.   Dizziness

8. Identify the correct influencing factors related to gastric emptying **during labour:**
    a.   Administration of opioid drugs
    b.   Fear and pain
    c.   Intake of food containing high levels of fibre
    d.   Intake of food containing high levels of fat
    e.   All of the above

9. Identify the incorrect statement/s relating to gastric activity in labour:
    a.   Gastric motility is decreased.
    b.   Gastric motility is increased.
    c.   Gastric emptying is mildly delayed during labour (with or without epidural analgesia).
    d.   Gastric emptying is unaffected with epidural analgesia.
    e.   An increase in gastric acidity and relaxation of the cardiac sphincter leads to oesophageal reflux and increases the risk of aspiration pneumonitis.
    f.   Aspiration pneumonitis is also known as Mendelson's syndrome.

10. Identify the correct statement/s about maternal metabolism before labour:
    a.   There is a degree of respiratory alkalosis.
    b.   There is a degree of metabolic acidosis.
    c.   There is reduced ability to use glucose to meet the main source of glucose for the fetus.
    d.   The provision of glucose (gluconeogenesis) from the metabolism of body fat (lipolysis) occurs, causing an increase in plasma ketones throughout pregnancy.
    e.   All of the above
    f.   a, b and d

11. Identify the incorrect statement/s about maternal metabolism during labour:

   a. Labour has no effect on maternal metabolism and plasma electrolytes.

   b. Compensatory lipolysis occurring to meet the body's energy requirements results in ketones being produced.

   c. The production of excess ketones may depress fetal pH and interfere with myometrial activity.

   d. The estimated metabolic cost of active labour is between 700 and 1100 calories per hour.

   e. Anaerobic metabolism causes lactate to accumulate which produces a small drop of maternal plasma pH to about 7.34 and a fall in PCO_2.

   f. All of the above

12. Identify the incorrect statement/s about the physiological changes relating to third stage of labour:

   a. On placental separation, blood clots seal off the torn blood vessels at the site to reduce blood loss.

   b. Within 24–48 hours, cardiac parameters fall to prelabour levels.

   c. Within 1 hour of birth, cardiac parameters fall to prelabour levels.

   d. After third stage, there may be cardiovascular instability caused by dramatic haematological changes taking place over this period.

   e. Cardiac parameters may take up to 6–8 weeks to return to prepregnancy levels.

FIRST STAGE OF LABOUR

Labour is a continuous and dynamic process and it remains unclear if normal labour has three distinct phases. For the purpose of this workbook, the traditional definitions of labour will be used until parameters are more clearly defined.

Stages of labour

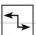 **Match**

13. Box 11.1 provides statements about the stages of labour (NICE 2017). To complete the table, draw a line to match and connect the stage of labour in column A with the correct statement in column B.

Box 11.1

A. Stage of labour	B. Statements
	Regular painful contractions confirmed
Latent first stage:	Active maternal effort is evident following confirmation of full dilatation of cervix in absence of expulsive contractions
Established first stage:	Expulsive contractions with a finding of full dilatation of the cervix or other signs of full dilatation of the cervix
	From birth of baby to the expulsion of the placenta and membranes
Second stage (Passive):	Baby is visible
	Period of time, not necessarily continuous there is some cervical change, including cervical effacement and dilatation up to 4 cm
Second stage (Active):	There is progressive cervical dilatation from 4 cm
	Finding of full dilatation of the cervix before involuntary expulsive contractions
Third stage:	Period of time, not necessarily continuous, when there are painful contractions

Short answers

14. Table 11.3 provides a list of descriptive statements related to labour. Complete the table by inserting the correct answer from the list provided.

Bandl's ring	Polarity	Cervical effacement	Lower uterine segment
Retraction ring	Show	Spurious labour	Upper uterine segment
Uterine contractions	Retraction	Operculum	Contraction and retraction

Table 11.3

	Statements	Answer
a.	This describes the gradual merging of the cervix into the lower uterine segment.	
b.	Dilatation and effacement of the cervix are absent.	
c.	Muscle fibres do not completely relax between contractions and fibres retain some shortening following contractions.	
d.	This thinner portion of the uterus is formed of the isthmus and the cervix.	
e.	This refers to the blood-stained mucoid discharge seen by the woman in early labour and the small loss of bright red blood during the transitional phase.	
f.	This thick, muscular portion of the uterus is mainly concerned with contraction and retraction.	
g.	This term refers to the cervical plug during pregnancy.	
h.	This physiological ridge occurs in uncomplicated labour and forms between the upper and lower uterine segments and become visible above the symphysis pubis.	
i.	This term describes the neuromuscular harmony between the two poles of the uterus throughout labour.	
j.	Intrauterine hydrostatic pressure can measure the pressure of these exerted on the amniotic fluid.	
k.	Uterine muscle has this unique property.	
l.	This exaggerated pathological ridge occurs in obstructed labour and develops between the upper and lower uterine segments.	

 Correct/incorrect

15. Table 11.4 provides statements related to the physiological process of labour. Complete the table by indicating the correct statements.

Table 11.4

	Statement	Correct
a.	Intact membranes in labour provide a barrier against ascending infection and maintain a good oxygen supply to the fetus.	
b.	From a physiological perspective, the moment for membranes to rupture is when the cervix is fully dilated and no longer able to support forewaters and the force of maximum contraction.	
c.	The term general fluid pressure refers to the pressure exerted on amniotic fluid by uterine contractions when membranes are intact.	
d.	In all women, the process of effacement always completes before the onset of labour and before dilatation of the external cervical os occurs.	
e.	The separation of the forewaters from the hindwaters keeps the membranes intact during first stage.	
f.	During each contraction, the force of the fundal contraction is transmitted to the upper pole of the fetus, down the long axis of the fetal spine, causing increasing flexion of the head (termed *fetal axis pressure*).	
g.	Transcutaneous electrical nerve stimulation (TENS) should be offered to women in established labour.	
h.	Either H2-receptor antagonists or antacids should be considered for women receiving opioids or who have or may develop risk factors making a general anaesthetic more likely.	
i.	In a fetus at term and with the vertex presenting, the diameter of the cervix would normally have to reach 10 cm.	
j.	A cervicograph plots the rate of cervical effacement in labour.	

Assessing progress

16. Box 11.2 revisits the terminology relating to fetal assessment. To complete the table, draw a line to match the terminology in column A and connect with the correct description in column B.

Box 11.2

A. Terminology	B. Description
Lie:	That part of the fetus which lies at the pelvic brim or in the lower pole of the uterus.
Presentation:	Relationship of the denominator to the six key points on the maternal pelvic brim.
Attitude:	This occurs when the widest presenting transverse diameter has passed through the brim of pelvis.
Denominator:	Relationship of the long axis of the fetus and the long axis of the uterus. It may be longitudinal, oblique or transverse.
Position:	This refers to that part of the fetus lying over the cervical os during labour.
Engagement:	Identifies the name of the part of the presentation used when referring to fetal position in relation to the pelvis.
Presenting part:	The relationship of the fetal head and limbs to its body. It may be fully flexed, deflexed or partially/completely extended.

Vaginal examination

 Complete

17. Table 11.5 provides statements relating to vaginal examination. Complete the table by indicating the correct statements.

Table 11.5

	Indications to perform vaginal examination	Correct
a.	Assess progress and delay in labour.	
b.	Confirm cervical effacement and dilatation of the cervix.	
c.	Antepartum haemorrhage.	
d.	Confirm full dilatation of the cervix.	
e.	Make a positive identification of presentation.	
f.	Determine whether the head is engaged (in case of doubt).	
g.	Abdominal pain.	
h.	Ascertain whether the forewaters have ruptured, or to rupture them artificially.	
i.	Vaginal bleeding.	
j.	Exclude cord prolapse after rupture of the forewaters especially if there is an ill-fitting presenting part or the fetal heart rate changes.	
k.	In multiple pregnancy: to confirm the axis of the fetus and presentation of the second twin and, if necessary, to rupture the second amniotic sac.	
l.	At the woman's request.	

Match

18. Box 11.3 provides information relating to the possible observations and findings from performing a vaginal examination. To complete, draw a line to match the maternal and fetal areas examined in column A and connect with the correct observation or finding in column B.

Box 11.3

A. Vaginal examination	B. Observations or findings
Labia:	Caput succudaneum
	Consistency (application to presenting part)
	Loaded or impacted
Perineum:	Discharge, bleeding
	Moulding
	Colour and odour
Vaginal orifice:	Cystocele (multiparous women)
	Length of canal
	Effacement and dilatation
Rectum:	Consistency (bulging, ease or difficulty in locating)
	Intact
	Oedema
Cervix:	Varicosities
	Position of fetal head (defined by occiput)
	Attitude (using sutures and fontanelles located)
Amniotic membranes:	Scars (previous episiotomy) or tears
	Cultural female genital mutilation (evidence)
Fetal head:	Warts and sores
	Descent estimation in relationship to maternal ischial spines (above or below spines)
Other observations:	Present or absent

Fetal heart rate (FHR)

Monitoring fetal well-being during labour involves measuring fetal heart rate (FHR) either through intermittent auscultations or continuous cardiotocography (CTG). The midwife needs to have sound knowledge and understanding of heart rate monitoring to interpret and recognize normal and abnormal recordings and the implications for fetus/baby.

True/false

19. Table 11.6 provides a range of statements relating to FHR. Complete the table by indicating if each statement is true or false.

Table 11.6

	Statement	True	False
a.	CTG should be offered in established labour to women at low risk of complications.		
b.	Intermittent periods of reduced baseline variability are regarded as normal, especially during periods of quiescence ('sleep').		
c.	Intermittent auscultation should be carried out immediately after a contraction for at least 1 min, at least every 15 min (record as a single rate).		
d.	The risk of fetal acidosis is low, if there is a stable baseline FHR between 110 and 160 beats/min and normal variability.		
e.	The presence of FHR accelerations, even with reduced baseline variability, is generally a sign that the baby is healthy.		
f.	Continuous monitoring of FHR should be offered in established first stage of labour to women at high risk of complications.		
g.	In the absence of other risk factors, women who have nonsignificant meconium should be offered continuous CTG.		
h.	Underlying causes of irregularities in FHR, such as hypotension or uterine hyperstimulation, need to be corrected.		
i.	Either pH or lactate should be used when interpreting fetal blood sample results.		
j.	If digital fetal scalp stimulation (during vaginal examination) leads to an acceleration in FHR, then this should be regarded as a sign that the baby is healthy.		
k.	If there are no other risk factors, then women who have nonsignificant meconium should not be offered continuous CTG.		
l.	Amniotomy alone for suspected delay in the established first stage of labour should be regarded as an indication to start continuous CTG.		
m.	Midwives should always use either a Pinard stethoscope or Doppler ultrasound to assess FHR in low-risk women.		

Short answers

20. Table 11.7 provides a range of incomplete statements relating to FHR monitoring. Complete the table by inserting short answers from the list provided.

Acceleration   Baseline rate   Nonreassuring   Presence/absence of decelerations
Abnormal   Bradycardia   Normal   Presence of accelerations
Baseline variability   Deceleration   Pathological   Reassuring
    Suspicious

Table 11.7

	Statements	Answer
a.	Identify the four features of FHR.	
b.	The feature of baseline FHR of 110–160 beats/min is described as being.	
c.	The feature of baseline FHR of 100–109 beats/min to 161–180 beats/min is described as being.	
d.	The feature of baseline FHR of <100 beats/min or >180 beats/min is described as being.	
e.	The CTG trace with one abnormal feature OR two nonreassuring features is categorized as being.	
f.	The CTG trace with one nonreassuring feature AND two reassuring features is categorized as being.	
g.	This refers to a drop in the FHR from the baseline of 15 beats for >15 s but <3 min.	
h.	This term refers to a deceleration of FHR lasting longer than 3 min.	
i.	The CTG trace with all features reassuring is categorized as being.	
j.	This term refers to a brief rise in FHR of at least 15 beats, for at least 15 s.	

Multiple choice questions (MCQ)

21. Identify the incorrect statement in relation to fetal blood sampling:
    a. Fetal blood sampling should never be performed during or immediately after a prolonged deceleration
    b. Take fetal blood samples with the woman in the right-lateral position
    c. Classification of pH is normal (≥ 7.25), borderline (7.21–7.24), abnormal (≤ 7.20)
    d. Classification of lactate is normal (≤ 4.1 mmol/L), borderline (4.2–4.8 mmol/L), abnormal (≥ 4.9 mmol/L)

22. Identify the incorrect categorization/s for FHR baseline variability:
    a. Reassuring category: 10 to 30 beats per minute
    b. Reassuring category: 5 to 25 beats per minute
    c. Nonreassuring category: <10 beats per minute for 20 to 40 minutes />35 beats per minute for 25 to 35 minutes
    d. Nonreassuring category: <5 beats per minute for 30 to 50 minutes />25 beats per minute for 15 to 25 minutes
    e. Abnormal category: <5 beats per minute for >50 minutes/>25 beats per minute for >25minutes/ sinusoidal
    f. Abnormal category: <10 beats per minute for >40 minutes/>45 beats per minute for >35 minutes

23. Identify the incorrect statement/s used when describing decelerations in FHR:
    a. Duration and timing in relation to the peaks of the contractions
    b. Whether or not the FHR returns to baseline
    c. How long the decelerations have been present
    d. Whether they occur with over 20% of contractions
    e. The presence or absence of a biphasic (W) shape and/or shouldering
    f. The presence or absence of reduced variability within the deceleration

24. Identify the correct statements to take into account when assessing decelerations in FHR:
    a. Early decelerations are uncommon.
    b. Early decelerations are benign and usually associated with head compression.
    c. Early decelerations with no nonreassuring or abnormal features on the CTG trace should always prompt further action.
    d. The longer and later the individual decelerations, then the higher the risk of fetal acidosis (particularly if accompanied by tachycardia or reduced baseline variability).

25. Identify the correct concerning characteristics of variable decelerations:
    a. Deceleration lasts more than 60 seconds
    b. Reduced baseline variability within the deceleration
    c. FHR fails to return to baseline
    d. Trace shows a biphasic (W) shape with no shouldering

26. Continuous CTG would be recommended if specific risk factors are present at initial assessment or arise during labour. Identify these risk factors from the following list:

a. Maternal pulse rate >120 beats per minute on two occasions 30 minutes apart

b. Maternal temperature ≥38°C (single reading), or ≥37.5°C on two consecutive occasions (1 hour apart)

c. Suspected sepsis or chorioamnionitis

d. The presence of either nonsignificant meconium or previous history of vaginal bleeding

e. Contractions lasting longer than 60 seconds (hypertonus) or >5 contractions in 10 minutes (tachysystole)

Physiological response to pain and pain pathways

Unlike most types of pain, the pain experienced in labour is not caused by a pathological process or trauma. Pain associated with labour is the result of an interaction between physiological and psychological factors. Midwives having a key role of managing pain experienced by women in labour, need to have knowledge of the physiological processes involved and how pain may impact on other body systems.

 Complete

27. Table 11.8 provides the physiological response to pain. Complete the table by removing the incorrect word/values so that the information reads correctly.

Table 11.8

	Physiological changes associated with pain in labour
a.	Pain may induce changes in the **sympathetic/parasympathetic** nervous system with release of **adrenaline (epinephrine)/noradrenaline (norepinephrine)** into the bloodstream resulting in changes in the body systems.
b.	*Associated changes in respiratory system:* **Increased/decreased** respiratory rate. This change may cause a **decrease/increase** in partial pressure of carbon dioxide ($PaCO_2$) level with a corresponding **increase/decrease** in pH. The fetus will be affected with a subsequent **rise/drop** in the fetal $PaCO_2$. This may be suspected by the presence of **late/early** decelerations on the CTG. **Hyperventilation/hypoventilation** may alter the acid–base equilibrium of the system. Resulting **acidosis/alkalosis** may then affect the diffusion of **oxygen/carbon dioxide** across the placenta leading to fetal **hypoxia/hyperemia**.
c.	*Associated changes in cardiovascular system:* **Increased/decreased** heart rate and blood pressure is associated with **sympathetic/nonsympathetic** response and **increase/decrease** in cardiac output. In the second stage, cardiac output **increases/decreases** by about **20%/50%**. Pain apprehension and fear may cause a **sympathetic/nonsympathetic** response producing more of an **increase/decrease** in cardiac output.
d.	*Other associated changes:* • **increase/decrease** in blood glucose levels; • **increase/decrease** in gastric motility leading to **delayed/accelerated** stomach emptying (possible nausea and vomiting); • **delay/acceleration** in bladder emptying; • **increase/decrease** cerebral and uterine blood flow caused by **vasoconstriction/vasodilation**; • **increase/decrease** in blood supply to the skin (causing sweating).

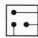 **Label**

28. Fig. 11.1 describes the sensory pathway showing the structures involved in the appreciation of pain. Label the figure using the list of structures and tissues provided.

Anterior aspect of spinal cord
Nerve cells in medulla oblongata
2nd neuron
Basal ganglia
Pons Varolii
Sensory nerve ending in skin receptor
3rd neuron
Cerebral cortex
Thalamus
Posterior root ganglion
1st neuron

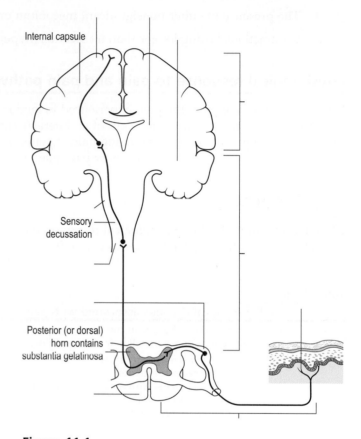

Figure 11.1

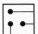

Label

29. Fig. 11.2 presents pain pathways showing the site at which pain may be intercepted by local anaesthetic techniques. Label the figure as detailed.

Label and shade

| Site for caudal epidural block |
| Site for epidural and spinal blocks |
| Site for paracervical block |
| Site for pudendal block |

Label

| Lumbar vertebrae 1–5 |
| Pudendal nerve |
| Sacral vertebrae |
| Thoracic vertebrae 11 and 12 |

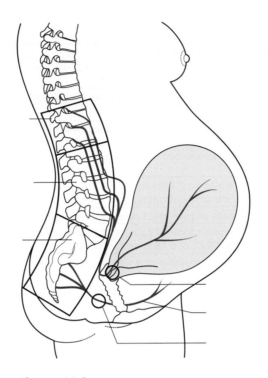

Figure 11.2

30. Fig. 11.3 shows a sagittal section of the lumbar spine with Tuohy needle in position.

Label

| Body of vertebra |
| Spinal cord |
| Subarachnoid space |
| Dura mater |
| Intervertebral discs |

| Ligamentum flavum |
| Epidural space |
| Spinal process |
| Inter- and supraspinous ligaments |

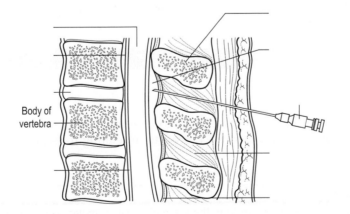

Body of vertebra

Figure 11.3

True/false

31. Table 11.9 provides a list of statements relating to the physiology of pain and pain in labour. Complete the table by indicating if the statements are true or false.

Table 11.9

	Statements	True	False
a.	The discomfort of pain is caused by the fetal head further descending into the pelvis, with descent causing pressure on the cervix, stretching of the vaginal walls and pelvic floor muscles.		
b.	Somatic sensation refers to the sensory function of the skin and body walls.		
c.	Sensory receptors that respond to pain are called *nociceptors*.		
d.	The gate-control theory declares that a neural or spinal 'gating' mechanism occurs in the substantia gelatinosa of the dorsal horns of the spinal cord. If the gate is open, then impulses pass through and pain is experienced. If the gate is closed, then pain signals are blocked.		
e.	Transcutaneous electrical nerve stimulation (TENS) stimulates the production of natural endorphins and enkephalins and obstructs incoming pain stimuli.		
f.	TENS should always be the first choice of pain relief offered to women in established labour.		
g.	Inhalation analgesia is the most common form of pain relief used in labour. It is a premixed gas made up of 50% nitrous oxide (N_2O) and 50% oxygen (O_2).		
h.	Nitrous oxide (N_2O) acts by limiting the neuronal and synaptic transmission within the central nervous system (CNS).		
i.	N_2O gas is heavier than O_2 gas. Therefore, safe storage of the gas cylinders involves keeping the cylinders stored on their side rather than upright to reduce the risk of administering a severely hypoxic mixture.		
j.	The maximum efficacy of inhalation analgesia occurs after 45–50 seconds which coincides with the height of the contraction providing maximum relief.		
k.	Opiate drugs are powerful analgesic properties. Their action lies in their ability to bind to receptor sites.		
l.	Opiate drugs do not have any side effects for either mother or baby.		
m.	Epidural analgesia does not provide any more effective pain relief than opioids.		
n	Epidural analgesia is not associated with long-term backache.		
o.	Epidural analgesia is not associated with a longer first stage of labour or an increased chance of a caesarean birth.		
p.	Epidural analgesia is associated with a longer second stage of labour and an increased chance of vaginal instrumental birth.		

SECOND STAGE OF LABOUR

 Definitions

32. Table 11.10 provides descriptive statements relating to definitions associated with the second stage of labour. Using your own knowledge, insert the correct term relating to each statement.

Table 11.10

	Descriptive statement	Related term
a.	This phenomenon occurs when pressure from the presenting part stimulates nerve receptors in the pelvic floor. The woman experiences the need to push which becomes increasingly, compulsive, overwhelming and involuntary. The secondary powers of expulsion are employed by the woman contracting her abdominal muscles and diaphragm.	
b.	A dome-shaped curve in the lower back is observed. This indicates posterior displacement of the sacrum and coccyx as the occiput progresses into the sacral curve.	
c.	This is a pigmented (purple-red) mark observed in the buttock cleft, which creeps up the anal cleft as labour progresses. It is also called the *purple line*.	
d.	This occurs during contractions when the uterus rises forwards and force of the fundal contraction is transmitted to the upper pole of the fetus, down the long axis of the fetus and applied by the presenting part to the cervix.	

Complete

33. Table 11.11 provides statements/activities relating to the soft tissue or structure displacement that may occur during second stage (a–e) and favourable maternal positions adopted during labour to promote descent and progress (f–g). Complete the table by inserting the correct response by either inserting the correct term or response.

Table 11.11

	Activity	Insert response
a.	Anteriorly, this anatomical structure is pushed upwards into the abdomen.	
b.	This anatomical structure is stretched and thins out so that the lumen of this structure is reduced.	
c.	Posteriorly, this anatomical structure becomes flattened into the sacral curve.	
d.	These muscles dilate, thin out and are displaced laterally.	
e.	This body is flattened, stretched and thinned.	
f.	List three favourable maternal positions encouraged in second stage of labour.	
g.	Consider these positions, list four **physiological** factors that make these more favourable.	

Mechanisms of labour

Knowledge and recognition of normal mechanism of labour enables the midwife to anticipate the next steps in the process of descent of the fetus through the birth canal. Mechanisms of labour is a collective term for the movements involved, as the fetus negotiates through the soft tissues and bony birth canal. The following activities relate to mechanisms of labour.

34. This activity relates to the principles common to all mechanisms. Complete the activity by inserting the correct word/s from the list provided to complete the three main principles.

Rotate   Symphysis pubis   Resistance
Pelvis   Pubic bone   Descent

i.   The activity involving _____ of the fetus takes place.

ii. Whichever part leads and first meets the _____ of the pelvic floor will _____

     forward until it comes under the _____.

iii. Whatever emerges from the _____ will pivot around the _____.

The mechanisms use a systematic stem, including common principles with information inserted relevant to each labour. The most common mechanism relates to the vertex presentation with either a right or left occipitoanterior position. Table 11.12 provides this completed mechanism as an example.

Table 11.12 (completed example)

a. **Lie is longitudinal**	d. **Attitude is one of good flexion**
b. **Presentation is cephalic**	e. **Denominator is the occiput**
c. **Position is right or left occipitoanterior**	f. **Presenting part is the posterior part of the anterior parietal bone**

Match

35. Table 11.13 relates to the main movements as the fetus descends through the birth canal. The aim is to provide the flow diagram of the sequence of events taking place in the birth canal. To complete this activity, draw a line to match the order of the movements in column A with the correct activity detailed in column B.

Table 11.13

A. Step		B. Activity
i.		Restitution
ii.		Extension of the head
iii.		Internal rotation of the shoulders
iv.	↓	Flexion
v.		Lateral flexion
vi.		Descent
vii.		Internal rotation of the head

 Complete

36. Table 11.14 provides a list of statements related to the seven key movements involved in the mechanism of labour. Complete the table by inserting the correct movement to match the statement. Use the list of seven key movements presented in column B (Q 35), noting that some movements are inserted more than one.

Table 11.14

	Statement	Insert movement
a.	This increases throughout labour and relates to the fetal spine being attached nearer to the posterior skull.	
b.	The twist in the neck is now corrected by a slight untwisting movement.	
c.	In multiparous women, this movement may not occur until labour actually begins.	
d.	Resistance of the pelvic floor is an important determinant in bringing this movement about.	
e.	The occiput slips beneath the subpubic arch and crowning occurs when the head no longer recedes between contractions.	
f.	The slope of the pelvic floor determines the direction of this movement.	
g.	Pressure exerted down the fetal axis will be more forcibly transmitted to the occiput than the sinciput.	
h.	During this movement, the fetal head pivots on the suboccipital region around the pubic bone.	
i.	The remainder of the body is born as the spine bends sideways through the curved birth canal.	
j.	The sinciput, face and chin are released and sweep the perineum.	
k.	In a well-flexed vertex presentation, the occiput leads and rotates anteriorly 1/8th circle causing a slight twist in the neck.	
l.	The occiput moves 1/8th of a circle toward the side of the head from which it started.	
m.	The anterior shoulder is the first to reach the levator ani muscle and rotates anteriorly to lie under the symphysis pubis.	

Perineal trauma

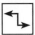 **Match**

37. Box 11.4 relates to classification of degrees of spontaneous tears. Complete the table by drawing a line to match the classification of tear (column A) and connect with the correct soft tissues involved (column B).

Box 11.4

A. Degree of tear:	B. Soft tissues involved:
First-degree:	Fourchette and superficial perineal muscles Main deep pelvic floor muscles - iliococcygeus muscle Comprises partial or complete disruption of the anal sphincter muscles Pubococcygeus muscles (in some cases)
Second-degree:	Skin of fourchette, perineum and perineal body (superficial and deep pelvic floor muscle), and external and internal anal sphincter with anal epithelium Either or both external and internal anal sphincter muscles
Third-degree:	Main superficial muscles - transverse perineal muscles Main superficial muscles - bulbospongiosus (bulbocavernosus) and transversus perineal muscles
Fourth-degree:	Fourchette only

Miscellaneous

 True/false

38. Complete the following statements in Table 11.15 by deciding if they are true or false by ticking the appropriate column.

Table 11.15

	Statement	True	False
a.	The widest diameter of the pelvic brim is the transverse		
b.	Caput succedaneum does not usually protrude through the cervix before full dilatation of the os		
c.	As the fetus descends, fetal oxygenation may be less efficient owing to either cord or head compression or to reduced perfusion at the placental site		
d.	External rotation of the head occurs at the same time as internal rotation of the shoulders		
e.	If flexion is maintained during descent, then it will be the suboccipitobregmatic diameter that distends the vaginal orifice		
f.	Contractions in second stage usually become weaker and longer with a longer resting phase		
g.	Left lateral position may aid fetal rotation		
h.	Epidural analgesia causes relaxation of the pelvic floor and delays internal rotation of the head		
i.	In the case of occipitoposterior positions, women report the 'all fours position' to be beneficial in reducing backache		
j.	Mediolateral episiotomy is the recommended technique which originates at the vaginal fourchette and usually directed to the right side. At time of episiotomy, the angle to the vertical axis should be between 45 and 60 degrees		

Multiple choice questions (MCQ)

39. Identify the incorrect statement relating to the prelabour rupture of membranes:

 a. Preterm prelabour rupture of membranes (PPROM) occurs <37 weeks' gestation when the fetal membranes rupture without the onset of spontaneous uterine activity and consequential cervical dilatation.

 b. Prelabour rupture of membranes (PROM) at term (>37 weeks' gestation) occurs with 60% of women with prelabour rupture of the membranes labouring spontaneously within 24 hours.

 c. A speculum examination should be carried out even if it is certain that the membranes have ruptured.

 d. Women presenting with PROM at term should be advised that the risk of serious neonatal infection is 1%, rather than 0.5% for women with intact membranes.

40. Breath-holding and attempting to exhale against closed airways is called:

 a. Valsalva manoeuvre

 b. McRobert's manoeuvre

 c. Rubin manoeuvre

 d. Ferguson's reflex

41. In the semi-recumbent or supporting sitting position:

 a. The pelvic outlet is increased

 b. The woman's weight is on her sacrum

 c. The coccyx is directed posteriorly

 d. All of the above

 e. None of the above

42. When the membranes remain intact this:

 a. Optimizes the oxygen supply to the fetus

 b. Helps prevent intrauterine and fetal infection

 c. Ensures the general fluid pressure is equalized throughout the uterus and over the fetal body

 d. a and c

 e. a, b and c

43. Identify the incorrect statement/s:

 a. Positive and dramatic effects on labour progress can be achieved by midwives encouraging the woman to change and adapt her position in response to the way her body feels.

 b. When the woman adopts a forward-facing position for birth (e.g., all-fours), then the midwife needs to reverse the mechanism of labour manoeuvres adopted to support the birth of the baby.

 c. Nulliparous women should be informed that the length of established labour varies between women with average duration of first stage lasting 8 hours and unlikely to be >18 hours.

 d. Women should be informed that the length of second and subsequent labours last on average 5 hours and are unlikely to last >12 hours.

 e. In multiparous women a perceptible cervical canal may remain.

REFERENCE

NICE Clinical guideline [CG190] Intrapartum care for healthy women and babies. Published 2014, reviewed 2017. https://www.nice.org.uk/guidance/cg190.

12 Third stage of labour

This chapter focuses on the normal physiological mechanisms of placental separation, descent and expulsion together with factors facilitating haemostasis and primary postpartum haemorrhage. The midwife has a key role to play in providing safe and effective care and to anticipate, recognize and act promptly and competently when haemorrhage occurs. The activities will test your knowledge in these areas.

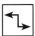 **Match and connect**

1. Box 12.1 provides activities relating to third stage of labour. To complete the activity, draw a line to match the two different types of management of third stage (column A) and connect with the accurate component (column B) for each stage.

Box 12.1

A. Management	B. Component of Care
Active management:	• Diagnosis: 'Prolonged' if incomplete >60 minutes from birth • No clamping of the cord (until pulsation has stopped) • Uterotonic drugs are not routinely used • Deferred cord clamping and cutting of the cord (not earlier than 1 minute from birth of healthy baby)
Physiological management:	• Uterotonic drugs • Controlled cord traction (CCT) after signs of placenta separation • Diagnosis: 'Prolonged' if incomplete >30 minutes from birth • Placental delivery by maternal effort • Also known as *expectant* management

Physiology of third stage

The following activities relate to the factors involved in separation and expulsion of the placenta and membranes, that is, mechanical and haemostatic factors. It is difficult to separate these two factors completely as they take place simultaneously during the process.

 Complete

2. Table 12.1 details the sequence of events involving physiological and mechanical factors in the separation of the placenta. Complete the sections by either inserting the missing word(s) from the list provided or removing the incorrect word/numerical value so that each stage in the separation process reads correctly.

accelerate	decidua basalis	spongy	tortuous
compressed	oblique	strongly	vagina

Table 12.1

	Sequence of events (physiological and mechanical factors)
a	The unique characteristic of uterine muscle lies in its power of **contraction/retraction**. During the second stage, the uterine cavity progressively empties, enabling the **contraction/retraction** process to _____. At the beginning of third stage, the **placenta/placental site** has already **increased/diminished** in area by about **20%/75%**.

↓

b.	As this occurs, the placenta becomes _____ and the blood in the **intervillous spaces/venous** return is forced back into the spongy layer of the _____. **Retraction/contraction** of the _____ uterine muscle fibres exerts pressure on the blood vessels so that blood does not drain back into the **maternal system/placenta**. The vessels during this process are termed '_____' as they become **relaxed/tense** and **emptied/congested** with blood.

↓

c.	With the next contraction, the **constricted/distended** veins burst and a small amount of blood seeps in between the thin septa of the _____ layer and the placental surface, stripping the placenta from its attachment. As the surface area for placental attachment **reduces/enlarges**, the relatively **non-elastic/elastic** placenta begins to detach from the uterine wall.

↓

d.	Once separation has occurred, the uterus contracts _____, forcing placenta and membranes to fall into the **upper/lower** uterine segment and finally into the _____ and emerging at the vulva.

Placental separation

 Complete

3. Fig. 12.1 shows the mechanism of placental separation. Consider the details of separation in the previous activity. Complete Fig. 12.1 by identifying the uterine wall in A, the fetal surface of the placenta in B and the maternal surface of the placenta in C.

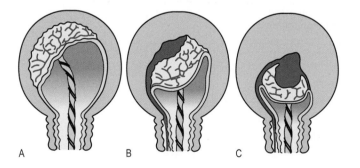

1 uterine wall
2 fetal surface of placenta
3 maternal surface of placenta

A   B   C

Figure 12.1

Complete Table 12.2 by describing the sequence of events in the mechanism of separation.

Table 12.2

	Description of the mechanism of separation
Fig. 12.1 (A):	
Fig. 12.1 (B):	
Fig. 12.1 (C):	

Complete

4. The following activities relate to the two recognized methods of expulsion of the placenta. Complete the activities with Fig. 12.2 as noted and complete the activities in Table 12.4.

Fetal surface
Maternal surface
Myometrium
Bleeding from site

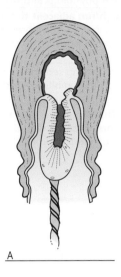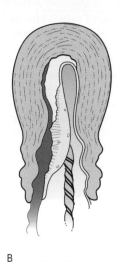

A _____   B _____

Figure 12.2A, B

a. *Label*

Identify and label the method of expulsion of placenta shown in Fig. 12.2A, B.

b. Complete the activities in Table 12.3.

Table 12.3

Activity related to two methods	Method of placental separation	
	Fig. 12.2A	**Fig. 12.2B**
a. Label method of placental separation		
b. Identify where separation begins on placental site		
c. Identify if a retroplacental clot is involved	Yes/no	Yes/no
d. Identify difference in duration	Shorter/longer	Shorter/longer
e. Identify difference in blood loss	More/less	More/less
f. Identify the placental surface first to appear at vulva		
g. List possible differences you can **observe** on examination		

h. Remove the *incorrect* words:
The majority of placentae are situated on the **anterior or posterior wall/lower uterine segment** of the uterus. In the majority of cases, separation usually starts from the **upper/lower** pole of the placenta and moves gradually **upwards/downwards**. Fundal placentae separate first at both poles followed by the fundal part. The length of the third stage may be **reduced by 2 minutes/increased by 5 minutes** when the placenta is located at the fundus.

Haemostasis and the role in placental separation

Complete

5. Table 12.4 provides information relating to haemostasis and the important role it has in placental separation. Complete the table by removing the incorrect word(s) so that the information reads correctly.

Table 12.4

	Haemostasis
	The normal volume of blood flow through a healthy placental site is **500–800/300–500** mL/min. Serious haemorrhage would occur at the time of placental separation if blood flow is not arrested within **seconds/minutes**. An interplay of the following **three factors** to control bleeding within the normal physiological processes is essential during this stage:
i.	The **tortuous/relaxed** blood vessels **intertwine through/run adjacent to** the **oblique/circular** uterine muscle fibres. **Retraction/relaxation** of the **oblique/longitudinal** uterine muscle fibres in the **upper/lower** uterine segment results in **thinning/thickening** of the muscles. This exerts pressure on the torn vessels, acting as clamps and securing these using this ligature action.
ii.	Presence of **vigorous/moderate** uterine contraction following separation brings the **placenta/uterine** walls into apposition so that **further/less** pressure is exerted on the umbilical **cord/placental site**.
iii.	Haemostasis is achieved by a transitory **deactivation/activation** of the coagulation and fibrinolytic systems during, and immediately following, placental separation. This protective response is especially **dormant/active** at the placental site so that clot formation in the **intact/torn** vessels is **diminished/intensified**. Following separation, the placental site is **gradually/rapidly** covered by a **platelet/fibrin** mesh and utilizing **5%–10%/15%–25%** of circulating **platelets/fibrinogen**.

Uterotonic drugs

 Match and connect

6. Box 12.2 relates to common uterotonic drugs used during the third stage of labour. To complete the box, draw a line to match the uterotonic drugs in column A and connect to the correct statement in column B.

Box 12.2

A. Uterotonic Drug	B. Statement
Ergometrine: Oxytocin:	• If ergometrine and oxytocin are combined, then 1 mL ampoule will contain 0.5 mg of this drug. • This drug is the synthetic form of a hormone (to stimulate smooth muscle contraction) produced in the posterior pituitary gland. • If ergometrine and oxytocin are combined, then 1 mL ampoule will contain 5 IU of this drug. • If this drug is administered as an IV bolus, it should be administered slowly because of profound and potentially fatal hypotensive side-effects. • If administered intramuscularly, then this drug will act within 6–7 minutes. • This drug is contraindicated if there is a history of hypertensive or cardiac disease. • If administered intramuscularly then this drug will act within 2.5 minutes.

 Short answers

7. Table 12.5 provides activities related to management of third stage. Complete the table by inserting the correct answer.

Table 12.5

	Activity	Answer
a.	List the signs of placental separation:	
b.	List the signs of placental descent:	
c.	Identify the commonly used brand name of oxytocin:	
d.	Identify the commonly used brand name of the combined drug ergometrine and oxytocin:	
e.	List the effects resulting from the combined action of ergometrine and oxytocin:	
f.	Identify the timing of administration of a uterotonic drug:	
g.	Identify side-effects of combined drug (ergometrine and oxytocin):	

Complications of the third stage

 True/false

8. Table 12.6 provides statements relating to third stage, management and complications. Complete the table by indicating if they are true or false.

Table 12.6

	Statement	True	False
a.	The unique characteristic of uterine muscle lies in its power of contraction.		
b.	Uterotonic drugs are always administered after the birth of the baby and before placental delivery.		
c.	In controlled cord traction (CCT), counter-traction must be provided to prevent inversion of the uterus.		
d.	The absence of oblique fibres in the lower uterine segment explains the greatly increased blood loss usually accompanying placental separation in placenta praevia.		
e.	The placenta always shears off the uterine wall during the final contraction.		
f.	In situations of haemorrhage caused by hypotonic uterine action, intravenous ergometrine is used as it secures a rapid contraction in 45 seconds.		
g.	Because of side-effects, only 1 dose of ergometrine (0.5 mg) should be routinely administered.		
h.	Prostaglandins are never recommended for use in third stage management.		
i.	Primary postpartum haemorrhage (PPH) is defined as excessive bleeding from the genital tract at any time following the baby's birth up to 48 hours following birth.		
j.	A disorder in blood clotting is one of the reasons why a primary PPH can occur.		
k.	Atonic uterus and retained placenta are common causes of PPH.		
l.	Secondary PPH is defined as any abnormal bleeding or excessive bleeding from the genital tract occurring between birth and 12 weeks postnatally.		

Atonic uterus

An atonic uterus relates to the failure of the myometrium at the placental site to contract and retract and to compress torn blood vessels and control blood loss by a living ligature action.

 Short answers

9. Table 12.7 provides activities related to the causes of atonic uterus. Complete the table by inserting the answer from the list provided.

Couvelaire	Multiple pregnancy	Placenta praevia	Precipitate labour	Relaxation
Incomplete	Placenta abruption	Polyhydramnios	Prolonged	Retained placenta
Placenta/membranes			Labour	Full bladder

Table 12.7

	Causes of atonic uterine action	Answer
i.	Identify two pregnancy-related conditions causing overdistension of the uterine muscles	
ii.	Identify the placenta-related condition either partly or wholly lying in the lower uterine segment	
iii.	Identify the placenta-related event resulting in blood seeping between the muscles fibres and interfering with effective muscle action	
iv.	In relation to iii, name the term referring to a severe case of this event occurring in the uterus	
v.	In relation to labour, identify two causes resulting in uterine inertia resulting from maternal exhaustion/sluggishness	
vi.	Identify two placental separation causes	
vii.	Identify one maternal mechanical reason	
viii.	Identify the uterine effect caused by a general anaesthesia, for example, halothane	

Primary postpartum haemorrhage

It is vital that students know the three basic principles of care applied immediately upon observing excessive bleeding. These are: 1) call for help; 2) stop the bleeding and 3) resuscitate the mother.

Completion

10. Fig. 12.3 provides a detailed flow of action to be taken in a primary PPH. Review the flow diagram and insert the missing words so that the flow reads correctly.

Apply pressure, repair the wound	In lower uterine segment	Placenta delivered
Controlled cord traction	Intravenous (IV) infusion syntocinong 40 u/L	Rub up a contraction
Empty the uterus	Lift the legs	Separated
Put the baby to the breast	Lower genital tract injury	Uterus atonic
Give an oxytocic	Measures fail to arrest bleeding	

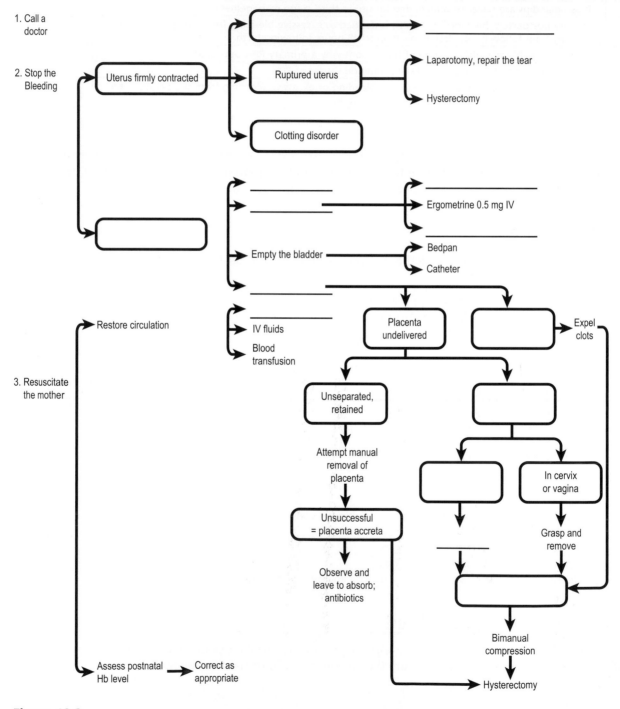

Figure 12.3

Bimanual compression

11. Table 12.8 provides information about interventions required to stem persistent bleeding from the uterus. Bimanual compression of the uterus may be required to apply pressure to the placental site. Ancillary or essential interventions are also included. Complete the activity in the following paragraph by removing the incorrect word(s) so that the information reads correctly.

Table 12.8

	Bimanual compression and other interventions
a.	The fingers of one hand are inserted into the vagina like a **fist/cone**; the hand is formed into a **cone/fist** and placed into the **posterior/anterior** vaginal **fornix/orifice**, the **wrist/elbow** resting on the bed. The other hand is placed behind the uterus **vaginally/abdominally**, the fingers pointing **away from/toward** the cervix. The **cervix/uterus** is brought **backwards/forwards** and **compressed/massaged** between the **back/palm** of the hand positioned **anteriorly/abdominally** and the **cone/fist** in the vagina.
b.	If bleeding is persistent: • The first action is to exclude a **cardiovascular/blood clotting** disorder. • Then an exploration of the vagina and uterus would be performed under **local anaesthetic/general anaesthetic**. • Compression balloons/may be used to provide pressure on the **placental site/vaginal walls**. • If bleeding continues, ligation of the **uterine/umbilical** arteries or **hysterectomy/salpingectomy** may need to be considered.

Miscellaneous

 True/false

12. Table 12.9 provides a range of statements relating to third stage of labour. Complete the table by indicating if each statement is true or false.

Table 12.9

	Statement	True	False
a.	Progressive formation of a haematoma may conceal a PPH		
b.	The main symptom of haematoma formation is increasingly severe maternal pain		
c.	One benefit of breastfeeding immediately following birth is the reflex release of prolactin from the posterior pituitary gland, which stimulates the uterus to contract		
d.	Haematoma formation only occurs in the perineum and lower vagina		
e.	On palpation, an enlarged uterus filling up with blood or blood clots feels soft, distended and lacking tone. The uterus is described as being 'boggy'		
f.	In placenta accreta, the placenta remains morbidly adherent to the uterine wall		
g.	To perform controlled cord traction (CCT) in active management, the cord is clamped before 5 minutes from birth		
h.	Cord blood sampling is usually taken when atypical maternal antibodies have been found during antenatal screening test		
i.	After administering oxytocin, the cord is only clamped immediately after birth where there is concern about the integrity of the cord or the baby's heart rate is <60 beats/min (and not getting faster)		
j.	Factors (not causal) increase the possibility of PPH include high parity, fibroids, anaemia, and previous history of PPH or retained placenta		
k.	The midwife must ensure that placental separation has occurred, and the uterus contracted before performing CCT. If CCT is performed without good uterine contractions, then this can result in the serious acute condition of uterine inversion		

REFERENCE

NICE Clinical guideline [CG190] Intrapartum care for healthy women and babies. Published 2014, reviewed 2017, https://www.nice.org.uk/guidance/cg190.

13 Complicated labour and birth

This chapter focuses on labour and birth complicated by a range of obstetric challenges and medical conditions. Obstetric challenges include preterm labour, prolonged labour, and malposition and malpresentation of the fetus. The midwife has a key role in the recognition and diagnosis of malposition and malpresentation during pregnancy and in the intrapartum period. This period can also be challenged with complications resulting from preexisting and new medical conditions arising over this period. The midwife needs to be prepared to appropriately deal with any complications and emergency situations. The activities will test your knowledge in the variety of related areas of practice and provide revision of some related pathophysiology.

Preterm labour

 True/false

1. Table 13.1 provides a range of statements relating to preterm labour. Complete the table by indicating of the statements are true or false.

Table 13.1

	Statement	True	False
a.	Antepartum haemorrhage (APH) is defined as bleeding from or into the genital tract, occurring from 28+0 weeks of pregnancy and before birth		
b.	Cervical trauma refers to physical injury to the cervix, such as surgical procedures, for example cone biopsy, large loop excision of the transformation zone (LLETZ) or radical diathermy		
c.	APH complicates 3%–5% of pregnancies and is a leading cause of perinatal and maternal mortality worldwide		
d.	Although not the most common causes, Royal College of Obstetricians and Gynaecologists (RCOG) report the most important causes of APH are placenta abruption and placental praevia		
e.	Preterm labour is always considered when the woman presents before 37+0 weeks reporting symptoms indicative of preterm labour, such as abdominal pain (with no clinical assessment at this point)		
f.	Preterm labour is suspected if the woman reports symptoms of preterm labour (e.g., abdominal pain) and clinical assessment (including speculum/digital vaginal examination) confirms the possibility but rules out established labour		
g.	A woman is in diagnosed preterm labour if she is in suspected preterm labour and has had a positive diagnostic test for preterm labour		
h.	A woman is in established preterm labour if she has progressive cervical dilatation from 4 cm with regular contractions		
i.	Preterm prelabour rupture of membranes (PPROM) is when the woman has ruptured membranes before 37+0 weeks but is not in established labour		
j.	Prophylactic cervical cerclage is considered for women in whom a transvaginal ultrasound scan carried out between 16+0 and 24+0 weeks reveals a cervical length <25 mm		
k.	Infection in women with PPROM is identified by a combination of both clinical assessment and tests (C-reactive protein, white blood cell count and measurement of fetal heart rate [FHR] using cardiotocography [CTG]) to diagnose intrauterine infection		
l.	Women with PPROM should be offered oral erythromycin 250 mg 4 times a day for a maximum of 10 days or until the woman is in established labour (whichever is sooner)		
m.	Maternal corticosteroids should be offered to women between 26+0 and 33+6 weeks of pregnancy who are suspected, diagnosed or established preterm labour, are having a planned preterm birth or have PPROM		
n.	Fetal blood sampling should not be carried out if the woman <38+0 weeks pregnant		

Prolonged pregnancy and induction of labour

Short answers

2. Table 13.2 provides a selection of activities related to pregnancy, complications and induction of labour (IOL). Using your own knowledge, complete the table by inserting short answers.

Table 13.2

	Activity	Answer
a.	Identify the legal age of fetal viability in most countries	
b.	In uncomplicated pregnancies, identify the gestational age range when IOL is offered to women	
c.	Name the term referring to artificial rupture of membranes to initiate or speed up labour	
d.	Remodelling takes place in the cervix before labour. List three changes in the cervix that need to be present before IOL	
e.	Identify the Bishop score indicating the cervix is ripe or 'favourable' for IOL	
f.	Identify the term used to describe difficult or slow labour and includes failure to progress and prolonged labour	
g.	In precipitate labour, identify the defined time (hour(s) from the onset of labour to birth	
h.	Name the term describing a large fetus or baby whose weight is ≥90th percentile for gestational age	
i.	List the risks associated with IOL	

Match and connect

3. Box 13.1 provides methods of inducing labour and related statements. To complete the activity, draw a line to match the method of inducing labour in column A and connect with the correct statement in column B.

Box 13.1

A. Inducing labour	B. Statement
	Separates the chorionic membrane from decidua leading to release of prostaglandins and onset of labour
	Uncertainties remain about how best to apply vaginal PGE2 in terms of dosage and timing
	Vaginal PGE2 is the preferred method
	This is appropriate method approximately 24 hours after prelabour rupture of membranes (term)
Membrane sweep:	Involves VE with examining finger passing through the cervix to rotate against the uterine wall
	This is an adjunct to IOL rather than an actual method of induction
	Procedure involves administration of a gel, tablet or controlled-release pessary.
	In this VE procedure, massaging around the cervix in the vaginal fornices may achieve a similar effect if the finger cannot be admitted into the cervix
Induction of labour:	Women informed of this option at 38 week antenatal visit (offered to nulliparous at 40/41 weeks; 41 weeks for parous) to promote spontaneous labour and reduce formal IOL
	Amniotomy, alone or with oxytocin, should not be used as this primary method
	Procedure may cause discomfort and vaginal bleeding
	Tocolysis should be considered if uterine hyperstimulation occurs during induction of labour

True/false

4. Table 13.3 provides a selection of statements relating to prolonged labour and IOL. Complete the table by indicating if each statement is true or false.

Table 13.3

	Statement	True	False
a.	Pharmacological prostaglandin E2 (PGE2) placed in the posterior fornix of the vagina is absorbed by the epithelium of vagina and cervix leading to relaxation and dilatation of the muscle of the cervix		
b.	Prostaglandins, naturally occurring female hormones, mediate a wide range of physiological functions, such as contraction and relaxation of smooth muscle		
c.	Vaginal PGE2 is not appropriate for use with specific clinical reasons because of the risk of uterine hyperstimulation		
d.	Prolonged pregnancy relates to the fetus and does not refer to a specific gestation		
e.	Prelabour rupture of membranes is not a maternal indication for IOL		
f.	From 42 weeks, women who decline IOL should be offered increased antenatal (AN) monitoring including biweekly CTG and ultrasound estimation of maximum amniotic pool depth		
g.	When offering PGE2 for IOL, healthcare professionals should inform women about the associated risks of uterine hyperstimulation		
h.	Healthcare professionals should inform women that the available evidence does not support herbal supplements, acupuncture, homeopathy, castor oil, hot baths, enemas or sexual intercourse for IOL		
i.	In the absence of any other indications, IOL should not be considered simply because the healthcare professional suspects a baby is large for gestational age		
j.	As the uterus continues to contract and retract in obstructed labour, the upper segment becomes progressively thinner and the lower segment becomes increasingly thicker		
k.	IOL using mechanical methods (amniotomy or Foley catheter) is associated with lower risk of scar rupture compared with induction using prostaglandins		

 Complete

5. Table 13.4 presents the inducibility features and scoring measured in the modified Bishop score. Complete the table by inserting the missing words and numerical values from the list provided.

consistency	ischial spines	firm	length	posterior
position	soft	dilatation	presenting part	−3
4	1	1–2	2–4	anterior

Table 13.4

Inducibility features	0	1	2	3
Cervix: _____ (cm)	<__	1–2	__–__	>__
Cervix: _____	_____	firm	medium	_____
Cervical canal: _____ (cm)	>4	2–4	__–__	<1
Cervix: _____	_____	middle	_____	N/A
_____ station (cm above or below) maternal _____	____	−2	−1, 0	+1, +2

Planning type of birth

 Correct/incorrect

6. Table 13.5 provides a range of statements related to planning birth (National institute for Clinical Excellence [NICE]), IOL (NICE, 2014), and the Royal College of Obstetricians and Gynaecologists (RCOG, 2015) guidance on vaginal birth after previous caesarean delivery (VBAC) and elective repeat caesarean section (ERCS). This evidence-based information is offered to women before birth. Complete the activity by indicating the statements providing the correct information.

Table 13.5

	Statements	Correct
a.	IOL to avoid a birth unattended by healthcare professionals should not be routinely offered to women with a history of precipitate labour	
b.	The success rate of planned VBAC is 72%–75%	
c.	Planned VBAC is associated with an approximately 1 in 200 (0.5%) risk of uterine rupture	
d.	IOL is generally recommended in breech presentation	
e.	The absolute risk of birth-related perinatal death associated with VBAC is extremely low and comparable to the risk for nulliparous women in labour	
f.	Planned VBAC is contraindicated in women with previous uterine rupture or classical caesarean scar	
g.	ERCS is associated with a small increased risk of placenta praevia and/or accreta in future pregnancies and of pelvic adhesions complicating any future abdominopelvic surgery	
h.	Epidural analgesia is contraindicated in a planned VBAC	
i.	There is a two- to threefold increased risk of uterine rupture and around 1.5-fold increased risk of caesarean delivery in induced and/or augmented labour compared with spontaneous VBAC labour	
j.	IOL using mechanical methods (amniotomy or Foley catheter) is associated with a lower risk of scar rupture compared with induction using prostaglandins	
k.	ERCS delivery should be conducted after 39+0 weeks of gestation	
l.	All women undergoing ERCS should receive thromboprophylaxis	
m.	Safety and efficacy of planned VBAC is uncertain in pregnancies complicated by postdates, twin gestation, fetal macrosomia, antepartum stillbirth or maternal age of ≥40 years	

Malpositions of the occiput

 True/false

7. Table 13.6 provides statements related to occipitoposterior (OP) position. Complete the table by indicating if each statement is true or false.

Table 13.6

	Statement	True	False
a.	OP positions are the least common type of malposition of the occiput		
b.	Interior rotation of an OP to an anterior position is unlikely to occur		
c.	Persistent OP position results from a failure of internal rotation or malrotation before birth		
d.	OP position may be associated with an abnormally shaped pelvis, for example, android pelvis has a roomier hindpelvis for the occiput to occupy		
e.	The oval shape of the anthropoid pelvis, with its narrow transverse diameter, favours a direct OP position		
f.	On inspection, the saucer-shaped depression at or just below the umbilicus is created by the dip between the fetal head and lower limbs and the outline created by the high unengaged head can look like a full bladder		
g.	On palpation, the limbs can be felt at both sides of the midline and the occiput and sinciput can be located on the same level		
h.	On auscultation, the fetal heart may be heard more easily at the flank on the same side as the back		
i.	On VE, locating the anterior fontanelle in the anterior part of the pelvis is diagnostic with the direction of the sagittal suture and location of the posterior fontanelle providing confirmation		
j.	The fetal spine straightens against the lumbar curve of the maternal spine and makes the fetus straighten its neck and adopt a more erect attitude		
k.	The fetal head is deflexed and smaller diameters of the fetal skull may present		
l.	The membranes tend to rupture spontaneously at an early stage of labour		
m.	The woman usually experiences backache during labour		

 Label and completion

8. The following activities relate to the diameters and dimensions of a deflexed head.
   a. Fig. 13.1 shows the engaging diameter of a deflexed head. Label the diameter and identify the length (cm) of the diameter.

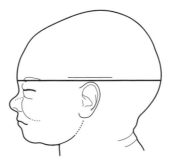

Figure 13.1 Engaging diameter of a deflexed head.

b. Fig. 13.2 shows the presenting dimensions of a deflexed head. Label the three diameters, identifying the length (cm) of the diameters and insert the numerical value (cm) of the circumference of the deflexed vertex.

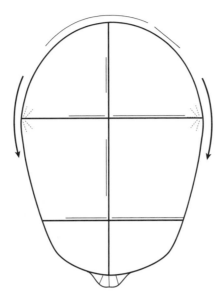

Figure 13.2 Presenting dimensions of a deflexed head.

 Complete

The occipitoposterior position of the occiput has two possible outcomes, that is, long rotation and short rotation. The following activities relate to the mechanism of labour in the right occipitoposterior position (Figs 13.3–13.6).

9. Table 13.7 provides an activity related to the mechanism of **right occipitoposterior position** (long rotation). Complete the table by either inserting the correct answer relating to the mechanism or removing the incorrect word/numerical value.

Table 13.7

Mechanism of right occipitoposterior position (long rotation)			
Lie:		Position:	
Attitude:		Denominator:	
Presentation:		Presenting part:	
(a) The **occipitofrontal/suboccipitofrontal** diameter (**11.5/10.5 cm**) lies in the **right/left** oblique diameter of pelvic brim.			
(b) The **occiput/sinciput** points to the right sacroiliac joint and the **occiput/sinciput** to the **left/right** iliopectineal eminence.			

Complete

10. Review the following Figs 13.3–13.6 showing the mechanisms of labour in right occipitoposterior position. Complete the activity in Box 13.2 in relation to flexion, descent and rotation movements.

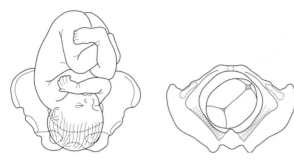

Figure 13.3

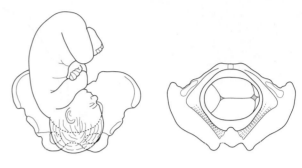

Figure 13.4

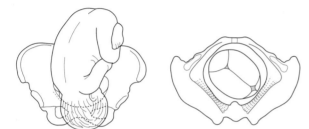

Figure 13.5

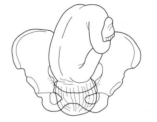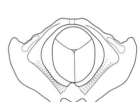

Figure 13.6

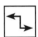

Match

11. Complete Box 13.2 in relation to flexion, descent and rotation movements in the right occipitoposterior position. To complete, draw a line to match each mechanism stage in column A and connect with the correct description of related component in column B.

Box 13.2

A: Mechanism (stage)	B: Description of component
Fig. 13.3 (Descent and flexion): Fig. 13.4 Internal rotation of head: Fig. 13.5: Fig. 13.6:	• Sagittal suture lies in the transverse diameter of the pelvis. • Occiput and shoulders have rotated 2/8th of a circle forwards • Sagittal suture now lies in the left oblique diameter of the pelvis • Occiput becomes the leading part • Occiput has rotated 3/8th of a circle forwards to lie under the symphysis pubis • Sagittal suture lies in the right oblique diameter of the pelvis • Occiput and shoulders have rotated 1/8th of a circle forwards • Position is right occipitoanterior • Sagittal suture lies in the anteroposterior diameter of the pelvis • Descent takes place with increasing flexion • There is a twist in the neck

Complete

12. Table 13.8a–f relates to the right OP position long rotation. This table continues on from the activities in Box 13.2. Complete the activities by removing the incorrect words in the description of the movements resulting in birth of the baby and by inserting the name of the mechanism at each stage (a–f).

Table 13.8

	Description	Mechanism
a.	The **occiput/sinciput** escapes under the symphysis pubis	
b.	The **occiput/sinciput**, face and chin sweep the **sacrum/perineum** and the head is born by a movement of **flexion/extension**	
c.	The **occiput/sinciput** turns 1/8th of a circle to the **right/left** and the head realigns with the shoulders	
d.	The shoulders enter the pelvis in the **left/right** oblique diameter; the **anterior/posterior** shoulder reaches the pelvic floor first and rotates 1/8th of a circle to lie under the symphysis pubis	
e.	At the same time the **occiput/sinciput** turns a further 1/8th of a circle to the **left/right**	
f.	The **anterior/posterior** shoulder escapes under the symphysis pubis, the **anterior/posterior** shoulder sweeps the perineum and the body is born by **extension/lateral flexion**	

13. Fig. 13.7 shows the 'persistent occipitoposterior position' <u>before</u> rotation of the occiput, and Fig. 13.8 shows 'persistent occipitoposterior position' <u>after</u> short rotation. Consider these two figures and then complete Box 13.3 by either removing the incorrect word or inserting the correct word (from your own knowledge) so that the paragraphs read correctly.

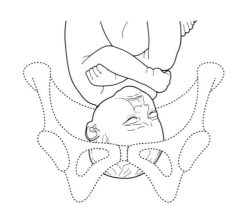

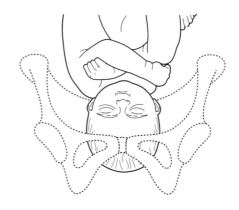

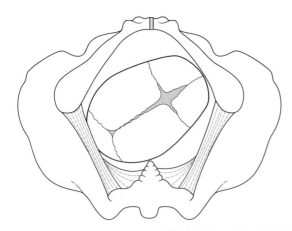

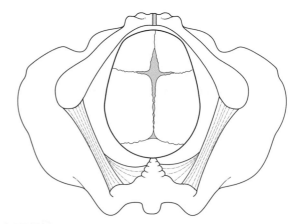

Figure 13.7   **Figure 13.8**

Box 13.3

Fig. 13.7: The position is **right/left** occipitoposterior. The _____ fails to rotate **backwards/forwards** in this situation. Instead the **occiput/sinciput** reaches the pelvic floor first and rotates **backwards/forwards**. The **occiput/sinciput** goes into the hollow of the sacrum.

Fig. 13.8: The position in now _____ occipitoposterior. The baby is born facing the _____. This is

termed a '_____ to _____' birth.

Fetal malpresentations

 Match

14. Box 13.4 provides an activity related to presentation (i.e., breech, brow, face). To complete the activity, draw a line to correctly match and connect the presentation in column A with the appropriate statements in column B.

Box 13.4

A. Presentation	B. Description
Breech:	Denominator: sacrum Occurs when head is completely extended May result in obstructed labour (C/S probable outcome) Presenting diameters: submentobregmatic (9.5 cm) and bitemporal (8.2 cm) Anencephaly can be a fetal cause Incidence at term is 3%–4%
Brow:	Denominator: mentum Presenting diameter: bitrochanteric (10 cm) Occurs when head is partially extended Submentovertical diameter (11.5 cm) will distend vaginal orifice Vaginal birth is rare if this presentation persists
Face:	Mentovertical diameter (13.5 cm) and bitemporal diameter (8.2 cm) present Incidence is ≤1:500 Fetal heart heard clearly above umbilicus (in non-engagement)

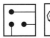 **Label and complete**

15. Fig. 13.9 shows the diameters involved in the delivery of face presentation. Complete the following activity on Fig. 13.9.

Label (name and length)

Engaging diameter
Diameter that sweeps the perineum

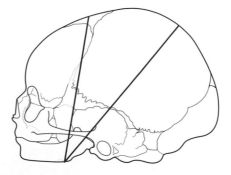

Figure 13.9 Diameters involved in delivery of face presentation.

Complete

16. Complete Table 13.9 by inserting the missing terms.

Table 13.9

Mechanism of a left mentoanterior position	
Lie:	Position:
Attitude:	Denominator:
Presentation:	Presenting part:

 Complete

17. Fig. 13.10 shows the diameter that lies at the back of the pelvic brim in a brow presentation. The length of this diameter exceeds all diameters in an average-sized pelvis.

Label

Name this diameter and identify the length (cm).

Moulding

As a result of moulding, the shape of the baby's head (after birth) gives an indication of the presentation during labour. The following activities relate to the types of moulding.

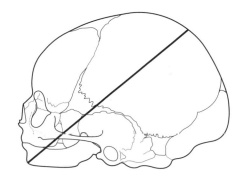

Figure 13.10

18. This activity relates to Figs 13.11–13.14. In activities a, b, c, d you are required to name the diameter(s), provide the length in cm and insert a dashed or dotted line to indicate moulding (where relevant).

    a. Fig. 13.11 shows the type of moulding in a vertex presentation.

Label

The two most common diameters and identify the length (cm) in a vertex presentation.

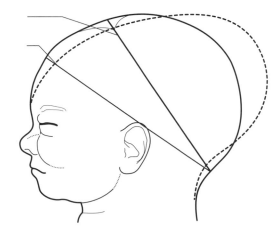

Figure 13.11

Label (b–d) and insert

b. Fig. 13.12 shows the head in a persistent occipitoposterior position. Label the diameter, identify the length (cm) and insert a dashed line to show the direction of moulding.

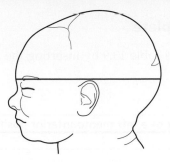

Figure 13.12 Upward moulding (dotted line) following persistent occipitoposterior position.

c. Fig. 13.13 shows the head in a face presentation. Label the diameters, identify the length (cm) and insert a dashed line to show the shape and direction of moulding.

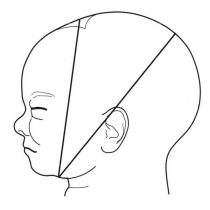

Figure 13.13 Moulding in a face presentation.

d. Fig. 13.14 shows the head in a brow presentation. Label the diameter, identify the length (cm) and insert a dashed line to show the direction of moulding.

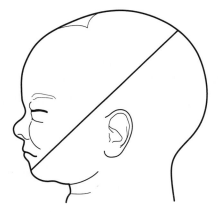

Figure 13.14 Moulding in a brow presentation.

Breech presentations

 Label

19. Figs 13.15–13.18 present the four different types of breech presentations. Label each Figure a–d.

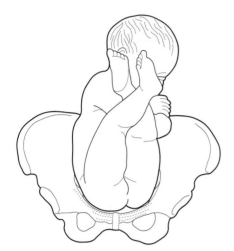

Figure 13.15

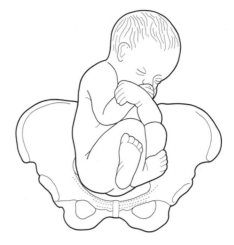

Figure 13.16

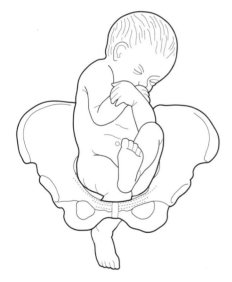

Figure 13.17

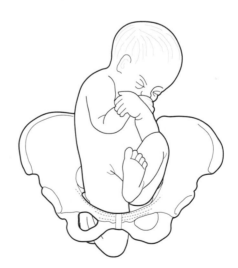

Figure 13.18

a. Fig. 13.15 _____

b. Fig. 13.16 _____

c. Fig. 13.17 _____

d. Fig. 13.18 _____

Complete

20. Table 13.10 relates to the mechanism of left sacroanterior position. Complete the table by either inserting the correct response or removing the incorrect word/numerical value.

Table 13.10

Mechanism of a left sacroanterior position			
Lie:		Position:	
Attitude:		Denominator:	
Presentation:		Presenting part:	
a. The **bitrochanteric/bisacral** diameter (**10.0/11.00 cm**) enters the pelvis in the **left/right** oblique diameter of the brim. The sacrum points to the **iliopectineal line/iliopectineal eminence**.			

Breech births and manoeuvres

Breech birth and manoeuvres involved are updated based on recent RCOG (2017) evidence as this updates the key textbooks (*i.e., Burns-Marshall technique is no longer advised because of concern of over extension of the fetal neck*).

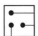 **Label and completion**

21. Tables 13.11 and 13.12 and Box 13.5 provide activities (a–c) related to movements involved in breech birth and manoeuvres involved to aid birth. Complete the activity by removing the incorrect word/s so that the information reads correctly.

    a. Table 13.11

Table 13.11

	Birth of the head (breech birth)
i.	On birth of the **shoulders/umbilicus** the baby is allowed to hang from the vulva **with/without** support. The baby's weight brings the **mentum/head** onto the pelvic floor on which the **mentum/occiput** rotates.
ii.	The **sagittal/coronal** suture is now in the anteroposterior diameter of the **inlet/outlet**. If the head does not **flex/rotate**, then two fingers should be placed on the **occiput/malar** bones and the **sacrum/head** rotated. The baby can hang for up to **1 or 2 minutes/15–20 minutes**. Gradually the **vertex/neck** elongates, the hairline appears and the **frontal/suboccipital** region can be felt.
iii.	Key methods used to achieve a controlled birth include: a) forceps applied to the after-coming head; b) Mauriceau-Smellie-Veit manoeuvre. Assistance is required for babies born with **flexed/extended** legs and **flexed/extended** arms. Controlled birth of the head is vital to avoid any sudden change in **intracranial/intraorbital** pressure.

b. Table 13.12

Table 13.12

	Mauriceau-Smellie-Veit manoeuvre (see Fig. 13.19 for information)
i.	Mauriceau-Smellie-Veit manoeuvre is mainly used when there is delay in **rotation/descent** of the head because of **flexion/extension**. The manoeuvre promotes jaw **extension/flexion** and shoulder **extension/traction**.
ii.	(A) in Fig. 13.19. The hands are in position **after/before** the body is lifted.
iii.	(B) in Fig. 13.19. This shows extraction of the **mentum/head**.
iv.	The manoeuvre involves the baby being laid astride the **fingers/arm** with the palm supporting the **head/chest**. One finger is placed on **occiput/each malar bone** to flex the **mentum/head**. The middle finger may be used to apply pressure to the **sinciput/chin**. Two fingers of the attendant's other hand are hooked over the **chest/shoulders** with the middle finger pushing up the **occiput/sinciput** to aid **extension/flexion**. Traction is applied to draw the head out of the vagina and, when the **frontal/suboccipital** region appears, the body is lifted to assist the head to pivot around the **sacrum/symphysis pubis**. The vault is delivered **quickly/slowly**.

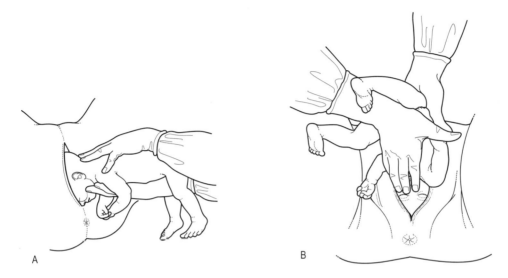

A   B

Figure 13.19 Mauriceau–Smellie–Veit manoeuvre for delivering the after-coming head of breech presentation: the hands are in position before the body is lifted. Extraction of the head.

c. Box 13.5

Box 13.5

EXTENDED LEGS (SEE FIG. 13.20 FOR INFORMATION)
When the popliteal fossae appear at the vulva, **four/two** fingers are placed along the length of one thigh with the fingertips **on the ankle/in the fossa**. The leg is swept to the side of the abdomen (**adducting/abducting** the **hip/knee**) and the knee is **deflexed/flexed** by the pressure on its under surface and the **upper/lower** part of the leg will emerge from the vagina. The process is repeated for the other leg.

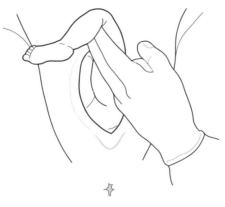

Figure 13.20

22. Table 13.13 presents a selection of statements relating to inducing labour and managing labour and birth with complications. Complete the activity by identifying the correct statements.

Table 13.13

	Statements	Correct
a.	Before membrane sweeping and before IOL, it is essential to confirm that there are no signs of a low-lying placental site	
b.	Of mode of delivery, the risk of maternal complications is lowest with emergency caesarean section	
c.	Caesarean section increases the risk of complications in future pregnancy, including the risk of an abnormally invasive placenta	
d.	Emergency caesarean section is needed in approximately 40% of women planning a vaginal breech birth	
e.	Caesarean section is associated with a small increase in the risk of stillbirth for subsequent babies (this may not be causal)	
f.	Term babies presenting by the breech have better outcomes than cephalic ones, irrespective of the mode of delivery	
g.	In induced and/or augmented labour compared with spontaneous VBAC labour, there is a two- to threefold increased risk of uterine rupture and around 1.5-fold increased risk of caesarean delivery	
h.	In a breech delivery, Loveset manoeuvre involves a combination of rotation and downward traction to deliver the arms and shoulders	
i.	In manoeuvres for breech birth, suprapubic pressure will aid flexion if there is delay because of an extended neck	
j.	A major breakthrough in the noninvasive detection of fetal anaemia is the use of Doppler ultrasound evaluation to measure the peak systolic velocity of the fetal middle cerebral artery (MCA)	
k.	Abnormal umbilical artery flow with absent or reversed end-diastolic velocity (AREDV) during pregnancy is a strong indication of placental insufficiency	
l.	Emergency caesarean section is indicated in prolapsed cord because of the risk of cord obstruction and fetal death or disability	

❓ Multiple choice questions (MCQ)

The following MCQs provide a selection of topics complicating the intrapartum period.

23. The most common cause of shoulder presentation is because of:
    a. Contracted pelvis
    b. Lax abdominal and uterine muscles
    c. Low uterine fibroid
    d. Cervical fibroid

24. If on abdominal examinations the lie tends to vary, then it is defined as unstable lie after:
    a. 30 weeks' gestation
    b. 32 weeks' gestation
    c. 34 weeks' gestation
    d. 36 weeks' gestation
    e. 38 weeks' gestation

25. Which of the following statements is **incorrect** about breech presentation:
    a. Occurs in 3%–4% of term deliveries
    b. More common preterm
    c. Less common in nulliparous women
    d. Associated with uterine and congenital abnormalities
    e. Has a significant recurrence risk

26. Routine caesarean section is routinely recommended in the following situation/s for:

    a. Breech presentation in spontaneous preterm labour at the threshold of viability (22–25+6 weeks' gestation)

    b. Twin pregnancy where the presenting twin is breech

    c. A breech first twin in spontaneous labour

    d. Breech presentation of the second twin in preterm deliveries

    e. Breech presentation of the second twin in term deliveries

27. Which of the following statements is **incorrect** about preterm breech labour:

    a. Routine caesarean section is recommended in spontaneous preterm labour (breech presentation).

    b. Labour with a preterm breech should be managed in the same way as a term breech labour.

    c. In situations where there is head entrapment, incisions in the cervix (vaginal birth) or vertical uterine incision extension (caesarean section) may be used, with or without tocolysis.

    d. None of the above

    e. b and c only

28. Identify the **correct** statement/s relating to timing of cord clamping for preterm babies (vaginal or caesarean section birth):

    a. If mother and baby are stable, wait at least 30 seconds before clamping the cord, but do not wait any longer than 3 minutes.

    b. Position the preterm baby at or below the level of the placenta before clamping the cord.

    c. In a situation immediately at birth when the baby needs to be removed from the mother (such as neonatal or maternal resuscitation), then consider milking the cord and clamp the cord immediately.

    d. All of the above

    e. a and c only

29. Identify the **incorrect** information about breech presentation:

    a. Occurs in 3%–4% of term deliveries.

    b. It is more common preterm and in nulliparous women.

    c. It is associated with uterine and congenital abnormalities.

    d. It has a low recurrence risk.

30. Which of the following statements about uterine hyperstimulation is/are **correct**:

    a. Relates to overactivity of the uterus as a result of IOL.

    b. Uterine tachysystole is defined as more than five contractions per 10 minutes for at least 20 minutes.

    c. Uterine hypersystole/hypertonicity is defined as a contraction lasting at least 2 minutes.

    d. Uterine tachysystole and hypersystole may or not be associated with changes in the fetal heart rate pattern (persistent decelerations, tachycardia or decreased short-term variability).

Intrapartum medical and obstetric complications

Obstetric and medical specialists will be responsible for treatment and pathways of care provided to women with pregnancies identified as being high risk because of obstetric or medical conditions. These may be preexisting conditions or new conditions arising during pregnancy. As midwives are involved in providing intrapartum care, it is important for them to have knowledge of related conditions, treatment and pathways of care during pregnancy and the intrapartum period.

31. Table 13.14 provides statements relating to medical and obstetric conditions during pregnancy and childbirth.

Table 13.14

	Statement	Correct
a.	Continuous CTG should be offered for all babies suspected to be small for gestational age (SGA) if there is concern about the baby's well-being	
b.	For women with mechanical heart valves and taking warfarin in the third trimester, their anticoagulation will be switched to low-molecular-weight heparin by 36+0 weeks of pregnancy or 2 weeks before planned birth (if this is earlier than 36+0 weeks)	
c.	Women with asthma should be offered the same options for pain relief during labour as women without asthma	
d.	Supplemental hydrocortisone in the intrapartum period is not contraindicated for women already taking inhaled or topical steroids	
e.	Prolonged labour in women with chronic kidney disease may lead to dehydration and acute kidney injury	
f.	In the SGA fetus where umbilical artery absent or reversed end-diastolic velocity (AREDV) is detected then delivery by caesarean section is recommended	
g.	Women with cardiac disease will be monitored in labour using continuous electrocardiogram (ECG) and pulse oximetry with continuous intra-arterial BP monitoring	
h.	Before woman with known immune thrombocytopenic purpura being admitted for birth, it is assumed that the baby will be at risk of bleeding irrespective of the woman's platelet count	
i.	Caesarean section is not recommended for women who are at high risk of cerebral haemorrhage	
j.	In women with bleeding disorders, maternal platelet count will be monitored weekly from 36 weeks, and steroids or intravenous (IV) immunoglobulin may be given to raise the maternal platelet count if platelet count is <50	
k.	Birth will be expedited if the source of sepsis is thought to be the genital tract	
l.	Under most circumstances, regional analgesia and anaesthesia will be avoided with a platelet count <50 $\times 10^9$/L	
m.	Nonsteroidal antiinflammatory drugs can add to the risk of bleeding with women with bleeding disorders	
n.	In labour women with a fever, a temperature of ≥38°C on a single reading or ≥37.5°C on two consecutive readings (1 hour apart), are offered paracetamol	

Pathophysiology

The following activity provides decision making, treatment and underlying pathophysiology of a range of conditions that can complicate pregnancy and labour.

 Multiple choice questions (MCQ)

32. Which of the following statements is incorrect relating to the SGA fetus:

    a. Ductus venosus Doppler has moderate predictive value for acidaemia and adverse outcome.

    b. In the preterm SGA fetus, middle cerebral artery (MCA) Doppler has limited accuracy to predict acidaemia and adverse outcome and should not be used to time delivery.

    c. In the term SGA fetus with normal umbilical artery Doppler, an abnormal middle cerebral artery Doppler (PI <5th centile) has moderate predictive value for acidosis at birth and should be used to time delivery.

    d. If MCA Doppler is abnormal, then delivery should be recommended no later than 37 weeks' gestation.

    e. Even when venous Doppler is normal, delivery is recommended by 32 weeks' gestation (i.e., 30–32 weeks' gestation).

33. Which of the following statements is incorrect relating to the large for gestational age (LGA) fetus:

    a. There is a higher chance of maternal medical problems, such as infection with emergency caesarean section.

    b. There is a higher chance of shoulder dystocia and brachial plexus injury with vaginal birth.

    c. There is a lower chance of instrumental birth and perineal trauma with vaginal birth.

    d. It can be difficult to confirm 'large for gestational age' until the baby is born.

34. In the intrapartum period, heart failure should always be considered if which of the following key signs and symptoms are present.

    a. Pale, sweaty, agitated with cool peripheries

    b. Heart rate persistently >110 beats per minute at rest

    c. Respiratory rate persistently >20 breaths per minute at rest

    d. Hypotension (systolic blood pressure <100 mmHg

    e. Normal oxygen saturation

    f. Elevated jugular venous pressure

    g. Added heart sound or murmur reduced air entry, basal crackles and wheeze, on listening to the chest

35. Which of the following investigations/actions are carried out when there is a clinical suspicion of heart failure in the intrapartum period:

    a. Electrocardiogram (ECG)

    b. Peripheral venous access is established

    c. Blood specimens for urea and electrolytes, and full blood count

    d. Arterial blood gases

    e. Chest x-ray

36. Heart failure is suspected if there is not another likely cause of which of the following symptoms:
    a. Breathlessness when lying down (ruling out aortocaval compression) or at rest
    b. Breathlessness and coughing (may be productive of pink frothy)
    c. Unexplained cough, particularly when lying down or which produces frothy pink sputum
    d. Palpitation (awareness of persistent tachycardia at rest)
    e. Paroxysmal nocturnal dyspnea
    f. All of the above

37. Identify the heart diseases for whom fluid balance is critical to cardiac function:
    a. Pulmonary arterial hypertension
    b. Hypertrophic cardiomyopathy
    c. Severe left-sided stenotic lesions (e.g., aortic stenosis and mitral stenosis)
    d. Cardiomyopathy with systolic ventricular dysfunction

38. Ergometrine is not indicated in the management of third stage with women with cardiac conditions; identify the correct reasons:
    a. Further deterioration in pulmonary arterial hypertension
    b. Drowsiness
    c. Because of risk of hypertension induced aortic dissection or rupture in cardiac conditions, such as bicuspid aortopathy and aortic dilatation, previous aortic dissection, Turner syndrome women with Loeys-Dietz syndrome
    d. Because of hypertension induced heart failure in cardiac conditions, such as severe valval stenosis and cynanotic heart disease
    e. Because of the risk of coronary ischaemia in coronary heart disease

39. Identify any **incorrect** statements about women with asthma and the safe use of drugs in labour:
    a. Prostaglandin E1 and prostaglandin E2 are options for inducing labour in women with asthma
    b. Prostaglandin E1 is an option for treating postpartum haemorrhage in women with asthma
    c. Administration of prostaglandin F2 alpha to women with asthma is not recommended because of risk of bronchospasm
    d. None of the above
    e. All of the above

40. For women with immune thrombocytopenic purpura or suspected immune thrombocytopenic purpura, take the following precautions to reduce the risk of bleeding for the baby:
    a. Do not carry out fetal blood sampling.
    b. Use fetal scalp electrodes with caution.
    c. Use ventouse, mid-cavity or rotational forceps with caution.
    d. Caesarean section may not protect the baby from bleeding.
    e. Measure platelet count in the umbilical cord blood at birth.

41. Which of the following statements is/are incorrect relating to intrapartum care for women classified as obese with a BMI >30 kg/m^2 at the booking appointment:

    a. Carry out an updated risk assessment in the third trimester taking changes in BMI into account.

    b. Women with adequate mobility should be managed in the second stage of labour in line with intrapartum guidelines for healthy women and babies.

    c. Women should be advised about using the lateral position in the second stage of labour.

    d. All obstetric units should have equipment needs (BMI >30 kg/m^2) and 'birthing beds' able to take a safe working load of 250 kg.

    e. Should routinely be offered a caesarean section.

42. Women in labour with sepsis are at higher risk of severe illness or death, identify which of the following signs does **not** indicate organ dysfunction:

    a. Alert and responsive

    b. Hypotension (systolic blood pressure <90 mmHg)

    c. Reduced urine output (<0.5 mL/kg/h)

    d. Need for 40% oxygen to maintain oxygen saturation >92%

    e. Tympanic temperature <36°C

    f. Altered consciousness

REFERENCES

https://www.nice.org.uk/guidance
- Intrapartum care for healthy women and babies, [CG190], 2014: updated: 2017
- Inducing labour, [CG70], 2008
- Preterm labour and birth, (NG 25), 2015
- Intrapartum care – high risk, (Draft September 2018)
Royal College of Obstetricians and Gynaecologists: https://www.rcog.org.uk/en/guidelines
- Management of Breech Presentation Green-top Guideline No. 20b, 2017
- Birth After Previous Caesarean Birth Green-top Guideline No. 45, 2015
- The Investigation and Management of the Small–for–Gestational–Age Fetus, Green–top Guideline No. 31, 2013: Minor revisions 2014

14 Midwifery and obstetric emergencies

> This chapter focuses on midwifery and obstetric emergencies. Assisted births will also be included. Assessing risk, recognizing signs and symptoms of the problem and immediate action is vital. Action taken may determine the outcome for the mother and fetus. The activities will test your knowledge in a variety of emergency situations, including the cause, underlying pathophysiology, management and complications where relevant.

 True/false

1. Consider the following statements in Table 14.1. Complete the table by deciding if the statements are correct by ticking the appropriate column.

Table 14.1

	Statement	True	False
a.	The management of placenta praevia accreta is associated with significant morbidity		
b.	Pelvic ultrasound may help to exclude the presence of retained products of conception (RPOC)		
c.	Bradycardia, and variable or prolonged decelerations of the fetal heart are associated with cord compression		
d.	Shoulder dystocia is a soft tissue dystocia		
e.	Infants of diabetic mothers have a two- to fourfold increased risk of shoulder dystocia compared with infants of the same birth weight born to nondiabetic mothers		
f.	The foot of the bed is raised in the Trendelenburg position		
g.	In shoulder dystocia, traction will promote attempts at delivery		
h.	Gaskin manoeuvre is another term for the 'all-four position'		
i.	Once cord prolapsed is diagnosed then an oxytocin infusion in progress should be stopped		
j.	Fetal macrosomia is not associated with shoulder dystocia		
k.	Maternal pushing may exacerbate impaction of the shoulders		

Cord prolapse

Cord prolapse has been defined as the descent of the umbilical cord through the cervix alongside (occult) or past (overt) the presenting part, in the presence of ruptured membranes. Cord presentation is the presence of the umbilical cord between the fetal presenting part and the cervix, with or without intact membranes.

 Short answers

2. This activity relates to the positions adopted in the emergency situation of 'cord prolapse' to alleviate pressure off the cord and allow the fetus to gravitate to the diaphragm. Figs 14.1 and 14.2 show two different positions. Complete the following related questions.

   a. Name the position adopted in Fig. 14.1: _____

   b. Name the position adopted in Fig. 14.2: _____

   Name another position adopted for cord prolapse:

   c. _____

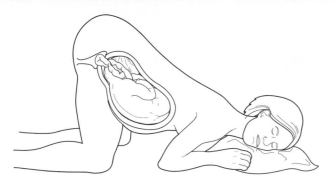

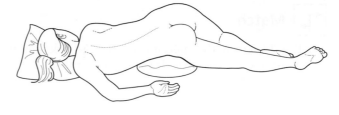

Figure 14.2

Figure 14.1

 Correct/incorrect

3. Table 14.2 provides statements relating to cord prolapse. Indicate the correct statements.

Table 14.2

	Statements	Correct
a.	Avoid performing artificial membrane rupture whenever possible if the presenting part is mobile and/or high	
b.	A routine vaginal examination is still indicated even if the fetal heart rate (FHR) monitoring is normal when spontaneous rupture of membranes occurs, and there are no risk factors for cord prolapse	
c.	The principal causes of asphyxia in cord prolapse following rupture of membranes are thought to be cord compression and umbilical arterial vasospasm preventing venous and arterial blood flow to and from the fetus	
d.	No evidence is available to support replacement of the cord into the uterus when prolapse occurs at or before the threshold of viability	
e.	To prevent vasospasm, there should be minimal handling of loops of cord lying outside the vagina	
f.	The presenting part can be elevated either manually or by filling the urinary bladder to prevent cord compression	
g.	Cord compression can be further reduced by the woman adopting the knee–chest or left lateral (preferably with head down and pillow under the left hip) position	
h.	If birth is likely to be delayed, tocolysis can be considered, while preparing for caesarean section if there are persistent FHR abnormalities after attempts to prevent compression mechanically.	
i.	During preparation for birth, time should be taken to use all the methods even if this delays birth.	

Match

4. Box 14.1 provides activities about the risk factors associated with cord prolapse (and cord presentation). To complete the activity, draw a line to match the general or procedure-related risks (column A) and connect with the correct associated risk factor (column B).

Box 14.1

A: Risk category	B: Associated risk factor
General:	Multiparity Vaginal manipulation of the fetus with ruptured membranes Low birthweight (<2.5 kg) External cephalic version (during procedure) Fetal congenital anomalies Breech presentation Stabilizing induction of labour Preterm labour (<37+0 weeks) Large balloon catheter induction of labour Transverse, oblique and unstable lie (after 37+0 weeks) Internal podalic version Second twin
Procedure-related:	Unengaged presenting part Insertion of intrauterine pressure transducer Low-lying placenta Polyhydramnios Artificial rupture of membranes with high presenting part

 Complete

5. The activity in Box 14.2 relates to the action of the midwife on diagnosis of the emergency situation of cord prolapse. Complete the statements (a–c) by inserting the missing word(s) from the list provided. Insert the correct birth management in (d) from your own knowledge.

Contraction	Fingers	Replaced	Temperature	Urgent
Drying	Presenting part	Spasm	Time	Vagina

Box 14.2

Actions of the midwife

a   Call for _____ assistance and note the _____ cord prolapse occurred.

b.   If the cord lies outside the vagina, then it should be gently _____ to prevent _____, to

maintain the _____ and prevent _____.

c.   The midwife may need to keep her _____ in the _____ and hold the

_____ off the umbilical cord, especially during a _____.

d.   Birth must be expedited with the greatest possible speed for a cord prolapse. What birth management would be done for the following circumstances?

• If the fetus is alive but vaginal birth is not imminent: _____ is required.

• If the presentation is cephalic the birth may be medically assisted through: _____ OR _____.

• If the cord prolapse is diagnosed in second stage (multiparous mother) birth may be expedited by:

_____.

Shoulder dystocia

Shoulder dystocia is defined as a vaginal cephalic delivery that requires additional obstetric manoeuvres to deliver the fetus, after the head has delivered and gentle traction has failed. The exact incidence remains uncertain. Significant perinatal morbidity and mortality is associated with the condition, even when the emergency is managed appropriately. The Royal College of Obstetricians and Gynaecologists recommend the use of the algorithm for the systematic management used to disimpact the shoulders. This is in preference to the use of mnemonic and eponyms. More detail of specific manoeuvres will be available in course manuals for obstetric emergency training.

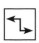   ## Match, short answers and complete

6. Box 14.3 provides a selection of activities related to shoulder dystocia. Complete the activities by inserting the correct word from the list provided, removing the incorrect words or inserting short answers from your own knowledge.

anterior	hollow	sacrum	symphysis pubis
behind	posterior	sacral promontory	

Box 14.3

Shoulder dystocia

a. Shoulder dystocia occurs more commonly when the _____ shoulder becomes trapped

 _____ or on the _____, while the _____ shoulder may be in the

 _____ of the _____ or high above the _____.

b. Identify three prelabour risk factors: _____

 _____

c. Identify three intrapartum risk factors: _____

 _____

d. Identify three signs: _____

 _____

 _____

e. Maternal and fetal morbidity is increased. Identify one maternal complication and one fetal complication:

 _____ _____

f. Complete the following terminology by removing the **incorrect** word.
 (i) The term 'adduct' means to pull or move something (e.g., arm or leg) **toward/away from** the midline of the body.
 (ii) The term 'abduct' means to pull or move something (e.g., arm or leg) **toward/away from** the midline of the body.

Complete

7. Fig. 14.3 provides the systematic approach in the management of shoulder dystocia. Complete the algorithm by addressing the activities as detailed.

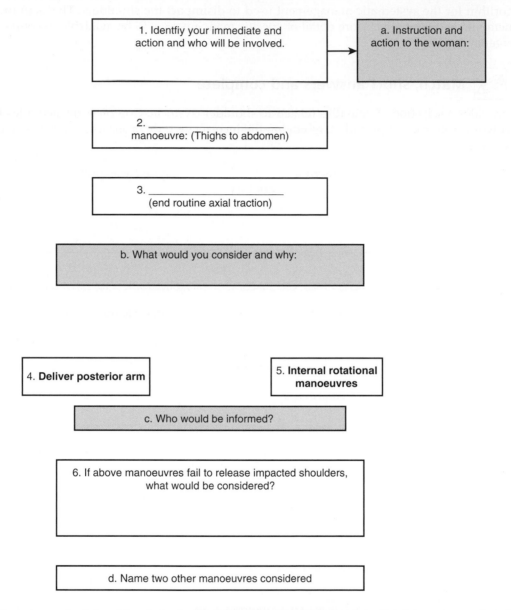

Figure 14.3 Management of shoulder dystocia (Cornthwaite et al: Training for obstetric emergencies - PROMPT and shoulder dystocia. © 2015 The Health Foundation.)

Positions and manoeuvres used in shoulder dystocia

Complete

8. Figs 14.4 and 14.5 show positions and noninvasive manoeuvres that may be involved in shoulder dystocia. Table 14.3 provides an activity related to noninvasive procedures. Complete the table by: (i) inserting the name of the manoeuvre, and (ii) removing the incorrect word(s).

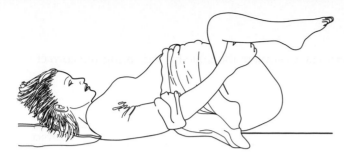

Figure 14.4

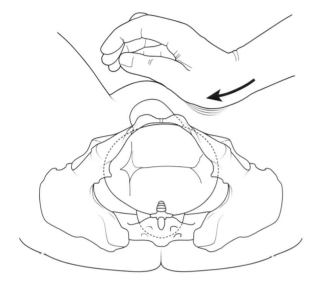

Figure 14.5

Table 14.3

	Noninvasive procedures
a.	Name of manoeuvre shown in Fig. 14.4
	This manoeuvre involves **flexion/extension** and **abduction/adduction** of the maternal hips. It straightens the **lumbosacral/symphysis pubis** angle, **rotates/diminishes** the maternal pelvis toward the mother's head and **decreases/increases** the relative anterior-posterior diameter of the pelvis. The legs should be **hyperflexed/hyperextended**. Apply routine traction (as in normal delivery) in an axial direction (in line with fetal spine).
b.	What manoeuvre does Fig. 14.5 demonstrate? Pressure should be exerted on the side of the fetal **chest/back** and toward the fetal **chest/back**. This manoeuvre may help to **adduct/abduct** the shoulders (**increase/reduce** the fetal bisacromial diameter) and push the **anterior/posterior** shoulder away from the **sacral promontory/symphysis pubis** into the wider **anterior or posterior/oblique or transverse** diameter.

9. If the first line simple and noninvasive measures fail to release the impacted shoulders, then individual circumstances guide the healthcare professional as to whether to try the 'all fours' technique before or after attempting internal rotation and delivery of the posterior arm. Second line internal rotational manoeuvres were originally described by Woods and Rubin. Complete the activities in Table 14.4 a–d by removing the incorrect word/s.

Table 14.4

	'All fours' and internal rotational manoeuvres
a.	The 'all fours position' (**Gaskin/Gasgoine** manoeuvre) may be especially helpful if the **anterior/posterior** shoulder is impacted behind the **symphysis pubis/sacral promontory**, as this position optimizes space available in the **sacral/spinal** curve and may allow the **anterior/posterior** shoulder to be delivered first.
b.	Internal movements: Vaginal access uses the space available in the sacral hollow. The whole hand should be entered **anteriorly/posteriorly** to perform internal rotation or delivery of the **anterior/posterior** arm. Access is made easier by repositioning the women to the end of the bed. Rotation can be most easily achieved by pressing on the anterior or posterior aspect of the **anterior/posterior** shoulder. Applying pressure on the posterior aspect of the posterior shoulder has the additional benefit of reducing the shoulder diameter by **abducting/adducting** the shoulders. Delivery can be facilitated by **flexion/rotation** into **a transverse/an oblique** diameter or when possible by a full 180-degree rotation of the fetal trunk, or by delivery of the **anterior/posterior** arm. If pressure on the **anterior/posterior** shoulder is unsuccessful, an attempt should be made to apply pressure on the **anterior/posterior** aspect of the anterior shoulder to **abduct/adduct** and rotate the shoulders into the **transverse/oblique** diameter.
c.	Delivering the **anterior/posterior** arm reduces the diameter of the fetal shoulders by the width of the arm. The fetal wrist should be grasped and the **anterior/posterior** arm should be gently withdrawn from the vagina in a **straight line/upward curve**.
d.	Third line measures are rarely required and include: **cleidotomy/cleidostomy, symphysiotomy/symphostomy** and the **Zavanelli/Zavaronie** manoeuvre.

Correct/incorrect

10. Table 14.5 provides statements relating to shoulder dystocia. Complete the table by indicating the correct statements.

Table 14.5

	Statement	Correct
a.	An episiotomy is always required	
b.	The 'all-fours' position has been described as having a success rate of 83%	
c.	Cleidotomy involves the surgical division of the clavicle or bending with a finger	
d.	The incidence of humeral fractures associated with the delivery of the posterior arm is between 2% and 12%	
e.	Symphysiotomy is a potentially useful procedure in both the developing and developed world	
f.	Downward traction on the fetal head should be avoided in the management of all births to prevent Brachial plexus injury	
g.	Zavanelli manoeuvre involved vaginal replacement of the head and then caesarean section for delivery	
h.	Prophylactic McRoberts' positioning before delivery of the fetal head is not recommended to prevent shoulder dystocia	
i.	Symphysiotomy has a low incidence of serious maternal morbidity and poor neonatal outcome	
j.	Zavanelli manoeuvre may be most appropriate for rare bilateral shoulder dystocia, where both the shoulders impact on the pelvic inlet, anteriorly above the pubic symphysis and posteriorly on the sacral promontory	
k.	Symphysiotomy involves the division of the anterior fibres of symphyseal ligament	
l.	The posterior axillary sling is another technique used	
m.	Suprapubic pressure should not be attempted with the McRoberts' manoeuvre	
n.	Fundal pressure should not be used	
o.	McRoberts' manoeuvre is a simple, rapid and effective noninvasive intervention and should be performed first	
p.	Shoulder dystocia should be managed as carefully as possible to avoid hypoxic acidosis, and unnecessary trauma	
q.	Pressure on the posterior aspect of the posterior shoulder has the additional benefit of reducing the shoulder diameter by adducting the shoulders	

Rupture of the uterus and inversion of the uterus

 True/false

11. Rupture of the uterus is one of the most serious complications in midwifery and obstetrics. Complete the following Table 14.6 by ticking whether the statements are true or false.

Table 14.6

	Statements	True	False
a.	Complete rupture of the uterus involves tearing of the uterine but never expulsion of the fetus		
b.	Incomplete rupture of the uterus involves tearing of the uterus and the perimetrium		
c.	Dehiscence (bursting) of an existing scar involves rupture of the uterine wall but the fetal membranes remain intact		
d.	Complete rupture of the uterus in a nonscarred uterus may present with sudden collapse of the mother who complains of severe abdominal pain		
e.	The following can cause a ruptured uterus: uterine surgery, previous caesarean section, oxytocin use and high parity		
f	Because of a previous scar being fibrous and avascular, blood loss associated with an incomplete or dehiscence is profuse		
g	Key signs associated with a ruptured uterus are: abdominal pain or pain over previous caesarean section scar; abnormalities of the FHR and pattern; vaginal bleeding; maternal tachycardia; poor progress in labour		

True/false

12. Uterine inversion is classified based on its severity, for example, first, second, third or fourth degree and also according to the timing in which it occurs, for example, acute, subacute or chronic. Consider the statements related to inversion of the uterus in Table 14.7. Complete the table by indicating if the statements are true or false.

Table 14.7

	Statement	True	False
a.	A fourth-degree inversion is a total uterine and vaginal inversion		
b.	Acute inversion occurs after 24 hours but before 48 hours		
c.	A second-degree inverted uterus is where the body or the corpus of the uterus is inverted to the internal os		
d.	Subacute inversion of the uterus occurs after the first 4 weeks but within 12 weeks		
e.	A first-degree inverted uterus is where the fundus reaches the internal os		
f.	A third-degree inverted uterus is where the fundus protrudes to or beyond the introitus and is visible		
g.	Chronic inversion of the uterus occurs after 4 weeks and is a common occurrence		

Instrumental and operative births

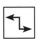 **Match and complete**

13. Table 14.8 provides statement relating to four types of instrumental assisted births (list provided). To complete the table, match and insert the correct instrument to each statement.

Wrigley's forceps   Keilland's forceps
Neville-Barnes or Simpson's forceps   Ventouse

Table 14.8

	Statements	Instrument
a.	These are generally used for a low or mid cavity delivery when the sagittal suture is in the anteroposterior diameter of the cavity/outlet of the pelvis	
b.	These are generally used for rotation and extraction of the head that is arrested in the deep transverse or in the occipitoposterior position	
c.	This is associated with more incidences of cephalohaematoma than other facial and cranial injuries	
d.	These are also used for the after-coming head of a breech delivery, or at a caesarean section	
e.	This involves positioning it over the flexion point along the sagittal suture in between the anterior and posterior fontanelles	
f.	These are designed to be used when the head is on the perineum	
g.	This cleaves to the baby's scalp by suction	
h..	These forceps have a much reduced pelvic curve to allow for the safe rotation of the fetus	

Complete

14. The following activity (Table 14.9) relates to the sequence of anatomical layers involved in the operative procedure of caesarean section. Complete the activity by inserting the correct sequence of layers from the list provided. This commences with the outer layer of skin.

abdominal peritoneum   subcutaneous fat
muscle (rectus abdominis)   pelvic peritoneum
rectus sheath   uterine muscle

Table 14.9

Skin	→	_____	→	_____
	→	_____	→	_____
	→	_____	→	_____

Shock—classification

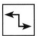 **Match**

15. Box 14.4 provides classifications of shock with possible causes and underlying pathophysiology. To complete the activity, draw a line to match the classification of shock in column A and connect with the accurate cause in column B for each classification.

Box 14.4

A: Classification of shock	B: Causes
Anaphylactic:	Caused by impaired ability of the heart to pump blood
Cardiogenic:	Results from an insult to the nervous system
Hypovolaemic:	Occurs with a severe generalized infection
Neurogenic:	Results from a reduction in intravascular volume
Septic or toxic:	May occur as a result of severe allergy or drug reaction

 Complete

16. The following activity relates to 'shock'. Complete the following paragraph by inserting the correct missing word from the list provided.

acute   complex   inadequate   organ
chronic   death   multisystem   tissues
circulatory   failure   recovery
collapse   fatal   reduction

Shock is a _____ syndrome. It involves a _____ in blood flow to the _____. This may

result in irreversible _____ damage and progressive _____ of the _____

system. If left untreated it will result in _____.

Shock can be _____ but prompt treatment results in _____ with little detrimental effect on

the woman. When there is _____ to initiate effective treatment or provide inadequate treatment this

can result in a _____ condition ending in _____ organ failure which may be

_____.

✎ Complete

17. Table 14.10 lists the classifications of 'shock'. Complete the table by inserting one example of shock related to obstetrics.

Table 14.10

	Type	Example
a.	Hypovolaemic:	
b.	Anaphylactic:	
c.	Neurogenic:	
d.	Septic or toxic:	
e.	Cardiogenic:	

18. Table 14.11 provides two activities relating to the physiological effects of 'shock'. Complete the activities by removing the incorrect word(s) so that the paragraphs read correctly.

Table 14.11

a.	**Compensatory stage of hypovolaemic shock:** The **rise/drop** in cardiac output produces a response from the **sympathetic/peripheral** nervous system through the activation of receptors in the **aorta and carotid arteries/renal arteries**. Blood is redistributed to the **vital organs/skin**. There is **constriction/dilatation** of the vessel in the gastrointestinal tract, kidneys, skin, and lungs. The response is seen as the skin becoming **pale/flushed** and **warm/cool**. Peristalsis **slows/increases**, urinary output is **increased/reduced** and exchange of gas is impaired as blood flow **increases/diminishes**. The heart rate **decreases/increases** and the pupils of the eyes **constrict/dilate**. Sweat glands are **stimulated/inactive** and the skin becomes **dry and warm/moist and clammy**. Adrenaline (Epinephrine) is released from the adrenal **medulla/cortex** and aldosterone from the adrenal **medulla/cortex**. Antidiuretic hormone (ADH) is secreted from the **anterior/posterior** lobe of the pituitary gland. Their combined effect is to cause **vasoconstriction/vasodilatation**, **decreased/increased** cardiac output and a **decrease/increase** in urinary output. Venous return to the heart will **increase/decrease**, but this will not be sustained unless the fluid loss is replaced.
b.	'Adult respiratory distress syndrome' (ARDS) *(because of physiological effects 'shock' on lungs)*. Gas exchange is **impaired/unaffected** as the physiological dead space **increases/decreases** within the lungs. Levels of carbon dioxide **rise/fall** and arterial oxygen levels **fall/remain unchanged**. **Ischaemia/increased blood flow** within the lungs alters the production of **surfactant/renin** and as a result of this, alveoli **collapse/enlarge**. Oedema in the lungs, caused by **increased/decreased** permeability, **exacerbates/reduces** the existing problem of diffusion of oxygen. Atelectasis, oedema and **reduced/increased** compliance impair ventilation and gaseous exchange. This leads ultimately to respiratory **failure/improvement**.

Amniotic fluid embolism

 Complete

19. Box 14.5 provides activities relating to amniotic fluid embolism. Complete the activities by inserting the missing word from the list provided and by removing the incorrect word(s) so that the paragraphs read correctly.

Cardiovascular	Compromise	Hypoxia	Pulmonary
Coagulation	Haemorrhage	Placental	

Box 14.5

Amniotic fluid embolism
a. Amniotic fluid embolism (AFE) occurs when amniotic fluid enters the **maternal/fetal** circulation via the _____ or _____ site. Maternal collapse can progress **rapidly/insidiously**. The body's initial response is pulmonary **vasospasm/vasodilation** causing hypoxia, **hypertension/hypotension**, _____ oedema and _____ collapse.
b. Secondly with AFE, there is the development of **left/right** ventricular failure, with maternal bleeding and _____ disorder and further uncontrollable _____.
Mortality and morbidity are **high/low**. Because of maternal **hypotension/hypertension**, there is uterine **hypertonus/hypotonus** and this will induce fetal _____ in response to uterine _____.

20. Table 14.12 relates to maternal signs and symptoms of amniotic fluid embolism. Using the list provided, complete the table by inserting the correct response for the signs and symptoms of each body systems.

Abnormal	cyanosis	haemorrhage	respiratory arrest
cardiac arrest	death	hypotension	respiratory distress
compromise	disseminated intravascular coagulation (DIC)	pale clammy skin	restlessness
convulsions	dyspnoea	panic	shivering tachycardia

Table 14.12

Maternal signs and symptoms of amniotic fluid embolism			
Cardiovascular system		**Respiratory system**	
Pulse rate:		Colour:	
Blood pressure		Breathing:	
Peripheral circulation effects:		Deteriorating effects:	
Severe effects:		Severe effects:	
Haematological system		**Neurological system**	
What happens at placental site:		Mother's demeanour:	
Coagulation disorders:		Mother's behaviour:	
What about the fetus:		Severe effects experienced:	

Basic life support measures

21. Box 14.6 relates to basic life support measures, Complete the activities by inserting the missing words and numerical values from the list provided. *N.B. Always refer to updated resuscitation guidelines.*

2	breath	chin lift	left-lateral tilt	pillows
30	breathing	experienced	movements	pulse
airway	circulation	head tilt	obstruction	safe
aortocaval	chest	help	perimortem caesarean section	shout
				supine

Box 14.6

Basic life support measures

---

i.   Adopt a _____ approach to the woman. Shake and _____ to check conscious level. Call for

_____ to get appropriate assistance.

ii. Remove any _____ and position the woman _____, on a _____ to prevent

_____ compression.

iii. A – _____

Position the head in a _____, _____. Remove any _____ in the mouth (e.g.,

dentures or vomit). Check for chest _____.

iv. B – _____. Listen and feel for _____.⁻

v.   C – _____. Check for a _____.

vi. Commence chest compressions if _____ absent or if _____ is absent or abnormal.

vii.. Ratio is _____ compressions: _____ breaths.

viii. Continue until _____ arrives or more _____ staff take over

ix. A _____ may be performed to assist with the resuscitation.

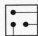 **Label and colour**

22. Fig. 14.6 shows cricoid pressure and the related structures. Label as indicated to complete the activity.

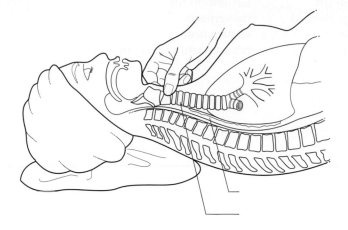

Label and shade/colour

Adam's apple
Oesophagus
Cricoid cartilage
Trachea
Trachea

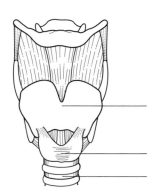

Figure 14.6

 Definitions: Match

23. Box 14.7 provides an activity related to emergency situations involving the umbilical cord. The aim is to construct the related definitions in column A from the statements provided in column B. Draw a line to match and connect the statements with the correct emergency situation.

Box 14.7

A: Emergency (umbilical cord)	B: Partial definition:
Occult cord prolapse:	and the fetal membranes are ruptured lies in front of the presenting part occurs when the umbilical cord
Cord prolapse:	with the fetal membranes still intact occurs when the umbilical cord lies alongside
Cord presentation:	occurs when the umbilical cord lies in front of the presenting part but not in front of the presenting part

Postpartum haemorrhage

Primary postpartum haemorrhage (PPH) is the most common form of major obstetric haemorrhage. The traditional definition of primary PPH is the loss of ≥500 mL of blood from the genital tract within 24 hours of birth. PPH can be minor (500–1000 mL) or major (>1000 mL). Major can be further subdivided into moderate (1001–2000 mL) and severe (>2000 mL). Secondary PPH is defined as abnormal or excessive bleeding from the birth canal between 24 hours and 12 weeks postnatally.

 Match

24. The causes of PPH relate to abnormalities of one or more of four basic processes termed *'the four Ts'* (tone, trauma, tissue and thrombin). The most common cause is resulting from uterine atony. Box 14.8 provides an activity related to 'the four Ts'. To complete the activity, draw a line to match up one of 'the four T's (column A) and connect with the correct risk factor (column B).

Box 14.8

A: 'The four Ts'	B: Risk factor
	Multiple pregnancy
Trauma:	Preeclampsia
	Placenta accreta
	Retained placenta
Tone:	Episiotomy
	Fetal macrosomia
	Failure to progress (third stage)
Tissue:	Previous PPH
	Perineal laceration
	Failure to progress (second stage)
Thrombin:	General anaesthetic

  Match and complete

25. Table 14.13 relates to the main therapeutic goals of the management of massive blood loss as maintaining. Complete the activity by inserting the correct numerical value from the list provided.

$> 50 \times 10^9/L$ >2 g/L   <1.5 times normal   >80 g/L   <1.5 times normal

Table 14.13

Hb:	Activated partial thromboplastin time (APTT):
Fibrinogen:	Prothrombin time (PT)
Platelet count:	

 Short answers

26. Table 14.14 provides activities about postpartum bleeding. Complete the table by providing short answers.

Table 14.14

	Possible causes of bleeding
a.	Identify four causes of PPH:
b.	Identify three causes of secondary PPH:

True/false

27. The risk of massive haemorrhage is associated with placenta-related conditions, such as placenta praevia and placenta accreta spectrum. Table 14.15 provides a range of statements relating to emergency treatment of massive bleeding. Complete the table by indicating if each statement is true or false.

Table 14.15

	Statement	True	False
a.	First-line management of PPH is the simple mechanical and physiological measures of 'rubbing up the fundus' and emptying the bladder to stimulate uterine contraction		
b.	During ongoing PPH, platelets should be transfused at a trigger of 75×10^9/L to maintain a level >50×10^9/L		
c.	Cryoprecipitate should not be used for fibrinogen replacement		
d.	Maternal complications in placenta accreta spectrum are primarily the result of massive haemorrhage		
e.	Placenta increta and placenta percreta are at the abnormally invasive ends of the accreta spectrum and these usually have the best clinical outcomes		
f.	Compression of the aorta may be a temporary but effective measure to allow time for resuscitation to catch up with the volume replacement and appropriate surgical support to arrive		
g.	The risk of massive haemorrhage with possible need for blood transfusion is estimated to be approximately 12 times more likely in caesarean section for placenta praevia than for other indications		
h.	In women presenting with secondary PPH, high vaginal and endocervical swabs should be performed to initiate appropriate antimicrobial therapy when endometritis is suspected		

? Multiple choice questions (MCQ)

28. In a cord prolapse, the bladder can be filled with 500 to 700 mL of sterile saline, which elevates the presenting part above the ischial spines by approximately:

    a. 1 cm

    b. 2 cm

    c. 3 cm

    d. 4 cm

29. The incidence of acute inversion of the uterus is approximately:

    a. 1 in 5000 births

    b. 1 in 10,000 births

    c. 1 in 20,000 births

    d. 1 in 30,000 births

30. Central venous pressure (CVP) is the pressure in the:

    a. Right atrium or superior vena cava

    b. Left atrium or inferior vena cava

    c. Pulmonary artery

    d. Pulmonary vein

31. The normal central pressure varies between:

   a.   20 and 25 cm of H_2O

   b.   15 and 20 cm of H_2O

   c.   10 and 15 cm of H_2O

   d.   5 and 10 cm of H_2O

32. In shock, the CVP pressure will be persistently:

   a.   Low and below 5 cm of H_2O

   b.   Low and below 10 cm of H_2OT

   c.   High and above 15 cm of H_2O

   d.   High and above 25 cm of H_2O

33. The stages of shock are:

   a.   Irreversible, compensatory, progressive, initial

   b.   Initial, progressive, compensatory, irreversible

   c.   Initial, compensatory, progressive, irreversible

   d.   Progressive, irreversible, compensatory, initial

34. Which of the following statements is/are incorrect?

   a.   Uterus preserving surgery is not possible in placenta percreta.

   b.   Surgical approach includes bilateral ligations of the anterior division of the iliac arteries before removing the placenta.

   c.   Antenatal diagnosis of placenta accreta spectrum reduces maternal peripartum haemorrhage and morbidity.

   d.   In placenta accreta spectrum, median blood loss is estimated between 2000 and 7800 mL with an average of 5 units of blood transfusion needed.

   e.   Attempts at removing placenta accreta at caesarean section can lead to massive haemorrhage, high maternal morbidity and maternal death.

REFERENCES

Royal College of Obstetricians and Gynaecologists: https://www.rcog.org.uk/en/guidelines
   • Prevention and Management of Postpartum Haemorrhage Green-top Guideline No. 52, 2016
   • Placenta Praevia and Placenta Accreta: Diagnosis and Management Green-top Guideline No. 27a, 2018
   • Umbilical Cord Prolapse Green-top Guideline No. 50, 2014
   • Shoulder Dystocia Green–top Guideline No. 42, 2012
   • Blood Transfusion in Obstetrics Green-top Guideline No. 47, 2015

15 The puerperium

This chapter focuses on the physiology of the puerperium, anatomy of the breasts and the physiology of lactation. Maternal physical and psychological complications are also included. Midwives as the lead professionals need to be vigilant during this period. They will be supported from the wider maternity and primary care teams depending on maternal needs and circumstances. The activities will test your knowledge in these areas.

  ## Complete and short answers

1. Table 15.1 provides questions/activities related to the puerperium (in the absence of complications). Complete the table by providing short answers.

Table 15.1

	Question/activity	Answer
a.	When does the puerperium start and what is the typical duration?	
b.	In general, what is the physiological expectation by the end of the puerperium?	
c.	Identify the four circulating hormones involved in the puerperium:	
d.	What term refers to the physiological process returning the uterus to prepregnant state?	
e.	What hormone/endocrine gland is involved in the process?	
f.	What symptom is caused by involuntary contraction of the uterus?	
g.	What term refers to vaginal blood loss?	
h.	List four constituents of vaginal blood loss:	

N.B. Professionally, it is recognized that some women will continue to experience problems related to childbirth extending well beyond the defined puerperium period. The possibility of a longer duration is now accepted alongside the range of initial morbidity.

Uterine changes

 ## Complete

2. Table 15.2 relates to the stages involved in the physiological processes occurring in the uterus at the end of third stage. Complete the activity by removing the incorrect word so that the physiological processes described are correct.

Table 15.2

a.	After birth of the baby, the separation and expulsion of placenta and membranes is assisted by the hormone **prolactin/oxytocin** acting on the contraction of the **uterine muscles/decidua**. This hormone is secreted from the **anterior/posterior** (lobe) of the **thyroid/pituitary** gland. Once placenta and membranes are expelled, this exposes ends of **minor/major** blood vessels and the uterine **cavity/perimetrium** collapses **inwards/laterally**. The collapse of uterine **walls/decidua** and muscle layers of the **endometrium/myometrium** simulating the action of ligatures, compress and occlude the exposed sinuses of the blood vessels. This action **reduces/increases** blood loss.

Continued →

Table 15.2 continued

b.	**Vasoconstriction/vasodilation** of the uterine blood supply results in the tissues receiving reduced **blood/nerve** supply. This leads to de-oxygenation and a state of **ischaemia/coagulation** arising in the uterine **tissues/nerve supply**. The overall muscles fibres **increase/reduce** in size through the process of **autolysis/regeneration**, involving autodigestion of the **ischaemic/hyperaemia** muscle fibres by proteolytic **toxins/enzymes**. Phagocytic action of **polymorphs/endomorphs** and macrophages in the blood, and lymphatic systems upon the waste products of **autolysis/regeneration**, which are then excreted in the urine via the **renal/hepatic** system. **Coagulation/ thrombocytopenia** takes place through platelet aggregation and the release of thromboplastin and **fibrin/Factor III**.
c.	With the exception of the placental site, the remains of the inner surface of the uterine lining regenerates **slowly/rapidly** to produce a covering of **epithelium/connective tissue**. Partial covering occurs within **2–5 days/7–10 days** after birth; total coverage is complete by the **10th day/21st day**. Once the placenta has separated, there is a **reduction/increase** in the circulating levels of pregnancy-related hormones. This leads to further physiological changes in muscle and connective tissue, as well as having a **minor/major** influence on the secretion of **oxytocin/prolactin** from the anterior **thyroid/pituitary** gland.
d.	To ensure that physiological processes are beginning to take place, the initial abdominal palpation is usually performed **before/soon after** expulsion of placenta and membranes. On abdominal palpation, the fundus should be located **laterally/centrally**. Fundal position is usually at the same level or slightly **above/below** the umbilicus and should feel **boggy/firm** to confirm a state of contraction.

Correct/incorrect

3. Table 15.3 provides a range of statements. Complete the table by identifying the correct statements.

Table 15.3

	Statement	Correct
a.	Just after birth, blood products are the major constitutes of vaginal loss	
b.	The midwife should place involution of the uterus into context alongside the colour, amount and duration of vaginal fluid loss and maternal general health	
c.	The production of oxytocin does not influence contraction of the uterus leading to afterpains	
d.	Afterpains and uterine tenderness on palpation should not be defined as separate issues	
e.	Retained placental fragments and other products of conception are likely to inhibit the process of involution	
f.	Urinary and bowel symptoms normally resolve within the first 2 weeks following birth	
g.	Morbidity associated with perineal injury and repair is a major health problem or women globally	
h.	In the first day following birth, many women experience an increase in urine output (diuresis) because of the body reabsorbing a quantity of excess fluid following birth	
i.	Detecting maternal morbidity (e.g., sepsis) can be assisted by the midwife combining uterine involution findings with other observations such as offensive lochia, raised or lowered temperature and abdominal tenderness	
j.	The sphere of midwifery practice includes advising women on how to manage their fertility	
k.	A minimum of one blood pressure measurement should be carried out and documented within 6 hours of the birth	
l.	The rate of involution is unaffected in circumstances where there has been over distension of the uterus (e.g., multiple pregnancy)	

Puerperal infection

Complete

4. Box 15.1 provides a range of infection-related statements the midwife may note or record on postnatal assessment. Complete the activity by drawing a line to correctly match and connect general infection signs/ symptoms and those specific to puerperal infection sites in column A with the statements in column B.

Box 15.1

A	B
Puerperal infection (signs/symptoms/recordings):	Respiratory collapse
	Blood clots may be passed
	Headaches and rigours possible
	One segment may be flushed or reddened
	Inflammation/tenderness around the area
	Blood loss may be fresher and heavier or scanty but foul smelling (compared with previous assessment)
	Virulent clear or purulent exudate
	Dysuria
	Blood cultures may be positive
Genital tract:	Slow healing or gaping at the skin edges
	One or both nipples have sore, broken or discoloured skin
	May be tenderness on palpation
	Haematuria
	Nausea and vomiting
Wounds:	Vagina loss heavier and fresher (or scant but offensive)
	Pain and tenderness in the renal angle (also along line of ureter)
	Fundus may be deviated to one side and not progressively reducing in size
Renal system:	Pale
	Pain felt deeper in the wound area
	Urine—cloudy, offensive with pus
	May be severe breathlessness
Breasts:	Pyrexia >38°C
	Palpation—may be subinvoluted uterus, poorly contracted/feel wide/'boggy'
	Feels tight and tender
	Tachycardia >100 beats per minute
	Listless, unwell with flu-like symptoms

True/false

5. Table 15.4 provides a range of statements. Complete the table by indicating if each statement is true or false.

Table 15.4

	Statement	True	False
a.	Emergency action is required if maternal temperature remains above 38°C on the second reading or there are other observable symptoms and measurable signs of sepsis		
b.	Every woman who is nonsensitized Rh-D-negative should be offered anti-D immunoglobulin within 72 hours, following birth of an RhD-positive baby		
c.	All women found to be sero-negative on antenatal screening for rubella should be offered an MMR (measles, mumps, rubella) vaccination following birth and before discharge (if hospital admission)		
d.	The most common species associated with puerperal sepsis is the ß-haemolytic *Streptococcus pyogenes* (Lancefield group A)		
e.	Women should be asked by their health practitioner about resumption of sexual intercourse and possible dyspareunia 2–6 weeks after the birth		
f.	Postnatal women should be advised to avoid getting pregnant for 1 month after receiving MMR. Lactating women can be advised to continue breastfeeding		
g.	Hormonal influences seem to be implicated in the postnatal 'blues', which is the least common complication of the puerperium		
h.	Psychiatric disorders are associated with a decrease in fertility		
i.	In almost all incidents of puerperal psychosis, the onset is rapid and involves a mood disorder with features such as loss of contact with reality, hallucinations and abnormal behaviour		

Multiple choice questions (MCQ)

6. National guidance recommends that women in the puerperium should be offered information and assurance on:

   a. The physiological process of recovery after birth (within the first 24 hours)

   b. The normal patterns of emotional changes and reassurance that these usually resolve within 10 to 14 days of giving birth (within 3 days)

   c. The common health concerns as appropriate (within 2–8 weeks)

   d. All of the above

   e. b and c

7. Expulsion of placenta and membranes initiates pregnancy-related changes including removal of hormones dependent on their half-life. Changes include:

   a. Within 24 hours, plasma estradiol decreases to levels that are less than 2% of pregnancy levels

   b. Oestrogen levels return almost to prepregnant levels by 7 days

   c. Basal metabolic rate returns to normal with the thyroid hormones reducing to normal levels within 4 weeks

   d. Progesterone levels take up to 21 days to reduce to prepregnancy levels

   e. All of the above

   f. a, b, c

8. Following birth and expulsion of placenta and membranes, the following physiological changes occur:

   a. Plasma volume and haematocrit rapidly return to normal values

   b. Cardiac output and blood pressure return to nonpregnant levels

   c. Oxygen demands, blood CO_2 levels return to normal and the tendency to hyperventilate disappears

   d. All of the above

   e. a and c

9. Over the period of the puerperium, the following physiological changes occur:

   a. Reduced levels of progesterone lead to the smooth muscles tone throughout the body returning to normal including resolution of renal tract dilatation

   b. The minor pregnancy-related conditions such as constipation and heartburn disappear

   c. The kidneys need to cope with excretion of excess fluid and increased in the breakdown products of protein

   d. The bladder and urethra are unaffected by pregnancy and the birth process

   e. All of the above

   f. a, b and d

   g. a, b and c

10. Which of the following infective organisms are endogenous (i.e., already present in/on the body):

    a. *Chlamydia trachomatis*

    b. *Escherichia coli*

    c. *Clostridium welchii*

    d. *Streptococcus faecalis*

    e. a and b

    f. b, c and d

11. In the puerperium, women should be evaluated immediately in the following circumstances:

    a. In the event of sudden or profuse blood loss, blood loss is accompanied by any of the signs and symptoms of shock

    b. Maternal complaint of unilateral calf pain, or signs of redness or swelling, which could indicate deep venous thrombosis

    c. Women experiencing shortness of breath or chest pain which could indicate pulmonary thromboembolism

    d. All of the above

    e. a and c

    f. b and c

The breasts and breastfeeding

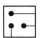 **Label**

12. Fig. 15.1 shows the anatomy of the breast. Label the figure from the list provided.

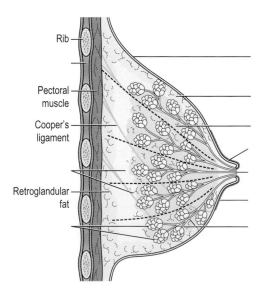

Label

| Intercostal muscle |
| Lobes |
| Lobules |
| Skin |
| Lactiferous ducts |
| Areola |
| Subcutaneous fat |
| Intra-glandular fat |
| Nipple |
| Nipple duct |

Rib

Pectoral muscle

Cooper's ligament

Retroglandular fat

Figure 15.1

Complete

13. Table 15.5a,b provides a range of activities related to the anatomy and physiology of the breasts and lactation. Complete the activities in the tables by inserting the short responses from the list of words provided.

acini cells
anterior lobe of the pituitary
    gland
areola
autocrine inhibitory factor
    (feedback inhibitor of
    lactation)
embryogenesis

lactiferous ducts
lactiferous tubules
lactogenesis
let down or milk ejection reflex
mammogenesis
milk removal
myoepithelial cells
neuromuscular control

nipple
oxytocin
posterior lobe of pituitary gland
prolactin
smooth
touch
whey

Table 15.5a

	Activity	Insert
a.	The term referring to the embryonic development of the mammary organs is:	
b.	The term referring to the growth and development of the mammary glands is:	
c.	The term referring to the initiation and production of milk is:	
d.	The alveoli contain milk-producing cells (lactocytes) are called:	
e.	These cells are surrounded by another type of cell which contract and propel the milk out. The cells are called:	
f.	The type of muscle these cells are composed of is:	
g.	These cells propelling milk are under the influence of the hormone called:	
h.	This hormone is secreted from which endocrine gland:	
i.	Milk is carried from the alveoli in small ducts called:	
j.	These ducts unite to form larger ducts conveying milk from one or more lobes. These ducts are called:	
k.	When these ducts emerge on the surface of the structure, they are called the:	
l.	The pigmented skin containing Montgomery's glands is called:	

Table 15.5b

	Activity	Insert
a.	In general, milk production is kept in abeyance until 30–40 hours following birth (until placental hormones decrease). The hormone responsible for milk production is:	
b.	The endocrine gland secreting this hormone is the:	
c.	Continual production of this milk-producing hormone is caused by:	
d.	As lactation progresses, the hormonal response to suckling diminishes and the main driving force for milk production becomes:	
e.	Identify the protein known to be present in secreted milk that is able to inhibit the synthesis of milk constituents:	
f.	The protein (above) collects in the breast as milk accumulates. This exerts a negative feedback control on continued milk production. Removal of milk in breasts allows milk production to accelerate. Name this feedback:	
g.	Identify the type of control for milk release:	
h.	Identify the reflex which allows milk release to the baby:	

True/false

14. Table 15.6 provides statements related to anatomy and physiology of breasts and physiology of breastfeeding. Complete the activity by deciding if the statements are true or false by ticking the appropriate column.

Table 15.6

	Statement	True	False
a.	Mammary tissue is divided into two areas: parenchyma (glandular tissue) is the functional component of the breast, whereas stoma provides the supportive tissue including the skin		
b.	During pregnancy, hormones oestrogen and progesterone induce alveolar and ductal growth, and stimulate the secretion of colostrum		
c.	Prolactin seems to be much more important to the continuation of lactation than to the initiation of lactation		
d.	The nipple is covered with epithelium and contains smooth muscle and elastic fibres		
e.	Montgomery's glands produce a sebum-like substance, which acts as a lubricant during pregnancy and breastfeeding		
f.	In early days of lactation, the 'let down' or 'milk ejection' reflex is a conditioned reflex		
g.	Prolactin is not involved in the suppression of ovulation		
h.	Milk production is affected by fluctuations in the mother's fluid intake		
i.	All lactating mothers will remain anovular until lactation ceases		
j.	Tactile stimulation of the breast stimulates oxytocin release		
k.	Expressed human milk can be stored for up to 12 weeks in the freezer compartment of a household fridge		
l.	With mastitis, the red area on the breast is often the outer, upper area, which may be painful to touch		
m.	All the vitamins required for good nutrition and health are supplied in breastmilk		
n.	Although rare, mastitis can develop into sepsis which needs urgent medical treatment		
o.	Human immunodeficiency virus cannot be transmitted to babies in breastmilk		

Breastmilk

 Complete

15. Table 15.7 provides statements about breastmilk. Remove the incorrect words so that the information is correct.

Table 15.7

a.	Colostrum has a **higher/lower** fat and protein content than mature milk. Foremilk (at the beginning of the feed) is of a high volume of relatively **low fat/high fat** milk. Hindmilk (as the feed progresses) **increases/decreases** in volume with an **increase/decrease** in the proportion of fat sometimes by as much as **five/fifty** times the initial value.
b.	It is the **fat/protein** content and not the **fat/protein** content that has particular significance for the **rapidly/slowly** growing brain of the newborn. The fat content is **highest/lowest** in the morning and **highest/lowest** in the afternoon.
c.	The main carbohydrate component is provided by **lactose/fructose** (which provides the baby with about **10%/40%** calorific requirements). This enhances the absorption of **calcium/sodium** and promotes the growth of *lactobacilli*, which **increase/decrease** intestinal acidity thus **increasing/reducing** the growth of pathogenic organisms. Whey, the dominant protein, forms soft, flocculent curds when **acidified/alkalized** in the stomach.

Match and connect

16. Box 15.2 provides information about factors in breastmilk. Draw a line to correctly match and connect the factors in column A with the correct statement in column B.

Box 15.2

A	B
Immunoglobulins:	*Lactobacillus bifidus* specifically discourages multiplication of pathogens. It is essential for synthesis of blood clotting factors. This binds to enteric iron, preventing pathogenic *E.coli* from obtaining the iron needed for them to survive.
Bifidus factor:	These are present to provide protection. This promotes the growth of gram-positive bacilli in the gut flora.
Vitamin K:	This is fat soluble and present in milk. IgA is the most important for the baby.
Lactoferrin:	It is present in greater concentrations in colostrum and in the high fat hindmilk. IgA covers intestinal epithelium and protects mucosal surfaces against pathogenic bacteria and enteroviruses.

Breastfeeding complications

Matching

17. Consider the statements related to breast problems in Table 15.8. Complete the table by matching the statements to the most likely breast problem.

Breast abscess
Engorgement
Sore and damaged nipples

Blocked ducts
Epithelial overgrowth
White spots

Candida albicans (thrush)
Mastitis (noninfective)
Mastitis (infective)

Table 15.8

	Statements	Condition
a.	Typically, one or more adjacent segments of the breast are inflamed and appear as a wedge-shaped area of redness or swelling. This occurs through milk being forced into the connective tissue of the breast. It is mainly noninfective.	
b.	Breasts are hard, often oedematous, painful and sometimes appear flushed. Condition occurs around day 3 or 4.	
c.	A fluctuant swelling may develop in a previously inflamed area. Pus may be discharged from the nipple.	
d.	A ductal opening in the tip of the nipple is obstructed by a white granule or by epithelial growth. This is not common.	
e.	The mother feels lumpy areas in the breast because of distended glandular tissue. Breasts may be firm, tender and possibly flushed.	
f.	This is a more common cause of a physical obstruction. A white blister is evident on the surface of the nipple closing off one of the exit points in the nipple.	
g.	This condition can become infective. This occurs when the milk is forced back into the bloodstream with maternal signs including pyrexia, tachycardia and flu-like symptoms.	
h.	The cause is almost always caused by trauma from the baby's mouth and tongue.	
i.	This condition is uncommon in the first week. The nipple and areola appear inflamed and shiny. Sudden onset of pain in a trouble-free period of feeding. Pain persists through the feed.	

Multiple choice questions (MCQ)

18. In addition to oestrogen and progesterone, other hormones involved in governing the complex sequence of events preparing the breasts for lactation include:

    a. Human placental lactogen

    b. Growth hormone, insulin-like growth factor, epidermal growth factor, fibroblast growth factor

    c. Prolactin

    d. Parathyroid hormone-related protein

    e. All of the above

    f. a, b and c

19. Colostrum is present in pregnancy from:

    a. 6th week

    b. 16th week

    c. 20th week

    d. 24th week

20. If breastfeeding (or expressing) is delayed, lactation can still be initiated (because of high prolactin levels) for at least:

    a. 4 days

    b. 7 days

    c. 14 days

    d. 21 days

21. Which of the following statements are signs that the baby is well attached to the breast:

    a. The chin is firmly touching the breast, the mouth is wide open and baby has a large mouthful of breast

    b. More dark skin (areolar) is seen above baby's top lip than below baby's bottom lip

    c. Baby's cheeks stay rounded during sucking and there is rhythmically long sucks and swallows (with pauses)

    d. It is not painful to the mother and there is no change in nipple shape/colour following feeds

    e. All of the above

22. Calcium is more efficiently absorbed from human milk because of the:

    a. Higher calcium: phosphorus ratio

    b. Higher phosphorus content

    c. Lower calcium: phosphorus ratio

    d. None of the above

23. Which of the following fact/s relate/s to mastitis:

    a. First sign is a red, swollen, usually painful, area on the breast

    b. Redness and swelling is not necessarily a sign of infection

    c. Harmful bacteria are not always present

    d. Antibiotics are always required to treat mastitis

    e. All of the above

24. Which of the following fact/s accurately support/s national guidance on safe storage and usage of breastmilk:

 a. Breast milk can be stored for up to 3 days in a fridge running below 10°C

 b. Breast milk can be stored between 4 and 8 days in a fridge between 0°C and 4°C

 c. Breast milk can remain at room temperature for 6 hours

 d. Breast milk can remain safe in a freezer for 6 months below −18°C or lower

 e. Previously frozen breast milk can be defrosted in the fridge for 12 hours

 f. Previously frozen breast milk defrosted outside the fridge should be used within 8 hours

25. Which method of contraception is not recommended for lactating mothers:

 a. Combined oral contraception

 b. Progestogen oral pill

 c. Progestogen implants

 d. Progestogen-releasing intrauterine system (IUS)

Perinatal psychiatric conditions

Mental illness can affect obstetric outcomes, the transition to parenthood and emotional well-being and health problems in the infant. The incidence of psychiatric disorders is increasing and in recent decades has become one of the leading causes of maternal mortality in the UK. Therefore, the emotional health and well-being of women during and following pregnancy is of primary importance to midwives.

 Correct/incorrect

26. Table 15.9 provides a range of statements related to psychiatric and perinatal psychiatric disorders. Complete the table by indicating the correct statements.

Table 15.9

	Statement	Correct
a.	The two classifications of mental health disorders include neuroses and psychoses	
b.	Perinatal psychiatric disorders only include disorders arising from conception and over the perinatal period	
c.	The term 'mental health problem' describes all types of emotional difficulties from transient and temporary states of distress to severe and uncommon mental illness	
d.	Schizophrenia and bipolar illness are psychotic disorders classified as minor mental illnesses	
e.	Adjustment reactions include distressing reactions to life events, including death and adversity	
f.	Personality disorders describe individuals who have persistent severe problems throughout their adult life dealing with stresses and strains of normal life. Examples include dysfunctional relationships, unawareness of consequences of their actions and persistently causing distress to themselves and others	
g.	Nonpsychotic and neurotic conditions, such as anxiety disorders, phobias and posttraumatic stress disorder are termed mild to moderate psychiatric disorders	

Continued →

Table 15.9 continued

	Statement	Correct
h.	Prevalence of psychiatric disorders (current or previous) in young women in early pregnancy is approximately 20%	
i.	Women with a previous postpartum (puerperal) psychosis (the most severe form of postpartum affective disorder) are at significant risk of developing a future postpartum (puerperal) psychosis	
j.	Provision of maternity care does not need to involve multidisciplinary and multi-agency teams	
k.	The onset of postpartum (puerperal) psychosis is often rapid and typically presents in the early postpartum period (usually first month)	
l.	The 'baby blues' is a normal reaction to childbirth. Physiological changes following pregnancy are thought to be responsible. Emotional symptoms are transient, occur by day 3 and resolved in 1 week	
m.	Postnatal depression describes a sustained depressive disorder in women following childbirth. It has an insidious onset and is a serious chronic disorder	
n.	Puerperal (postnatal) psychosis is the most severe form of postpartum affective (mood) disorder. It is an acute early onset condition presenting in the first 14 days from birth. Puerperal psychosis steadily deteriorates and will usually require admission to a psychiatric unit	

REFERENCES

Visit the following websites:

National Institute for Health and Care Excellence (NICE) for up to date guidance, standards and pathways (postnatal care, maternal and infant nutrition): https://www.nice.org.uk/

Breastfeeding Network for up to date guidance: https://www.breastfeedingnetwork.org.uk/

16 Miscellaneous topics

This chapter covers a range of miscellaneous topics, including pharmacology in pregnancy and childbirth, infertility, nutrition and metabolic-related issues and the fundamentals of complementary therapies. The midwife needs to have knowledge of current practice in these areas and the impact on the woman/fetus to provide appropriate evidence-based guidance and support. Activities will test your basic knowledge in these specialist areas.

PHARMACOLOGY ISSUES IN CHILDBIRTH

  Complete and short answers

1. Table 16.1 provides a range of activities related to pharmacology and pregnancy. Complete the activities by inserting the correct short answer from the list of words provided.

pharmacokinetics	metabolism	pharmacodynamics	teratogenic
ectoderm	excretion	endoderm	distribution (translocation)
absorption	larger size	smaller size	mesoderm

Table 16.1

	Activities	Answer
a.	Organogenesis, the process by which three germ layers turn into the internal organism, occurs between ~18 and 55 days postconception. Name the three layers:	Inner: Middle: Outer:
b.	Identify the term referring to the way the body handles drugs:	
c.	Identify the four major stages involved in way the body handles drugs:	
d.	Identify the term referring to the effect drugs have on the body function:	
e.	Identify the term that refers to a substance (if present during organogenesis) leading to a malformed baby:	
f.	In relation to size, which molecules do not cross the placenta?	
g.	In relation to size, which molecules easily cross the placenta?	

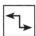 **Match**

2. Box 16.1 presents the physiological changes of pregnancy and how these may influence the way the mother's body handles drugs administered. To complete the activity, draw a line to match and connect the physiological change in column A with the correct possible effect in column B.

Box 16.1

A. Physiological changes (pregnancy)	B. Possible effects
a. Gastric motility is reduced (prolonged time in gut): b. Increased circulating plasma volume: c. Increase in blood flow to the kidneys: d. Increased amounts of total body water and fat: e. Some metabolic pathways in the liver increase: f. Major changes in levels of plasma proteins to which some drugs bind:	• Increase in excretion rate of the drug • May alter distribution of the drug • Amount of the drug available is affected • Metabolism is quicker • This decreases plasma concentration • May change absorption rate (oral drugs), that is, slows down, increases or no change

Possible adverse effects on the fetus

Drugs administered to the mother at different stages of pregnancy can be teratogenic to the fetus and infant. The prime example is the tragedy of thalidomide use by pregnant women (early pregnancy) in the 1960s (caused major reduced limb formation).

  Complete: match

3. This question focuses on the possible adverse effects on the fetus and infant. Box 16.2a–c provides activities related to adverse effects, timing of drug administration during pregnancy and drug groups. Complete the activities by drawing a line to match the drugs listed in column A with the correct adverse effect in column B.

Box 16.2a

	A. Drugs (teratogenic)	B. Adverse effects
a.	ß-blockers (<28 weeks):	• Premature closure of ductus arteriosus and oligohydramnios
b.	Angiotensin-converting enzyme (ACE) inhibitors (2ⁿᵈ/3ʳᵈ trimester):	• Folate metabolism interference
c.	Iodine (early-late):	• Reduced fetal growth
d.	In 3ʳᵈ trimester, nonsteroidal antiinflammatory drugs (NSAIDs) (e.g., ibuprofen/diclofenac):	• Fetal renal failure
e.	In 1ˢᵗ trimester, commonly used antibiotic, trimethoprim:	• Fetal thyroid function

Box 16.2b

	A. Drug (teratogenic)	B. Adverse effects
a.	Lithium or benzodiazepines:	• Most of this drug group are teratogenic
b.	Warfarin:	• Vaginal carcinoma, urogenital abnormalities, reduced fertility (females)/increased risk of hypospadias (males)
c.	Sodium Valproate:	• Craniofacial, cardiac and central nervous system (CNS) abnormalities
d.	Phenytoin:	• Cardiac defects (e.g., increased risk of Ebstein's anomaly)
e.	Retinoic acid derivatives:	• Neural tube defects (minor/major)
f.	Androgens:	• Facial anomalies, CNS anomalies
g.	Diethylstilbestrol (1ˢᵗ trimester):	• Craniofacial abnormalities (e.g., oral deformities)
h.	Cytotoxic drugs:	• Masculinization of female fetus

Box 16.2c

	Drugs (antibiotics)	Possible adverse effect
a.	Tetracyclines (e.g., tetracycline, oxytetracycline, doxycycline)	• Haemolysis in fetus at term–avoid during labour/birth
b.	Aminoglycosides (e.g., gentamicin, netilmicin)	• Arthropathy in fetus
c.	Chloramphenicol	• No adverse effects
d.	Nitrofurantoin	• Risk of ototoxicity but often used in severe maternal infection
e.	Quinolones (e.g., ciproflaxin, ofloxacin)	• Discolouration and dysplasia of fetal bones and teeth when used in 2ⁿᵈ/3ʳᵈ trimester
f.	Polar drugs (e.g., penicillin, cephalosporins)	• 'Gray (Grey) baby syndrome' when used in 2ⁿᵈ/3ʳᵈ trimester

Miscellaneous

 Correct/incorrect

4. Table 16.4 provides statements related to drugs in pregnancy and childbirth. Complete the table by indicating the correct statements.

Table 16.2

	Statement	Correct
a.	Teratogenic drugs do not interfere with normal development	
b.	The fetus and neonate have much reduced ability to handle drugs because of the immaturity of liver enzyme systems	
c.	Oxytocin should not be given within at least 3–6 hours of prostaglandin because of the risk of uterine hyperstimulation	
d.	Heparin is a large molecule and cannot cross the placenta	
e.	A mother taking a largely fat-soluble drug will pass more to the baby who feeds for prolonged periods (because of amount of hindmilk consumed)	
f.	In women with long-term use of opiate analgesics, there is no risk of neonatal withdrawal after birth	
g.	Drugs that affect the central nervous system will readily cross the placental barrier	
h..	Paracetamol is the recommended first-line analgesic agent in pregnancy	
i..	Warfarin is contraindicated for breastfeeding	
j..	Corticosteroids are used in pregnancy for fetal lung maturation	
k.	Local anaesthesia accidentally injected intravenously (IV) is a common cause of maternal collapse in midwifery/obstetric practice	
l.	The antibiotic chloramphenicol is avoided in newborns/premature babies as they lack the necessary liver enzymes to metabolize the drug	
m.	Antipsychotic medication dose in pregnancy is reduced to the minimum for clinical effectiveness as this medication freely passes to developing fetus and fetal brain	
n.	All anticonvulsive medication is safe to administer in pregnancy and is not associated with increased risk to the fetus	
o.	All psychotropic medication passes across the placenta to the fetus and into breastmilk	
p.	Drugs, mainly excreted from the body by the kidneys, can also be excreted in expired air, perspiration, faeces and breastmilk	

? **Multiple choice questions (MCQ)**

5. The recommended daily dose of folic acid for all women planning a pregnancy and throughout the first trimester is:

   a. 400 µg

   b. 500 µg

   c. 400 mg

   d. 500 mg

6. Women at risk of neural tube defects should receive a daily dose of folic acid supplementation of:

   a. 5 mg

   b. 7 mg

   c. 10 mg

   d. 12 mg

7. Which of the following statements are correct?
   a. Modern antacids are safe for use during pregnancy because they are relatively nonabsorbable
   b. Paracetamol relieves pain and reduces temperature but has no antiinflammatory action
   c. Ibuprofen reduces the inflammation, relieves pain and reduces temperature
   d. Hydralazine is usually administered intramuscularly

8. Which of the following drugs affects milk production and contraindicated for breastfeeding mothers?
   a. Beta blockers
   b. Bromocriptine
   c. Nonsteroidal antiinflammatory drugs (NSAIDs)
   d. Methyldopa

9. Which of the following statements about continued use of lithium throughout pregnancy are correct?
   a. Lithium in early pregnancy is not associated with an increased risk of neural tube abnormalities
   b. Lithium is associated with increased risk of diabetes insipidus
   c. Lithium is associated with increased risk of fetal hypothyroidism and fetal macrosomia
   d. Lithium is associated with increased risk of neonatal cyanosis and hypotonia

10. Which of the following statements are correct?
    a. Alcohol may interfere with the let-down response and milk yield.
    b. Alcohol takes up to 2 hours to clear 1 unit from breastmilk.
    c. Smoking during lactation does not result in reduced milk supply
    d. Nicotine replacement therapy does not reduce the amount of nicotine in breastmilk

Infertility

Midwives need to understand infertility, causes and treatment as they will increasingly come into contact with families who require assistance to conceive. The following activities will test your knowledge in this area.

  Complete: match

11. Box 16.3a,b provides the causes of male and female infertility. To complete the boxes, draw a line to match the main causes in column A with the correct associated physiological or physical disorders in column B.

Box 16.3a

A: Male causes	B: Disorders
Defective spermatogenesis: Defective sperm transport: Ineffective sperm delivery:	• Drug induced problems • Physical anomalies • Impotence (psychosexual problems) • Obstruction or absence of seminal ducts • Systemic disease (e.g., diabetes mellitus) • Testicular disorders (trauma/environmental) • Impaired secretions from accessory glands • Endocrine disorders (dysfunction of hypothalamus, pituitary, adrenal and thyroid glands)

Box 16.3b

A: Female causes	B: Disorders
Defective ovulation:	• Ovum (tubal obstruction or fimbrial adhesions) • Sperm: because of thick cervical mucus or loss of tubal patency • Endocrine disorders (dysfunction of hypothalamus, pituitary, adrenal and thyroid glands)
Defective transport:	• Because of hormone imbalance, congenital anomalies, fibroids or infection • Ovarian disorders: hormonal, PCOS, endometriosis
Defective implantation:	• Systemic disease (e.g., renal disease)

 True/false

12. Table 16.3 provides statements related to infertility. Complete the activity by indicating if the statements are true or false.

Table 16.3

	Statements	True	False
a.	Polycystic ovarian syndrome (PCOS) is the most common cause of infertility		
b.	Infection of the uterine tubes is called 'salpingitis'		
c.	Chlamydial infection and gonorrhoea are the most common organisms causing pelvic inflammatory disease (PID)		
d.	Features of PCOS include obesity and insulin resistance		
e.	Women with endometriosis respond well to ovarian hyperstimulation		
f.	Superovulation involves using drugs to stimulate development of a single ovum		
g.	Diagnosis of PCOS is confirmed by the presence of hyperandrogenism, menstrual irregularity and polycystic ovaries		
h.	Women have a finite number of oocytes resulting in fecundity decreasing with age		
i.	In vitro fertilization treatment consists of a series of steps including superovulation, egg recovery, fertilization and embryo transfer		

Nutrition and metabolic-related issues

Adequate nutrition during pregnancy has both short and long-term impacts on the well-being of the mother and growing fetus. It is important for midwives to have good knowledge in this area to provide good nutritional advice.

13. Table 16.4 provides nutrition-related activities. Complete the activities by providing short answers from the list provided.

facilitated diffusion	fats	glucose	iodine
sucrose	carbohydrates	potassium	starch
cholesterol	zinc	adenosine triphosphate (ATP)	vitamin C and most of vitamin B complex
protein	calcium	mitochondria	vitamins A, D, E and K

Table 16.4

	Activities	Answer
a.	Name the main source of energy in the diet	
b.	Identify one monosaccharide	
c.	Identify one disaccharide	
d.	Identify one polysaccharide	
e.	Identify the physiological process by which the body cells take up glucose circulating in blood (under the influence of insulin)	
f.	Name the specific part of the body cell where glucose is oxidized to form energy (Kreb's cycle)	
g.	Name the high-energy phosphate bonds needed for the body's energy	
h.	Name the highest-density energy source for the body	
i.	Name the fat-related compound vital for human metabolism	
j.	Name the part of the diet necessary for forming new cells and the manufacture of enzymes, hormones and antibodies	
k.	Name two of the seven minerals required by the body	
l.	Name two of the 18 trace elements in the body	
m.	Name the water-soluble vitamins	
n.	Name the fat-soluble vitamins	

 Match

14. Box 16.4 provides a selection of vitamins and related effects of vitamin deficiencies. To complete the activity, draw a line to match the vitamin in column A and correctly connect with the effects in column B.

Box 16.4

Vitamin	Deficiency
Vitamin A:	• Compromises blood clotting as a result of anticoagulant or antibiotic therapy
Vitamin B6:	• Causes poor digestion, gum disease and poor resistance to bacterial infections.
Vitamin B12:	• May result in spontaneous abortion, preterm labour and still birth
Vitamin C:	• Can cause premenstrual depression, anaemia and convulsions
Vitamin D:	• (If severe) may lead to blindness, skin disorders, tooth decay and gastrointestinal disorders
Vitamin E:	• Can cause pernicious anaemia and neurological symptoms
Vitamin K:	• May cause rickets in children and osteomalacia in adults. May be poor muscle tone, restlessness and irritability

Correct/incorrect

15. Table 16.5 provides a range of statements about vitamins. Complete the table by indicating these statements that provide correct information.

Table 16.5

	Statements	Correct
a.	Vitamin K has a role in blood clotting, easy bruising and bleeding occurs in severe deficiency	
b.	Vitamin C helps to maintain body tissues (e.g., collagen) and to form haemoglobin	
c.	The contraceptive pill can increase the absorption of vitamin E	
d.	Folic acid is essential for the formation of erythrocytes. Perinatal supplementation does not protect against neural tube defects	
e.	Vitamin D has no role to play in activating absorption of calcium, or the mineralization of bone	
f.	Deficiency in vitamin B2 (riboflavin) involves poor wound healing with typical signs including cracks on lips, corners of mouth and tongue	
g.	Vitamin B1 (thiamine) deficiency causes the disease 'beri-beri' with pain, weakness, degeneration of muscles and poor movement coordination	
h.	Deficiency in vitamin B6 (pyridoxine) can cause abdominal pain in children and dermatitis and depression in adults	
i.	The disease pellagra is caused by a deficiency in vitamin B3 (niacin)	

COMPLEMENTARY THERAPIES

Complementary therapies are classified into three groups. Group 1 therapies are professionally organized, with national standards of education, statutory or voluntary self-regulation, disciplinary codes of practice and a reasonable body of evidence. Group 2 therapies are complementary or supportive to other healthcare, with less available evidence and many therapies in the process of regulatory development. Group 3 therapies are alternative, largely unregulated therapies with little or no body of evidence and divided into two subgroups: a. traditional systems; b. diagnostic therapies.

 Short answers

16. Table 16.6 provides a list of statement describing a selection of complimentary therapies. Complete the activity by inserting the accurate name of the therapy from the list provided.

Acupuncture	Traditional Chinese medicine (TCM)	Reflexology	Shiatsu
Homeopathy	Mindfulness	Reiki	Yoga

Table 16.6

	Complimentary therapy	Answer
a.	Involves using extremely diluted (watered down) natural substances to treat physical and mental health problems	
b.	Rebalance of the body's energy systems, and involves acupuncture, tuina (a form of massage), as well as herbal remedies	
c.	Stimulates nerves and muscles which may release natural pain-relieving chemicals (involves inserting fine needles into body)	
d.	Involves focusing individual's attention to what is happening in the present moment—to become more aware of thoughts and feelings and react calmly	
e.	A Japanese technique involving the 'laying of hands' on different areas of the body including the head, shoulders, stomach and feet. Aim is to restore life force energy to heal and maintain well-being	
f.	Involves spiritual and physical practices to increase self-awareness, such as posture work, breathing exercises, mediation and visualization	
g.	Based on the idea that different points on feet, hands, face and ears are linked to other parts of the body through the central nervous system	
h.	This is a holistic approach to a physical therapy supporting and strengthening the body's natural ability to heal and balance itself	

Complete: match

17. Box 16.5 presents a selection of classified complementary or alternative therapies regularly used in health care. To complete the activity, draw a lie to match and connect the therapy classification group in column A with the correct therapy in column B.

Box 16.5

A. Classification	B. Therapies
Group 1 (regulated profession):	• Acupuncture • Massage • Alexander technique • Aromatherapy • Indian Ayurvedic medicine • Crystal therapies • Homeopathy • Iridology • Chiropractic
Group 2 (compliments healthcare):	• Hypnotherapy/hypnosis • Mindfulness • Herbal medicine • Oesteopathy • Reflexology
Group 3 (a. traditional and b. diagnostic):	• Traditional Chinese medicine (TCM) • Shiatsu • Reiki • Tibetan medicine • Yoga

Complementary therapies in pregnancy and childbirth

 ## True/false

18. Table 16.7 provides statements relating to complementary therapies in pregnancy and childbirth. Complete the table by indicating if the statements are true or false.

Table 16.7

	Statement	True	False
a.	Ginger biscuits should be advised as a remedy for nausea		
b.	Essential oils and pharmaceutical drugs are absorbed, metabolized and excreted via separate biochemical pathways		
c.	Moxibustion, a traditional Chinese medical intervention, may be an effective treatment for the correction of nonvertex presentation. It uses heat from burning herbal preparations containing Artemisia vulgaris (mugwort) to stimulate acupuncture points		
d.	Pregnant women often have very rapid and very profound reactions to reflexology		
e.	Culinary use of herbs and herbal teas are generally safe in normal amounts		
f.	Raspberry leaf tea is thought to facilitate normal uterine action		
g.	Essential oils can be administered via the skin, respiratory tract, mucus membranes and the gastrointestinal tract		
h.	The use of essential oils is contraindicated with neonates as it may interfere with the mother/infant bonding process		
i.	Homeopathic remedies interfere with breastfeeding		
j.	When inhaled, essential oil molecules reach the limbic centre in the brain, the circulation and major organs		
k.	The physiological process of osmosis underpins the use of cabbage leaves to ease engorgement of the breasts		

17 The baby at birth

This chapter focuses on the baby at birth and their ability to adapt to extrauterine life. As the key professional, the midwife must have a sound knowledge of the physiological processes taking place at this time and how to support the baby through this profound transitional phase. The activities will test your knowledge in this area.

Uterine hypoxia

 Complete

1. The following activity relates to the fetal response to intrauterine hypoxia. Complete the activity by inserting the correct word(s) (14 in total) from the extended list provided.

accelerating	glycogen reserves	relaxes	respiration
anaerobic glycolysis	meconium	vessels	constricts
aspiration	meconium-stained	decelerating	swelling
bradycardia	metabolic acidosis	metabolic alkalosis	acidotic
gasping	oxygen		

The fetus responds to hypoxia by _____ the heart rate in an effort to maintain

supplies of _____ to the brain. If hypoxia persists, glucose depletion will stimulate

_____. This results in a _____. Cerebral

_____ will dilate and some brain _____ may occur.

_____ develops as the fetus becomes more _____ and

cardiac _____ are depleted. The anal sphincter _____ and

the fetus may pass _____ into the liquor. Hypoxia triggers

_____, breathing movements which may result in the _____

of _____ liquor into the lungs.

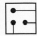 **Match and label**

2. Fig. 17.1 shows the factors predisposing to intrauterine hypoxia. This relates to maternal, fetal or placental issues. Complete the figure by matching the number with the correct label from the list provided.

Table 17.1

Cord prolapse or compression, true knot in cord	
Maternal hypertension and vascular disease	
Placental disease, dysfunction or separation	
Fetal compromise impacting upon normal growth and development.	
Maternal hypoxia, cardiopulmonary disease	

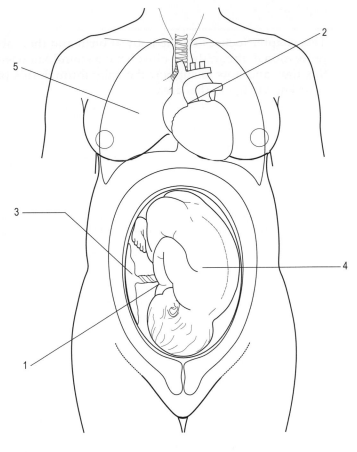

Figure 17.1

Initial assessment of the newborn

 Complete

3. The Apgar score is an initial assessment of the baby's condition at birth. The midwife assesses the baby at 1 minute and 5 minutes after birth. Table 17.2 shows the signs and possible scores. Using your own knowledge, complete the table by inserting the missing word(s) and numerical values.

Table 17.2

Score	Indicator				
	Heart rate	Respiratory effort	Muscle tone	Reflex response to stimuli	Colour
0		Apnoeic	Limp	No response	
1	<100 beats per minute				
2					Pink

4. Complete the following mnemonic for the Apgar score (and the sign it relates to on the APGAR scoring checklist).

A: _____ (relates to _____).

P: _____ (relates to heart rate).

G: Grimace (relates to _____).

A: _____ (relates to _____).

R: _____ (relates to breathing).

Adaptation to extrauterine life

 Complete

5. Table 17.3 provides activities relating to the healthy term baby's pulmonary and cardiovascular adaptation to extrauterine life. Complete the table by removing the incorrect word(s) and completing the statements as noted.

Table 17.3

	Pulmonary and cardiovascular adaptation to extrauterine life
a.	Pulmonary adaptation: Respiration is stimulated by mild **hypercapnia/hypocapnia**, hypoxia and **alkalosis/acidosis**. There is a change in the rhythm of respiration from **episodic/regular, shallow/deeper** fetal respiration to **episodic/regular, shallow/deeper** breathing. This is caused by a combination of chemical and neural stimuli, notably a **fall/rise** in pH level, a **fall/rise** in partial pressure of oxygen (PaO$_2$) and a **fall/rise** in partial pressure of carbon dioxide (PaCO$_2$). Considerable **negative/positive** intrathoracic pressure of up to 9.8 kPa (**50 cm/100 cm** water) is exerted as the first breath is taken. The pressure exerted to effect **exhalation/inhalation increases/diminishes** with each breath taken until only **5 cm/30 cm** of water is required to **deflate/inflate** each lung. This is caused by surfactant.
b.	Surfactant is a complex of **proteins** and **lipoproteins/carbohydrate substrates**. In utero, the amount of surfactant **decreases/increases** until the lungs are mature at **34 to 37 weeks'/30 to 34 weeks'** gestation. It is produced by **type 2/type 1** epithelial cells in the lungs and lines the **alveoli/trachea** to **increase/reduce** the **surface tension/surface area** within the **alveoli/trachea**. This permits **dead air space/residual air** to remain in the **alveoli/trachea** between breaths and prevent them from **deflating/collapsing** at the **beginning/end** of each expiration. Surfactant **increases/reduces** the work or effort of breathing.
c.	Cardiovascular adaptation: At birth, the lungs expand and pulmonary vascular resistance is **lowered/raised**. This results in the majority of cardiac output being sent to the lungs. **Deoxygenated/oxygenated** blood returning to the heart from the lungs **increases/decreases** the pressure within the **right/left** atrium. At the same time, pressure in the **right/left** atrium is **raised/lowered** because blood ceases to flow through the cord. This brings about functional closure of the **foramen ovale/ductus venosus**. Contraction of the walls of the **ductus venosus/ductus arteriosus** occurs almost immediately after birth. This is thought to occur because of the sensitivity of the muscle of the **ductus venosus/ductus arteriosus** to **decreased/increased** oxygen tension and **increased/reduction** in circulating prostaglandins. There is usually functional closure of the **ductus venosus/ductus arteriosus** within **8 to 10 hours/24 to 36 hours** of birth with complete closure taking place within **several months/12 months**. The remaining temporary structures of the fetal circulation—**umbilical vein/umbilical veins, ductus venosus/ducutus arteriosus** and hypogastric **arteries/veins**—close functionally within a few **minutes/hours** after birth and constriction of the cord. Anatomical closure of fibrous tissue occurs within **2 to 3 months/12 months**.

Thermal adaptation

6. Complete the following statements in relation to thermal adaptation.

   a. Intrauterine temperature is: _____ °C

   b. Birthing room average temperature is between: _____ and_____°C

   c. The baby will lose heat in the following ways:

      i. _____ of amniotic fluid from the skin.

      ii. _____ when the baby is in close contact with cold surfaces.

      iii. _____ to cold objects.

      iv. _____ caused by currents of cool air passing over the surface of body.

   d. The baby's _____ surface area: body mass ratio potentiates heat loss, especially from the large

      _____.

   e. The subcutaneous tissue is _____.

   f. The baby has limited ability to _____.

   g. The baby is unable to increase _____ voluntarily to generate heat.

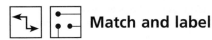 **Match and label**

7. Fig. 17.2 shows the modes of heat loss in the neonate. Complete the figure by correctly inserting the following graphics:

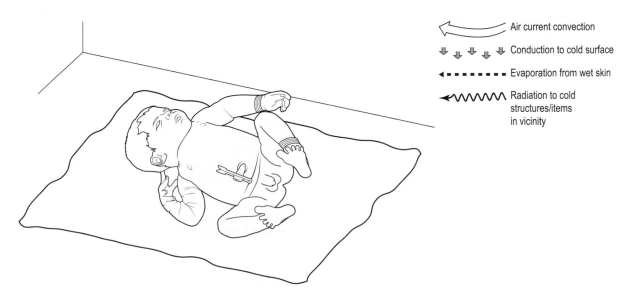

Figure 17.2

Complete

8. Complete Fig. 17.3 by shading or colouring in all the sites of brown fat in the neonate.

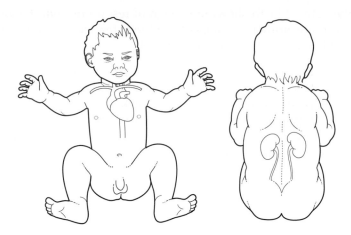

Figure 17.3 Sites of brown fat.

 Complete

9. The activity in Box 17.1 relates to cold stress and transient tachypnoea of the newborn. Complete the activity by inserting the missing word(s) (10 in total) from the extended list provided.

acidosis	rapid	caesarean section	pulmonary
cyanosed	respiratory rate	ventouse extraction	three
decrease	rib cage	vasodilation	five
increases	tachypnoea	apnoea	seven
grunt	vasoconstriction	slow	

Box 17.1

Cold stress causes _____, thus reducing pulmonary perfusion. Respiratory

_____ as the pH and PaO_2 of the blood _____ and the $PaCO_2$

_____ leading to respiratory distress exhibited by _____. This

condition is characterized by _____ respirations of up to 120/min. It is common after a

caesarean section. The baby may be _____ but maintains normal blood gases apart from PaO_2.

There is little or no recession of the _____ and there is minimum, if any,

_____ on expiration. The _____ may remain elevated for up to

5 days.

Neonatal resuscitation

 Complete

10. This activity relates to the baby at birth showing no sign of respiratory effort. Complete Table 17.4 by inserting the missing word(s) or numerical values from the extended list provided. Word(s) may be used more than once whereas other words may not be required.

aerate	dried	radiant heater	oesophagus
neutral	head	shoulders	ventilate
airway	hypothermia	neck	ventilation
assisted ventilation	hypoglycaemia	sustained	40 to 50
chest movement	inflation	towel	30 to 40
clock timer	nose and mouth	trachea	50 to 60

Table 17.4

---

a. The baby is _____ quickly. The _____ is started.

The_____ is switched on to prevent _____.

↓

---

b. The head should be put in the neutral position to maintain the _____ and keep the

_____ straightened. If necessary, a small _____ can

be put under the baby's _____ to cause slight extension of the

_____. Review for signs of respiratory effort.

↓

---

c. If the baby fails to respond then _____ is necessary. Place a correctly fitting mask

to cover the _____ and ensure a good seal. Use a 500 mL self-inflating bag to

_____ the lungs, deliver five _____ inflations (each breath is for 2 to 3 seconds).

↓

---

d. Review for _____.

If YES- this is present: continue to _____ at a rate of _____

___ respirations per minute (ventilation breaths).

If NO- this is not present: then review the _____ position and re-commence the five

_____ breaths. Move to _____ breaths once

_____ is confirmed.

Complete

11. This activity relates to external cardiac massage. Complete the following statements by inserting the correct numerical values.

 a. Chest compressions should be performed if the heart rate is <_____ beats per minute and only

   following 30 seconds of ventilation breaths.

 b. The chest is depressed at a rate of _____ to_____ times per minute, at a ratio of _____ compressions

   to _____ ventilation and at a depth of _____ to _____ cm of the baby's chest. **Note: For resuscitation**

   guidance, always refer to the most current resuscitation guidelines.

 True/false

12. Consider the following statements in Table 17.2. Complete the table by deciding if the statements are correct by ticking the appropriate column.

Table 17.5

	Statement	True	False
a.	Before birth, the fetal lung is full of fluid		
b.	The closure of the foramen ovale can be reversed and re-opened		
c.	The stimuli for respiration results from normal labour, partially because of the intermittent cessation of maternal perfusion with contractions		
d.	Nonshivering thermogenesis refers to the process involving brown adipose tissue that assists in the rapid mobilization of heat resources from free fatty acids and glycerol in times of cold stress		
e.	The two-finger method of chest compression is haemodynamically more effective		
f.	Brown fat uses the same amount of oxygen as other tissues		
g.	During primary apnoea, the circulation and heart rate are maintained		
h.	The body has a high capacity to store vitamin K		

? **Multiple choice questions (MCQ)**

13. During birth the fluid leaves the alveoli of the lungs via the:
 a. Thoracic duct or to the lung capillaries
 b. Alveolar walls into the pulmonary lymphatic vessels
 c. Airway and out of the mouth and nose
 d. All of the above
 e. b and c only

14. During fetal life, the percentage of the cardiac output circulated to the fetal lungs through the pulmonary artery is.
 a. 10%
 b. 15%
 c. 20%
 d. 25%
 e. 50%

15. What percentage of the body mass does the head of the newborn comprise?
    a. 10%
    b. 15%
    c. 20%
    d. 25%
    e. 40%

16. The newborn has sufficient brown fat to meet minimum heat needs after birth for between:
    a. 12 and 24 hours
    b. 2 and 4 days
    c. 4 and 6 days
    d. 6 and 7 days

17. Which of the following statements is correct about vitamin K:
    a. It can only be absorbed from the intestines in the presence of bile salts
    b. It is water-soluble
    c. The body has a high capacity to store vitamin K
    d. All of the above

18. Which immunoglobulin (Ig), transferred to the fetus in utero, provides the newborn with passive immunity to specific viral infections which the mother has been exposed:
    A. IgG
    B. IgM
    C. IgE
    D. IgA

19. Intrauterine growth restriction (IUGR), which occurs in the first trimester, caused by a combination of intrinsic and extrinsic factors, results in which type of fetal growth:
    A. Appropriate fetal growth
    B. Symmetrical fetal growth
    C. Asymmetrical fetal growth
    D. None of the above

18 The newborn baby

This chapter focuses on a variety of situations relating to the newborn baby. This includes the healthy baby, the ill baby and babies who have experienced birth trauma. The activities will test your knowledge in these areas.

 Complete

1. The following activity relates to the normal newborn baby at term. Complete the statements by inserting the correct word(s) or numerical values from the extended list provided.

15	30	40	60	100
23.5	36.0	37.8	72	110
20	36.5	48	85	160
24	37.3	50	90	180

a. The normal core temperature is generally considered to be between _____°C and _____°C.

b. The respiratory rate is between _____ and _____ breaths per minute.

c. The heart rate is between _____ and _____ beats per minute.

d. The average haemoglobin level at term is between _____ and _____ g/dL, of which _____% to ____% is

   fetal haemoglobin.

e. Meconium is passed within _____ hours of birth and is totally excreted within _____ to ___ hours.

f. The six inherited inborn errors of metabolism routinely screened for (newborn blood spot test) include:

   _____

   _____

   _____

Definitions

2. Complete the following definitions related to the classification of babies by weight and gestation

   a. Low birthweight (LBW) babies weigh below _____ g at birth.

   b. Very low birthweight (VLBW) babies weigh below _____ g at birth.

   c. Extremely low birthweight (ELBW) babies weigh below _____ g at birth.

   d. A preterm baby is one born before completion of the _____th gestational week, regardless of

       birthweight.

 True/false

3. Table 18.1 presents statements relating to the newborn. Complete the table by deciding if the statements are true or false.

Table 18.1

	Statement	True	False
a.	Vernix caseosa is a white sticky substance present on the baby's skin at birth and flakes off within the first 7 days		
b.	At birth, the muscles are complete with subsequent growth occurring by hyperplasia rather than hypertrophy		
c.	Ortolani's test is carried out as a component of screening for developmental dysplasia of the hip (DDH)		
d.	The lower pH of the baby's skin creates an 'acid mantle' which protects against infection		
e.	Epithelial pearls (Epstein's pearls) are not commonly observed in the mouth		
f.	Vasomotor instability causes the harlequin colour change noted on the skin		
g.	Moro reflex occurs in response to a sudden stimulus		

Match

4. Table 18.2 describes a range of skin-related observations the midwife may note on routine examination. Match these correctly to the most likely cause or condition (1–14) and insert to complete the table.

   1. Bruising   2. Cyanosis   3. Erythema toxicum   4. Herpes simplex
   5. Jaundice   6. Milia   12. Staphylococcal   14. Umbilical sepsis
   8. Pallor   10. Plethora   11. Skin rashes   9. Petechiae or purpura rash
   13. Thrush   7. Miliaria

Table 18.2

	Statement relating to skin observations	Conditions/causes
a.	Babies are usually described as being beetroot red. The colour may indicate an excess of circulating red blood cells	
b.	A pale, mottled baby is an indication of poor peripheral perfusion	
c.	The mucous membranes are the most reliable indicators of central colour in all babies. This indicates low oxygen saturation levels in the blood	
d.	These are common but most are benign and self-limiting	
e.	Early onset of this condition (presenting in the first 24 hours) is abnormal	
f.	These are white or yellow papules over the cheeks, nose and forehead. These disappear in the first weeks of life	
g.	These are clear vesicles on the face, scalp and perineum, caused by the retention of sweat in unopened sweat glands	
h.	This can occur extensively following assisted births	
i.	These can occur in neonatal thrombocytopenia	
j.	This rash occurs in 30%–70% of babies. It consists of white papules on an erythematous base and is benign	
k.	This is a fungal infection of the mouth and throat. It is common in neonates	
l.	This is a most serious viral infection. It presents as a rash with vesicles or pustules	
m.	Severe infections of this bacteria make the skin look as though it has been scalded. It can lead to bullous impetigo	
n.	This can be caused by a bacterial infection at the base of the cord	

Warning signs

 Complete

5. The general assessment of warning signs indicates a possible underlying problem in the baby. Complete the text boxes in Fig. 18.1 by inserting the correct words or numerical values related to the warning signs of problems with the baby.

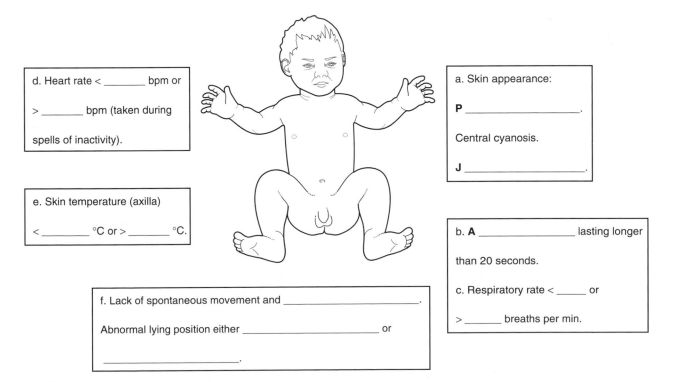

d. Heart rate < _____ bpm or

> _____ bpm (taken during

spells of inactivity).

e. Skin temperature (axilla)

< _____ °C or > _____ °C.

f. Lack of spontaneous movement and _____.

Abnormal lying position either _____ or

_____.

a. Skin appearance:

P _____.

Central cyanosis.

J _____.

b. A _____ lasting longer

than 20 seconds.

c. Respiratory rate < _____ or

> _____ breaths per min.

Figure 18.1

6. Table 18.3 presents statements of the warning signs of congenital cardiac disease. Complete the table by inserting the correct word(s) (13 in total) from the extended list provided.

breathless	eyelids	scrotum	tachypnoea
cardiac	feet	sweaty	apnoea
cyanosis	gain	systolic	diastolic
liver	oedema	tachycardia	bradycardia

Table 18.3

	Statements
a.	Persistent _____
b.	_____ (this is often out of proportion to the degree of respiratory distress)
c.	Persistent _____ at rest.
d.	Poor feeding: infants may be _____ and _____ during feeds.
e.	A sudden _____ in weight leading to clinical signs of _____: this is usually noted in the baby having puffy _____ or _____ and in males, the _____ may be swollen.
f.	Enlargement of the _____.
g.	Evidence of _____ enlargement on x-ray, persisting beyond 48 hours of life.
h.	A very loud _____ murmur is invariably significant.

Neonatal problems and conditions

 True/false

7. Table 18.4 presents statements relating to the newborn. Complete the table by deciding if the statements are true or false.

Table 18.4

	Statement	True	False
a.	Necrotizing enterocolitis (NEC) is an acute inflammatory change affecting the small and large bowels in predominantly premature neonates		
b.	Hypothermia is defined as a core temperature below 35.5°C		
c.	Hirschsprung's disease should be suspected in term babies with delayed passage of meconium		
d.	Respiratory distress syndrome occurs as a result of the insufficient production of surfactant		
e.	The term hypotonia describes an increase of body tension and tone		
f.	Hyperthermia is defined as a core temperature above 38.5°C		
g.	Preterm infants below 30 weeks' gestation have a resting position that is usually characterized as hypertonic		
h.	Posseting is unrelated winding and overhandling of the baby after feeding		
i.	At 36–38 weeks' gestation, the resting position of a healthy newborn is one of total flexion with immediate recoil		

Matching

8. Table 18.5 presents statements related to the signs of respiratory compromise. Complete the table by inserting the correct term to match each statement.

Apnoea   Asynchrony   Grunting
Nasal flaring   Recessions   Tachypnoea

a. Grunting. b. Asynchrony. c. Nasal flaring. d. Tachypnoea. e. Recessions. f. Apnoea.

Table 18.5

	Statement	Response
a.	This is an audible noise heard on expiration	
b.	The breathing has a see-saw pattern as the abdominal movements and the diaphragm work out of unison	
c.	This occurs with the nares when the body tries to attempt to minimize the effect of the airways resistance by maximizing the diameter of the upper airways	
d.	This is a compensatory rise in the respiratory rate initiated by the respiratory centre. The rise aims to remove hypercarbia and prevent hypoxia	
e.	Chest distortions occur because of an increase in the need to create higher respiratory pressures in a compliant chest. They appear across the thorax	
f.	This is the absence of breathing for more than 20 seconds	

 Definition

9. Complete the following definition by inserting the three missing word(s).

> A neutral _____ environment is defined as the ambient air temperature at which
>
> _____ consumption or heat production is minimal, with body temperature
>
> _____ within the normal range.

The remainder of the main activities in this chapter relates to birth traumas.

Caput succedaneum and cephalohaematoma

 Short answers

10. Complete Table 18.6 by providing short answers to the following conditions.

Table 18.6

Condition	Caput succedaneum	Cephalhaematoma
What is this?		
When does it occur?		
What is the cause?		

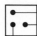 **Colour and label**

11. Fig. 18.2 shows a caput succedaneum. Colour and label as noted.

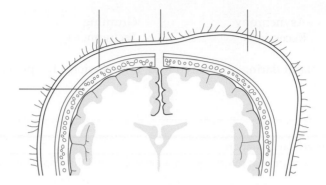

Figure 18.2

Label

| Skull |
| Periosteum |
| Scalp |

Label and colour/shade
Blood and serum

12. Fig. 18.3 shows a cephalohaematoma. Label and colour as noted.

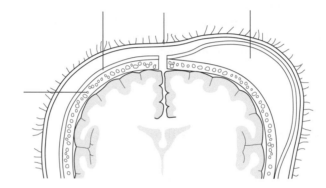

Figure 18.3

Label

| Skull |
| Periosteum |
| Scalp |

Label and colour/shade
Blood

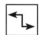 **Match**

13. Box 18.1 presents a list of statements relating to either caput succedaneum or cephalhaematoma. Complete this activity by drawing a line to match and connect each statement to the correct condition. An example is provided.

Box 18.1

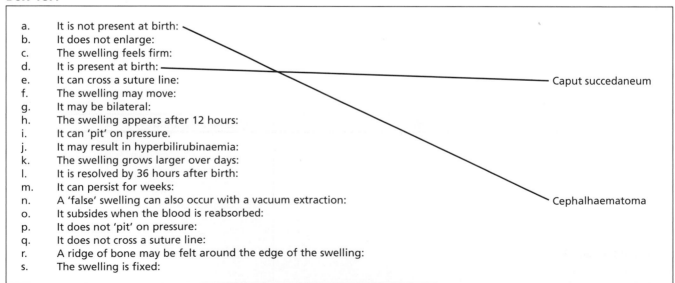

a. It is not present at birth:
b. It does not enlarge:
c. The swelling feels firm:
d. It is present at birth:
e. It can cross a suture line:
f. The swelling may move:
g. It may be bilateral:
h. The swelling appears after 12 hours:
i. It can 'pit' on pressure.
j. It may result in hyperbilirubinaemia:
k. The swelling grows larger over days:
l. It is resolved by 36 hours after birth:
m. It can persist for weeks:
n. A 'false' swelling can also occur with a vacuum extraction:
o. It subsides when the blood is reabsorbed:
p. It does not 'pit' on pressure:
q. It does not cross a suture line:
r. A ridge of bone may be felt around the edge of the swelling:
s. The swelling is fixed:

Caput succedaneum

Cephalhaematoma

Birth injuries

14. Table 18.7 presents statements relating to birth injuries. Consider the statements and correctly match to the injury from the list provided. Complete the table by inserting the injury.

Brachial plexus	Erb palsy	Klumpe palsy
Skin damage	Total brachial palsy	Subdural haemorrhage
Subarachnoid haemorrhage	Torticollis	Umbilical haemorrhage

Table 18.7

	Statement	Injury
a.	This injury may occur to the fetal head if excessive compression or abnormal stretching tears the tentorium cerebella	
b.	This results from poorly applied cord ligature	
c.	i. Trauma results from excessive lateral flexion, rotation or traction of the head and neck during vaginal breech or shoulder dystocia: ii. Three main types of this nerve injury include:	
d.	Damage to this organ is often iatrogenic, resulting from instrumental births	
e.	Preterm babies who suffer hypoxia resulting in disruption of cerebral blood flow may suffer from this injury	
f.	Damage is caused by excessive traction or twisting causing tearing to muscle(s) during birth of the anterior shoulder or rotation of shoulders in a breech or C/S. The most common is the sternomastoid muscle	

 Miscellaneous multiple choice questions (MCQ)

15. Weight loss is normal in the first few days but is deemed to be abnormal if the weight loss is more than:

a. 5%

b. 10%

c. 15%

d. 20%

16. The Moro reflex is present in the newborn for the first:

a. 4 weeks

b. 6 weeks

c. 8 weeks

d. 10 weeks

17. Pseudomenstruation in the first days of life is caused by the withdrawal of:

a. Progesterone

b. Relaxin

c. Oestrogen

d. All of the above

e. None of the above

18. During a convulsion the baby may have:
    a. Tachycardia
    b. Hypertension
    c. Raised cerebral blood flow
    d. Raised intracranial pressure
    e. All of the above

19. The percentage of all births affected with a cardiac defect is approximately:
    a. 1%
    b. 3%
    c. 5%
    d. 7%

20. In relation to newborn, the consensus on the lowest safe level of blood glucose is:
    a. 2.4 mmol/L
    b. 2.6 mmol/L
    c. 2.8 mmol/L
    d. 3.0 mmol/L

21. Nephrogenesis in the neonate is complete by:
    a. 33 weeks' gestation
    b. 34 weeks' gestation
    c. 35 weeks' gestation
    d. 36 weeks' gestation

22. Postnatal maturation of the gut is stimulated by an increase in which of the following peptide hormones:
    a. Gastrin
    b. Prolactin
    c. Oxytocin
    d. Motilin
    e. Leptin

19 Jaundice and blood group incompatibility

The main focus of this chapter is jaundice and blood group incompatibility. These are conditions that midwives deal with on a regular basis and a sound understanding is required for both. The activities will test your knowledge in these areas.

JAUNDICE

Physiological jaundice

 Complete

1. Conjugation changes the end-products of red cell breakdown so they can be excreted in faeces or urine. Haemoglobin from these cells is broken down to the by-products of haem, globin and iron. Complete the following related statements using the list provided.

   amino acids   biliverdin   red blood cells   urobilin
   stercobilinogen   body   proteins   unconjugated
   bilirubin

   a. Haem is converted to _____ and then to _____. _____.

   b. Globin is broken down into _____ and used by the body to make _____.

   c. Iron is stored in the _____ or used for new _____.

2. The following activity relates to the two main forms of bilirubin in the body. Complete the two sentences by removing the incorrect word(s) so that these read correctly.

   a. **Unconjugated/conjugated** bilirubin is **fat soluble/water soluble** and cannot be excreted easily in bile or urine.

   b. **Unconjugated/conjugated** bilirubin has been made **fat soluble/water soluble** in the liver and can be excreted in faeces and urine.

Match

3. The following activity involves the bilirubin pathway (Fig. 19.1) Label the missing stages by inserting the correct statement from the extended list provided.

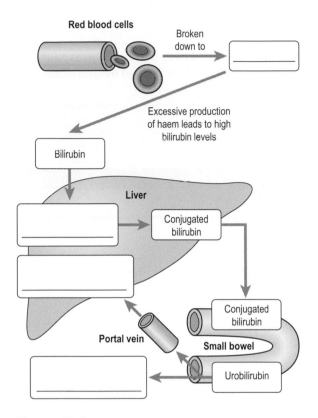

Haem + globin.
Bilverdin and globin.
Urobilirubin conjugated to glucuronic acid in hepatocytes.
Conjugated with glucuronyl transferase in hepatocytes.
85% of bile salts reabsorbed, 15% of urobilirubin.
95% of bile salts reabsorbed, 10% of urobilirubin.
5% of bile salts excreted, 90% of urobilirubin.
90% of bile salts excreted, 5% of urobilirubin.

Figure 19.1

Neonatal physiological jaundice

 Complete

4. Box 19.1 provides statements relating to neonatal physiological jaundice. Using your own knowledge, complete the following statements by inserting the correct word(s) and numerical values.

Box 19.1

a. Neonatal _____ jaundice occurs when unconjugated (____ soluble) bilirubin is deposited in the _____ instead of being taken to the _____ for processing into conjugated (_____ soluble) bilirubin that can be excreted from the body in _____ or _____.

b. This is a normal transitional state affecting up to ___ % of term babies and ___% of preterm babies who have a progressive rise in _____ bilirubin levels with jaundice on day ___.

c. Physiological jaundice *never* appears before _____ hours of life and usually fades by __ week, with bilirubin levels usually never exceeding _____ to _____ μmol/L (____ – ___ mg/dL) depending on the gestational age.

Match

5. Table 19.1 presents straightforward statements that relate to the causes of neonatal physiological jaundice. Match the statements correctly to the possible cause (i–iv).

i. Enzyme deficiency
iii. Increased enterohepatic reabsorption

ii. Decreased albumin-binding capacity
iv. Increased red cell breakdown

Table 19.1

	Statement	Causes
a.	When the baby is born and the pulmonary system becomes functional, then there is haemolysis of the large cell mass no longer required. This results in an increased level of unconjugated bilirubin	
b.	Newborns have lower concentrations and the decrease in capacity reduces the transport of bilirubin to the liver	
c.	Levels of activity are lower during the first 24 hours after birth and this reduces the conjugation of bilirubin in the liver	
d.	If all sites are used then levels of unbound 'free' fat soluble bilirubin rises in the blood and finds tissues with the affinity for fat	
e.	The newborn bowel lacks the normal enteric bacteria that breaks down conjugated bilirubin to urobilinogen	
f.	Drugs also compete for these sites and this leaves less capacity for bilirubin transport	

Pathological neonatal jaundice

Short answers

6. Complete the following activities relating to pathophysiology. Refer to the textbooks as required.

a. Kernicterus (bilirubin toxicity) is an _____ caused by deposits of

_____ bilirubin in the _____ ganglia of the _____.

b. Early signs can be _____ and include (identify at least two): _____

_____

_____

c. Long-term clinical features can include (identify at least four): _____

_____

_____

_____

7. Complete the following statements related to the criteria for diagnosis of jaundice in the newborn by inserting the correct numerical values from the list provided.

3	5	15	200
7	10	24	225
14	20	25	250

a. Pathological jaundice usually occurs within the first ____ hours of life.

b. A conjugated bilirubin of ____ μmol/L (or > ____ % of the total serum bilirubin) would indicate a pathological finding with further investigation required.

c. Persistence of jaundice beyond ____ days for the term infant requires investigation.

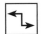 **Match**

8. Box 19.2 provides a selection of statements (column A), which will result in interference with the important processes (column B) identified in leading to pathological jaundice. Complete the activity by drawing a line to match and connect the correct statement with the process involved. An example is provided.

Box 19.2

A. Statement	B. Process
a. Blood type/group incompatibility:	• Conjugation
b. Drugs that compete with bilirubin for albumin-binding sites:	
c. Immaturity of the enzyme system:	
d. Hepatic obstruction:	• Excretion
e. Obstruction by 'bile plugs' (e.g., cystic fibrosis):	
f. Infection, idiopathic neonatal hepatitis:	
g. Acidosis, hypothermia or hypoxia:	• Production
h. Polycythemia:	
i. Spherocytosis:	
j. Metabolic or endocrine disorders that alter uridine diphosphate glucanosyltransferase (UDP-GT) enzyme activity:	• Transport
k. Extravasated blood (cephalhaematoma or bruising):	

BLOOD GROUP INCOMPATIBILITY

 Complete

9. The following activity relates to the causes of haemolytic jaundice through maternal blood group types. Complete the following two paragraphs by removing the incorrect word/s.

a. RhD **incompatibility/compatibility** can occur when a woman with **Rh-negative/Rh-positive** blood type is pregnant with a **Rh-negative/Rh-positive fetus**. The placenta acts as a barrier to fetal blood entering the maternal circulation. During pregnancy or birth, fetomaternal haemorrhage (FMH) can occur when small amounts of fetal **Rh-negative/Rh-positive** blood cross the placenta and enter the **Rh-positive/Rh-negative** mother's blood. The woman's immune system produces **anti-D/anti-O** antibodies. In subsequent pregnancies, these maternal antibodies can cross the placenta and destroy the red cells of any **Rh-negative/Rh-positive** fetus.

b. ABO **isoimmunization/immunization** usually occurs when the mother is blood **group O/group A** and the baby is blood **group A/group O** (or less often **group AB/group B**). Individuals with **type O/type A** blood develop antibodies throughout life from exposure to antigens in food, gram-**negative/positive** bacteria or blood transfusion. The woman usually has high serum **anti-A/anti AO** and **anti AO/anti-B** antibody titres by the time she is pregnant for the first time. Some women produce **IgA/IgG** antibodies that can cross the placenta and attach to the red cells and destroy them.

Miscellaneous

 True/false

10. Consider the statements presented in Table 19.2. Complete the table by indicating if each statement is true or false.

Table 19.2

	Statement	True	False
a.	Preterm babies are at risk of physiological jaundice because the shorter red cell life increases production of unconjugated bilirubin		
b.	Mothers should be advised to discontinue to breastfeed if the baby experiences prolonged jaundice		
c.	Anti-D antibodies are the most common type		
d.	In neonatal meningitis, very early signs may be nonspecific and then followed by meningeal irritation, signs of raised intracranial pressure and alterations to consciousness		
e.	In relation to Rhesus factor inheritance: the baby will always have Rhesus positive blood group if born to a Rhesus-negative (dd) mother and a Rhesus-positive (DD homozygous) father		
f.	ABO incompatibility is the most frequent cause of severe haemolysis in the neonate		
g.	Toxoplasmosis is a protozoan parasite found in uncooked meat and cat and dog faeces		
h.	Direct Coomb's test (DCT) is used to detect the presence of maternal antibodies on baby's red blood cells		
i.	Anti-D prophylaxis has a key role to play in Rh-D isoimmunization which can cause severe haemolytic disease in the newborn (often with adverse outcomes)		

? Multiple choice questions (MCQ)

11. Jaundice typically becomes visible in the newborn when serum bilirubin levels reach which level:

a. 75 μmol/L   b. 80 μmol/L   c. 85 μmol/L   d. 90 μmol/L

12. Which of the following is inhibited by substances found in breast-milk, causing jaundice to develop:

a. Stercobilinogen

b. Beta glucoronidase

c. Glucoronyl tranferase

d. Lipase

13. Which condition causes the neonate to develop a deep bronze jaundice in the second week of life, with putty coloured stools and dark urine:

a. Extrahepatic biliary atresia

b. Hydronephrosis

c. Rhesus isoimmunization

d. Hypothyroidism

14. Phototherapy, using blue light at a wavelength of 400 to 500 nm, converts conjugated bilirubin in their subcutaneous tissue to a nontoxic, water-soluble substance by inducing which of the following process/processes:

a. Photooxidation

b. Structural isomerization

c. Configurational isomerization

d. All of the above

20 Congenital abnormalities and metabolic disorders

This chapter is focused on congenital abnormalities and metabolic disorders. The midwife is often the first to notice an abnormality in a baby, either during the birth process or in the early postnatal period. It is essential to have knowledge of these conditions for early recognition and to provide appropriate care to the baby and support the parents. The activities will test your knowledge of the main abnormalities and disorders.

Inherited disorders

A congenital abnormality is any defect in form, structure or function.

 True/false

1. Table 20.1 presents statements relating to inherited disorders. Consider each statement and decide whether they are true or false.

Table 20.1

	Statements	True	False
a.	A dominant gene needs to be present on both chromosomes before producing its effect		
b.	Mitosis is cell division that occurs in somatic cells where each new cell gets a full set of chromosomes		
c.	The zygote should have one sex chromosome and 23 autosomes from each parent		
d.	Mitochondria are always inherited from the father		
e.	Meiosis is the type of cell reduction that occurs in the formation of gametes, in which one of each chromosome pair is lost		
f.	A recessive gene will produce its effect even if present in only one chromosome of a pair		
g.	Trisomy refers to a situation where a particular chromosome is represented 3 times in the nucleus		
h.	In an X-linked recessive inheritance, the condition affects almost exclusively females, although males can be carriers		
i.	Cystic fibrosis is an autosomal dominant condition		
j.	Duchenne muscular dystrophy is an example of an X-linked recessive inheritance		
k.	Trisomy 18 and 21 are examples of chromosomal abnormality		
l.	Haemophilia is an example of an X-linked dominant inheritance		
m.	Turner's syndrome is an example of a monosomal condition where there is only one sex chromosome		

Congenital defects and conditions

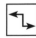 **Match and complete**

2. Table 20.2 presents statements about defects and conditions. Match the statements to the conditions from the list provided (1–13). Complete the table by inserting your answer.

1. Choanal atresia
2. Cleft lip and palate
3. Diaphragmatic hernia
4. Exomphalos
5. Gastroschisis
6. Hirschsprung's disease
7. Imperforate anus
8. Malrotation/volvulus
9. Meconium ileus (cystic fibrosis)
10. Oesophageal atresia
11. Pierre Robin sequence
12. Pyloric stenosis
13. Rectal atresia

Table 20.2

	Statement	Answer
a.	List five conditions suspected if the baby fails to pass meconium in the first 24 hours after birth	
b.	This condition occurs when there is herniation of the abdominal contents into the thoracic cavity	
c.	This condition arises from a genetic defect that causes hypertrophy of the muscles of the pyloric sphincter	
d.	There is an aganglionic section of the bowel	
e.	One characteristic of this condition is micrognathia (hypoplasia of the lower jaw)	
f.	This defect occurs where the bowel or other viscera protrude through the umbilicus	
g.	This defect may be unilateral or bilateral. It may affect the soft palate, hard palate or both	
h.	This condition involves a unilateral or bilateral narrowing of the nasal passages with a web of tissue or bone occluding the nasopharynx	
i.	In this condition, there is incomplete canalization of the oesophagus in early uterine development	
j.	This occurs because of a paramedian defect of the abdominal wall with extrusion of bowel that is not covered with peritoneum	

Cardiac defects

  Label and completion

3. Fig. 20.1 shows the normal heart. Label as indicated. Colour or shade (as preferred) the location of oxygenated and deoxygenated blood within the normal heart (refer to a coloured physiology textbook).

Label

Aorta
Right atrium
Left atrium
Pulmonary artery
Right ventricle
Left ventricle

Identify the direction of flow (colour as preferred)

Flow of blood through the aorta
Flow of blood through the pulmonary artery

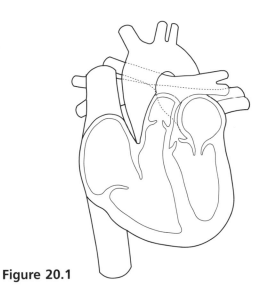

Figure 20.1

4. Box 20.1 Provides statements (i–iii) describing transposition of the great arteries. Complete the box by removing the incorrect word(s) so the statements read correctly.

Box 20.1

i. In this condition, the aorta arises from the **right/left** ventricle and the pulmonary artery arises from the **left/right** ventricle.
ii. **Oxygenated/deoxygenated** blood is circulated back through the lungs and **oxygenated/deoxygenated** blood is circulated back into the systemic circulation.
iii. A **patent ductus venosus/ductus arteriosus** needs to be maintained to provide opportunity for **oxygenated/deoxygenated** blood to access the systemic circulation. Otherwise the baby will die.

5. Fig. 20.2 shows tetralogy of Fallot (TOF). Compare with the normal heart structure in Fig. 20.1A to highlight the defects. Label from the list of terms provided.

Label

Aorta
Subpulmonary stenosis
Pulmonary artery
Right ventricular hypertrophy
Ventricular septal defect (VSD) with overriding aorta

Colour or shade (as preferred)

Oxygenated blood flow through vessels
Deoxygenated blood flow through vessels

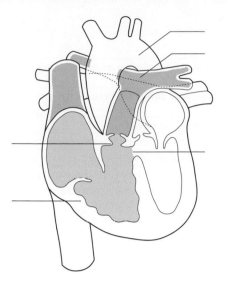

Figure 20.2

6. Complete the statement about tetralogy of Fallot defect by inserting the missing word(s).

In this condition there are four key cardiac defects. These include the following:

   i. Pulmonary outflow is _____

  ii. Ventricular septal defect (VSD)

 iii. Right ventricle is _____

 iv. An _____ aorta

7. There are a small number of cardiac defects that may not require medical/surgical treatment in early life. These will require careful follow-up of signs of developing heart failure at a later stage and may then require treatment. List three cardiac defects within this category:

   i. _____

  ii. _____

 iii. _____

8. Detailed examination of the newborn will reveal the following subtle signs of cardiac failure in situations involving ventricular septal defects. Complete the following statements.

   a. There will be increased respiration rate. This is known as _____.

   b. There will be increased heart rate. This is known as _____.

   c. There will be incipient _____ especially following exertion of crying or feeding.

   d. On auscultation _____ _____ may be heard.

Spina bifida

 Definitions

9. Complete the following definitions related to spina bifida.

   a. Spina bifida results from _____ of fusion of the _____ _____.

   b. A meningocele refers to the protrusion of the _____ through the defect. It does

      _____ contain _____ tissue.

   c. Meningomyocele refers to the protrusion of _____ through the defect and it involves

      the _____ _____.

   d. Encephalocele is the term used when the defect is at the _____ of the _____ of the skull.

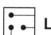 **Label**

10. Fig. 20.3 shows various forms of spina bifida. Label according to terms provided subsequently.

Label and colour/shade on the 'normal' vertebra

| Skin |
| Spinal cord |
| Dura |

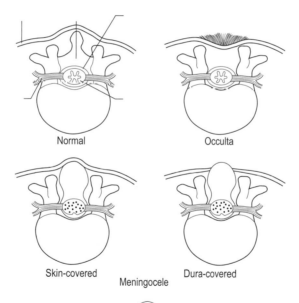

Normal   Occulta

Skin-covered   Dura-covered

Meningocele

Flat meningomyelocele

Label on the 'normal' vertebra

| Vertebral arch |
| Nerve |

Colour/shade on the other four figures

| Skin |
| Spinal cord |
| Dura |

Figure 20.3

Miscellaneous congenital defects

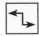 **Matching**

11. Table 20.4 provides statements relating to a variety of defects. Complete the activity by matching the statement to the correct congenital defects listed (1–9) and inserting in the table.

1. Cryptochordism
2. Achondroplasia
3. Fetal alcohol syndrome/spectrum
4. Port wine stain
5. Osteogenesis imperfecta
6. Hypospadius
7. Potter syndrome
8. Talipes equinovarus
9. Talipes calcaneovalgus

Table 20.4

	Statement	Condition
a.	This autosomal dominant disorder of collagen production leads to brittle bones	
b.	This is an autosomal dominant condition where the baby is small with a disproportionately large head and short limbs	
c.	This is a purple-blue malformation affecting the face. It is fully formed at birth and does not regress with time	
d.	The urethral meatus opens onto the under surface of the penis	
e.	This refers to undescended testes which may be unilateral or bilateral	
f.	The characteristics are a growth-restricted infant with microcephaly, close set eyes, small upturned nose, thin upper lip, close set ears. There are learning difficulties	
g.	In this foot deformity, the foot is dorsiflexed and everted	
h.	The baby's face has a flattened appearance, low set ears, and is incompatible with life because of lung hypoplasia	
i.	In this foot deformity, the ankle is bent downwards (plantarflexed) and the front part of the foot is turned inwards (inverted)	

Miscellaneous

 Complete

12. This activity relates to the baby born to a diabetic mother. Complete the paragraph by removing the incorrect words so that it reads correctly.

Infants born to a diabetic mother have **low/high** blood glucose concentrations because of the excess of **insulin/glucogen**. This is produced by the fetal **pancreatic gland/liver** as a result of stimulation by **increased/decreased** maternal **insulin/glucose** concentrations. The excess of **insulin/glucose** also acts as a **growth factor/growth inhibitor** and brings about **reduced/excessive** fat and glycogen deposition. The baby usually has a macrosomic appearance.

True/false

13. Table 20.5 presents statements relating to metabolic and other disorders. Consider the statements and decide if they are true or false.

Table 20.5

	Statement	True	False
a.	Hyponatraemia in the presence of weight gain suggests a defect in water excretion		
b.	Infants with galactosaemia will test positive for glucose in the urine		
c.	Hypocalcaemia can cause tremors, jitteriness, lethargy and poor feeding		
d.	Phenylketonuria (PKU) is an autosomal dominant disorder		
e.	Cocaine has harmful effects on the baby, including significant fetal growth restriction, brain injury caused by haemorrhage or infarction, abnormalities of brain development, limb reduction and gut atresias		
f.	Thyroid stimulating hormone (TSH) is produced by the anterior pituitary gland		
g.	Phenylketonuria (PKU) cannot be treated with a diet specifically restricted in phenylalanine		
h.	Galactosaemia is a disorder caused by the absence or deficiency of the enzyme galactose-1-phosphate uridyltransferase (Gal-1-P UT)		
i.	Infants with hypothyroidism tend to be large, postmature and have a large posterior fontanelle		
j.	Opiates cross the placenta and the fetus is likely to be exposed to the same peaks and troughs of drug exposure as the mother		

14. Which of the following conditions may result in cyanosis in the newborn:
    a. Transposition of the great arteries (TGA)
    b. TOF
    c. VSD
    d. Hydrocephalus
    e. Persistent pulmonary hypertension in the neonate (PPHN)
    f. Sepsis
    g. Atrial septal defect (ASD)

15. Complete the following statements regarding neurological reflexes by inserting the correct term:

    a. The _____ reflex may be absent following heavy sedation of hypoxemic ischaemic encephalopathy (HIE).

    b. The _____ reflex may be depressed in the preterm neonate or following maternal sedation during labour.

    c. Visual cues should normally replace the _____ reflex by 4 months age.

16. In relation to developmental dysplasia of the hip (DDH), which of the following statements are true?
    a. It is more common following a breech presentation.
    b. It is more common with polyhydramnios.
    c. The right hip is more affected than the left.
    d. It is more common in girls.
    e. A dysplastic hip may present as dislocated, dislocatable or with subluxation of the joint.

17. Look at the image in the subsequent Fig. 20.4 and identify which side of the newborn's face is exhibiting a facial palsy and what visible features confirm this diagnosis?

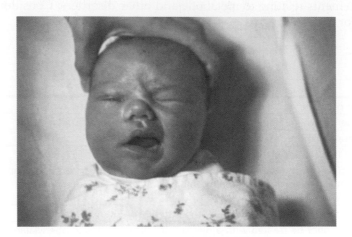

Figure 20.4

ANSWERS

1 The female pelvis and pelvic floor

ANSWERS

1. Correct: i, iii, iv, vi. Incorrect: ii (it is basin-shaped); v (it is the anterior walls), vii (it is only posterior).

2. Correct: i, ii, iv, v, vii, viii, ix, xi. Incorrect: iii (it is anterior); vi (it is posterior surface); x (it is triangular).

3.

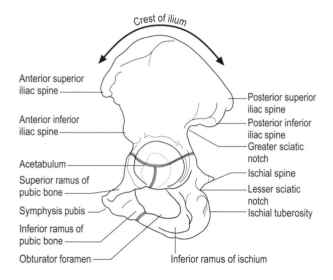

Figure 1.1

4. **i.** The **sacroiliac joints** join the sacrum to the ilium and as a result connect the spine to the pelvis. **ii.** The symphysis pubis is the midline cartilaginous joint uniting the <u>rami</u> of the <u>left</u> and <u>right pubic bones</u>. **iii.** The sacrococcygeal joint is formed where the <u>base</u> of the <u>coccyx</u> articulates with the <u>tip</u> of the sacrum.

5.

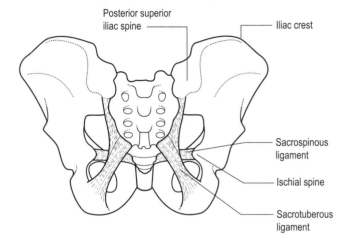

Figure 1.2

6.

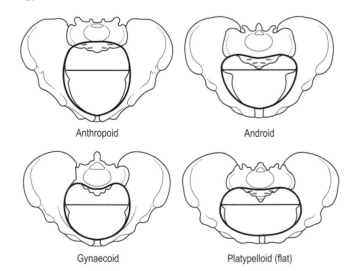

Figure 1.3

7.

Table 1.3

Features	Gynaecoid	Anthropoid	Android	Platypelloid
Brim	Rounded	Long oval	Heart-shaped	Kidney-shaped
Forepelvis	Generous	Narrowed	Narrow	Wide
Side walls	Straight	Divergent	Convergent	Divergent
Ischial spines	Blunt	Blunt	Prominent	Blunt
Sciatic notch	Rounded	Wide	Narrow	Wide
Sub-pubic arch	90 degrees	>90 degrees	<90 degrees	>90 degrees
Incidence	50%	25% (50% non-Caucasian)	20%	5%

8.

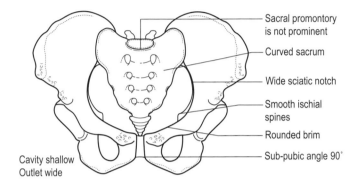

- Sacral promontory is not prominent
- Curved sacrum
- Wide sciatic notch
- Smooth ischial spines
- Rounded brim
- Sub-pubic angle 90°

Cavity shallow
Outlet wide

Figure 1.4

9. Gynaecoid: a, m.   Android: d, e, g, h, j, n.
   Anthropoid: c. f, i, k.   Platypelloid: b, l.

10. **1. a.** Pelvic brim,   **b.** Pelvic cavity,   **c.** Pelvic
    outlet.;   **2.** Anatomical structures forming the
    false pelvis include the <u>upper flared-out portions
    of the iliac bones</u>. The false pelvis protects the
    <u>abdominal organs</u>.

11. **a.** Sacral promontory   **b.** Sacral ala or wing
    c. Sacroiliac joint   **d.** Iliopectineal line (which is
    the edge formed at the inward aspect of the
    ilium)   **e.** Iliopectineal eminence (which is the
    roughened area formed where the superior ramus
    of the pubic bone meets the ilium)   **f.** Superior
    ramus of the pubic border   **g.** Upper inner border
    of the pubic bone   **h.** Upper inner border of the
    symphysis pubis

12.

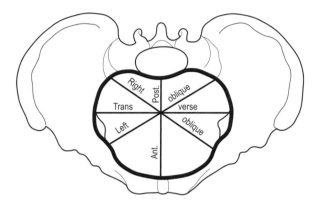

Figure 1.6

13. **1.** Transverse diameter.   **2.** Oblique diameter.
    3. The anteroposterior diameter extends from the
    <u>sacral promontory</u> to the <u>symphysis pubis</u>. The
    other term for this diameter is the <u>conjugate</u>
    diameter.

14.

	Anteroposterior	Oblique	Transverse
Brim	11	12	13
Cavity	12	12	12
Outlet	13	12	11

Figure 1.7

15. True: b, c, d, f, g, i.   False: a, e, h, j.

16.

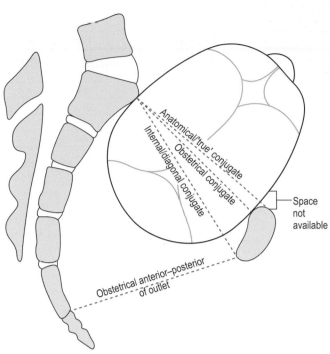

Anatomical 'true' conjugate

Internal/diagonal conjugate

Obstetrical conjugate

Space not available

Obstetrical anterior–posterior of outlet

Figure 1.8

17. 1. Engagement of the fetal head may necessitate <u>lateral</u> tilting, known as *asynclitism*, to allow the <u>biparietal</u> diameter to pass the narrowest <u>anteroposterior</u> diameter of the brim. **2.** In anterior asynclitism, the <u>anterior</u> parietal bone moves down behind the <u>symphysis pubis,</u> until the <u>parietal eminence</u> enters the brim. The movement is then reversed and the fetal head tilts in the opposite direction, until the <u>posterior</u> parietal bone negotiates the <u>sacral promontory</u> and the fetal head is engaged. **3.** In posterior asynclitism, the movements of anterior asynclitism are reversed. The <u>posterior</u> parietal bone negotiates the <u>sacral promontory</u> before the <u>anterior</u> parietal bone, moving down behind the <u>symphysis pubis</u>. Once the pelvic brim has been negotiated, descent progresses normally, accompanied by <u>flexion</u> and <u>internal</u> rotation.

18. Correct: d, e, f, h, j, k, l, m, n. Incorrect: a, b, c, g, i.

19. 1-b; 2-c, 3-c, 4-a.

20. 1-c, 2-d, 3-d, 4-e.

21. Rachitic pelvis: a, f. Osteomalacic pelvis: b, Naegle's pelvis: c, e. Robert's pelvis: c Spinal deformity: d.

22. The basin-shaped gynaecoid pelvis has a generous forepelvis, with a rounded brim and straight walls (suitable for childbirth). The bones in the rachitic pelvis are poorly ossified and soft. The bones will deform because of the weight of the upper body—the sacral promontory is pushed downwards and forwards; the ischium and ilium are drawn outwards; a flat pelvic brim results (similar to the platypelloid pelvis); the sacrum is usually straight; the coccyx bends acutely forward and pubic arch is wide because of the widened distance between the ischial tuberosities. Caesarean section may be required if severe contraction of the pelvis is evident. The fetal head will attempt to enter the pelvic brim by asynclitism.

23. a. It provides support for the pelvic organs; it is important in the maintenance of continence (bladder and bowels) as part of the anal and urinary sphincters and it has an important role in sexual intercourse. **b.** The pelvic floor influences the passive movements of the fetus through the birth canal and relaxes to allow the fetus to exit from the pelvis.

24. a.

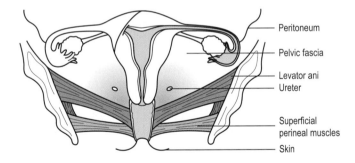

Peritoneum

Pelvic fascia

Levator ani

Ureter

Superficial perineal muscles

Skin

Figure 1.9

b.

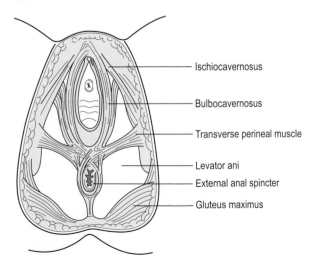

Ischiocavernosus

Bulbocavernosus

Transverse perineal muscle

Levator ani

External anal spincter

Gluteus maximus

Figure 1.10

c.

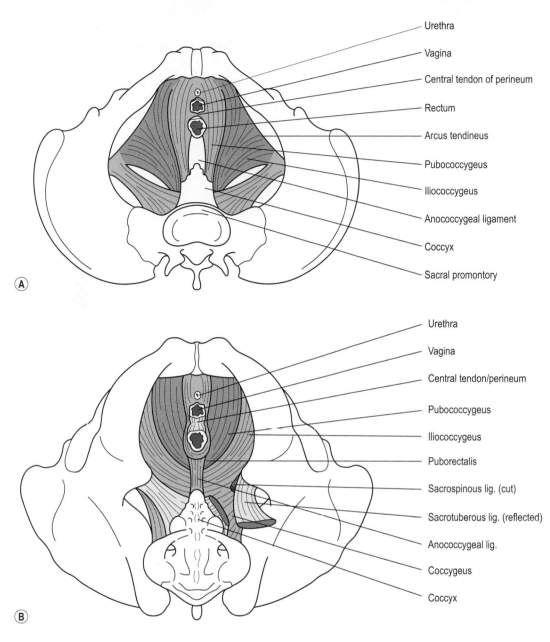

Urethra

Vagina

Central tendon of perineum

Rectum

Arcus tendineus

Pubococcygeus

Iliococcygeus

Anococcygeal ligament

Coccyx

Sacral promontory

Ⓐ

Urethra

Vagina

Central tendon/perineum

Pubococcygeus

Iliococcygeus

Puborectalis

Sacrospinous lig. (cut)

Sacrotuberous lig. (reflected)

Anococcygeal lig.

Coccygeus

Coccyx

Ⓑ

Figure 1.11

d.

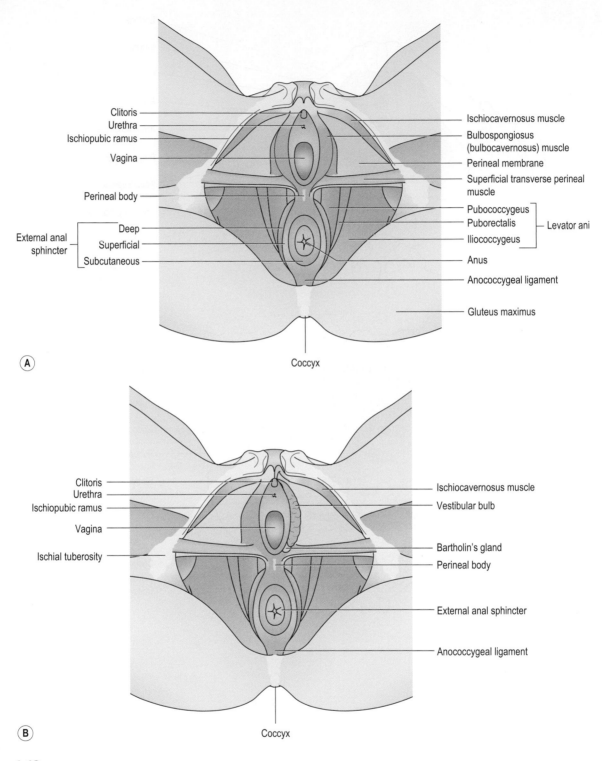

Figure 1.12

e.

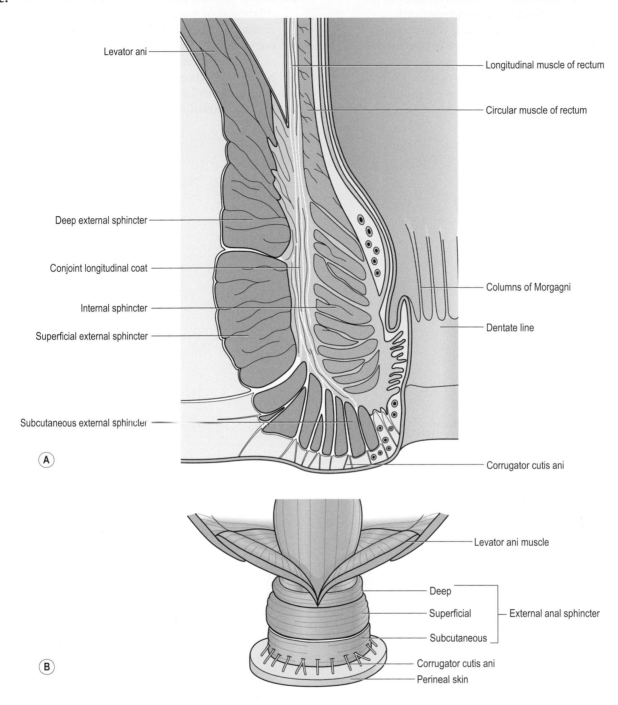

Levator ani

Deep external sphincter

Conjoint longitudinal coat

Internal sphincter

Superficial external sphincter

Subcutaneous external sphincter

(A)

Longitudinal muscle of rectum

Circular muscle of rectum

Columns of Morgagni

Dentate line

Corrugator cutis ani

Levator ani muscle

Deep
Superficial   — External anal sphincter
Subcutaneous

Corrugator cutis ani
Perineal skin

(B)

Figure 1.13

25. Correct: a, b, d, e, g, h.

26. True: b, d, e, g, i.   False: a (incomplete deep muscle groups and ischiocarvenosus is a superficial muscle); c (fascia is loosely packed); f (consists mainly of the paired levator ani muscles); h (has the ability).

27. **Cystocele:** herniation of the bladder. **Urethrocele:** is a displacement of the urethra with loss of the acute angle between it and the bladder. **Uterovaginal Prolapse:** prolapse of the pelvic organs often resulting in urinary and faecal incontinence. **Rectocele:** prolapse of the posterior middle vaginal wall allowing herniation of the rectum. **Enterocele:** herniation higher in the vagina (not palpable on examination).

Dyspareunia: painful sexual intercourse.

Procidentia: total prolapse of the uterus outside of the body (extremely rare).

Treatment for pelvic floor prolapse: normally surgical repair. Ring pessary for ill and frail.

28. Avoid women pushing in labour until full dilatation of the cervix is confirmed; prevent birth of the baby before full dilatation of the cervix; ensure second stage is not prolonged without obvious progress; avoid fundal pressure for placental delivery; early ambulation of women post birth and encourage pelvic floor exercises. Ensure careful repair of any perineal trauma.

2 The reproductive systems

ANSWERS

1.

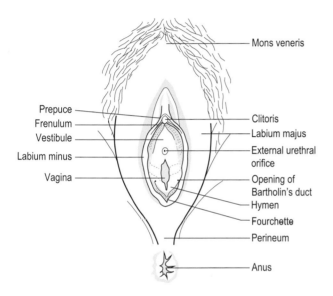

Mons veneris

Prepuce
Frenulum
Vestibule
Labium minus
Vagina

Clitoris
Labium majus
External urethral orifice
Opening of Bartholin's duct
Hymen
Fourchette
Perineum

Anus

Figure 2.1

2. i-Prepuce; ii-Bartholin's glands; iii-labia minora; iv-clitoris; v-vestibule; vi-mons veneris/mons pubis; vii-urethral orifice; viii-labia majora; ix-Skene ducts; x-hymen; xi-vaginal orifice.

3.

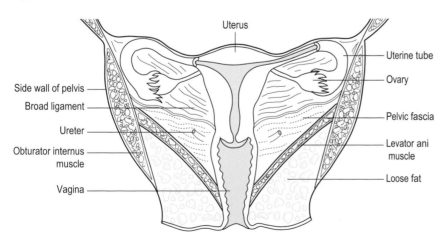

Uterus

Side wall of pelvis
Broad ligament
Ureter
Obturator internus muscle
Vagina

Uterine tube
Ovary
Pelvic fascia
Levator ani muscle
Loose fat

Figure 2.2

4.

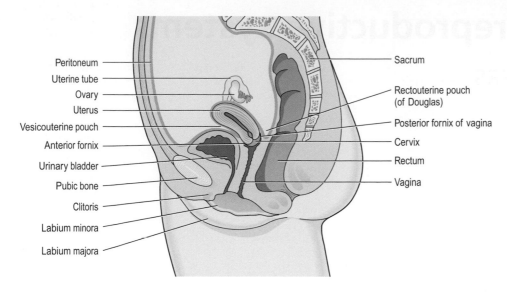

Peritoneum
Uterine tube
Ovary
Uterus
Vesicouterine pouch
Anterior fornix
Urinary bladder
Pubic bone
Clitoris
Labium minora
Labium majora

Sacrum
Rectouterine pouch (of Douglas)
Posterior fornix of vagina
Cervix
Rectum
Vagina

Figure 2.3

5.

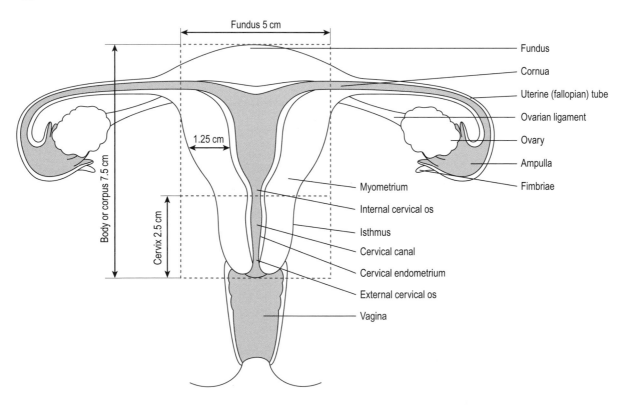

Fundus 5 cm
Body or corpus 7.5 cm
1.25 cm
Cervix 2.5 cm

Fundus
Cornua
Uterine (fallopian) tube
Ovarian ligament
Ovary
Ampulla
Fimbriae
Myometrium
Internal cervical os
Isthmus
Cervical canal
Cervical endometrium
External cervical os
Vagina

Figure 2.4

6.

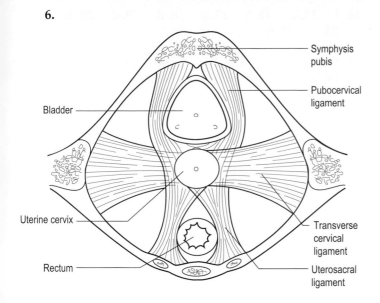

Figure 2.5

7. True: c, d. f, g, i, k, l, m, n, o, p.   False: a, b, e, h, j.

8. The uterus is a hollow **pear**-shaped **muscular** organ, described as being a **thick** organ, and is located in the **true** pelvis between the **bladder** and the **rectum**. The position of the uterus within the **true** pelvis is one of **ante**-version and **ante**-flexion. **Ante**-version means that the uterus leans forward and **ante**-flexion means that it bends forwards upon itself. When the woman is standing, the **anteverted** uterus is in an almost **horizontal** position with the **fundus** resting on the bladder. The uterus has three layers: endometrium, perimetrium and myometrium. The **endometrium** is the **inner** layer and the myometrium, the **middle** layer, is the **thickest** of the three layers.

9. i. a-10 cm; b-7.5 cm; c-2.5 cm.   **ii.** a-10 cm; b-1 mm; c. 2.5 cm; d-5 cm.   **iii.** a-7.5 cm; b-5 cm; c-2.5 cm; d-60 g; e-1.25 cm.   **iii.** pH 4.5.

10. a-lesser lips; b-greater lips; c-vault; d-mucosa, muscle and fascia; e-interstitial, isthmus, ampulla and infundibulum with fimbriae; f-goblet cells; g-plicae; h-oviduct, salpinges and fallopian tubes; i-Doderlein's bacilla, glycogen and lactic acid

11.

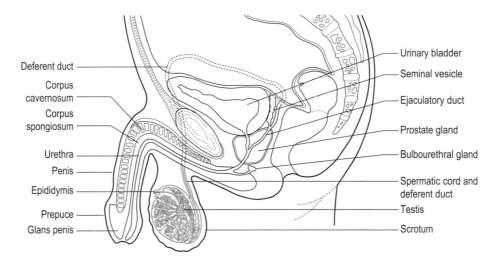

Figure 2.6

12. True: d, e, f, h, i.   False: a, b, c, g.

13.

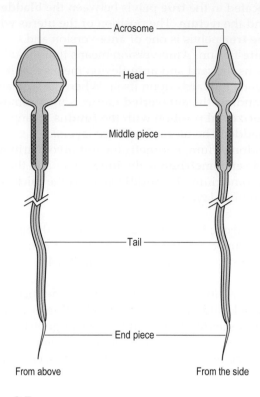

Figure 2.7

14. f.   **15.** d.   **16.** b.   **17.** e.   **18.** d.   **19.** d.   **20.** a.
21. e.   **22.** b.

23. Correct: a, c, d. e. h, i, j.   Incorrect: b (this should be in early embryonic life); f (this is rare); g (lower end).

3 The female urinary tract

ANSWERS

1.

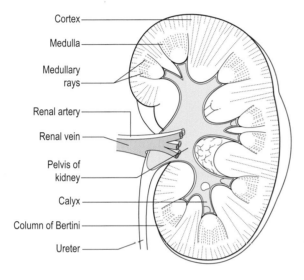

Cortex
Medulla
Medullary rays
Renal artery
Renal vein
Pelvis of kidney
Calyx
Column of Bertini
Ureter

Figure 3.1

2. Elimination of toxins; Elimination of waste materials; Regulation of pH of blood; Regulation of osmotic pressure of blood; Regulation of water content; Secretion of hormones.

3.

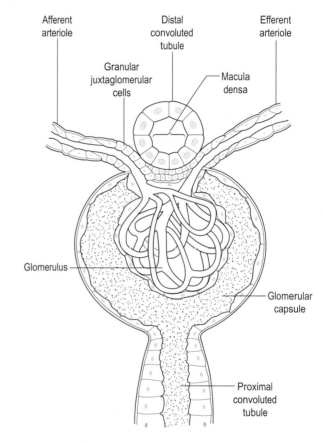

Afferent arteriole
Granular juxtaglomerular cells
Distal convoluted tubule
Macula densa
Efferent arteriole
Glomerulus
Glomerular capsule
Proximal convoluted tubule

Figure 3.2

4.

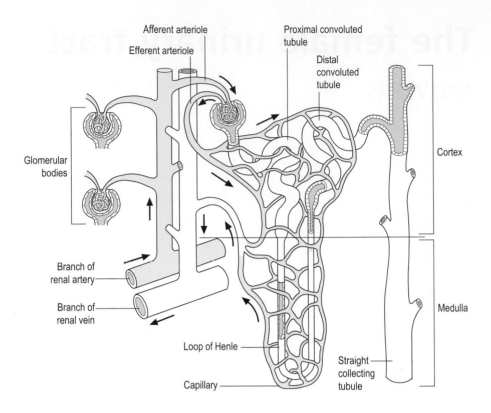

Figure 3.3

5. Three processes are involved in the production of urine: (i) **filtration**; (ii) **selective reabsorption**; and (iii) **secretion**. In **filtration**, fluid and solutes are forced through a **membrane** by **hydrostatic pressure**. Water and other small molecules pass through **easily.**
During **selective reabsorption,** removal of **two-thirds** of the filtrate takes place in the **proximal** tubule. **Aldosterone** increases reabsorption of **sodium** and water. **ADH** increases permeability of the tubules, **increasing** water reabsorption. **Secretion** is an important mechanism in clearing the blood of unwanted substances, for example, **drugs.**

6. b.   7. c.   8. c.   9. c.   10. e.   11. a.   12. a.
13. e.   14. d.   15. e.   16. b.

17. **Constituents in glomerular filtrate**: water, glucose, amino acids, mineral salts, hormones (some), ketoacids, creatinine, urea, uric acid, some small drugs.
Constituents remaining in glomerular capillaries: erythrocytes; platelets, leucocytes, plasma proteins and some large drugs.

18.

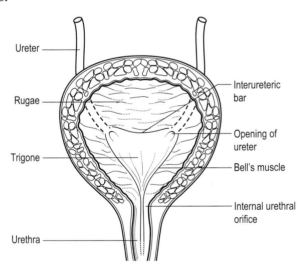

Figure 3.4

19. An important function of the renal system is electrolyte balance. pH is a measure of hydrogen [H⁺] ion concentration, and runs on a numerical scale of 1–14. More hydrogen [H⁺] ions result in an acidic solution demonstrated by a low pH. Less hydrogen [H⁺] ions result in an alkaline solution, demonstrated by a high pH value. A neutral pH value is 7. The typical pH of urine is between 5 and 6, compared with the pH of gastric juices which is 1 to 3.

20. Urachas (single fibrous band): Extends from the <u>apex of bladder</u> to the <u>umbilicus</u>.
Two pubocervical ligaments: Extend from the bladder neck anteriorly to the <u>symphysis pubis</u>.
Two lateral ligaments: Extend from the <u>bladder</u> to the <u>side walls of the pelvis</u>.

21. Correct: b, c, d, f, h, j, k, l, m, o.

22. **A**:i-Nephron, ii-Glomerular capsule (Bowman's capsule); iii-Afferent arteriole; iv-Efferent arteriole; v-Layers–Renal cortex and renal medulla; vi-Autoregulation; vii-Suprarenal (adrenal); viii-Adrenaline (epinephrine).   **B**: i-10 cm; ii-6.5 cm; iii-3 cm; iv-100 g.

23. **A**: i-Peristalsis; ii-Pramidal; iii-Globular; iv-Trigone; v-600 mL (500–1000 mL).
B. i-SG 1.010–1.030; ii-Average pH 6 (variation pH 4.5–8.0); iii-93%–97%; iv-1000/1500 mL/day.

24. True: iii, iv, vi, vii, viii.   False: i, ii, v.

25. d.   **26.** b.   **27.** d.   **28.** a.

29. i-Asymptomatic bacteruria (ABU); ii-Mid-stream specimen of urine (MSSU); iii-Cystitis; iv-Acute pyelonephritis; v-Cystoscopy or intravenous (IV) pyelography.

4 Hormonal cycles: fertilization and early development

ANSWERS

1. Phase one

In the **follicular** phase, low levels of ovarian hormones stimulate the **hypothalamus** to produce **gonadotrophin releasing hormone (GnRH)**. This hormone causes the production of **follicle stimulating hormone (FSH)** and **luteinizing hormone (LH)** by the **anterior** pituitary gland. Under the influence of this hormone, the Graafian follicle secretes **oestrogen** resulting in a surge in **LH**. The secretion of **FSH** is inhibited when hormone levels reach a certain peak. Eventually the largest and most dominant follicle secretes inhibin, which further suppresses **FSH**, and this follicle prevails and becomes competent to ovulate. The time from growth and maturity of the Graafian follicles to ovulation is normally around **1 week**, day **5 to 14** of a 28-day cycle of events.

Phase two

Ovulation is stimulated by a sudden **surge** in **LH**, which matures the **oocyte**. This surge occurs around day **12 to 13** of a 28-day cycle and lasts for **48 hours**.

Phase three

In the final **luteal** phase, the **corpus luteum** is formed by **proliferation** of the residual ruptured follicle. This is a **yellow** irregular structure producing **oestrogen** and **progesterone** for approximately **2** weeks. This develops the **endometrium** of the uterus, which awaits the fertilized oocyte. The **corpus luteum** continues its role, until the **placenta** is adequately developed to take over this role. If fertilization does not occur, then the **corpus luteum** degenerates and becomes the **corpus albicans**. There is a decrease in **oestrogen and progesterone** hormones and inhibin levels. These low hormone levels stimulate the **hypothalamus** to produce **GnRH**. These rising hormone levels stimulate the **anterior** pituitary gland to produce **FSH** and the cycle begins again.

2.

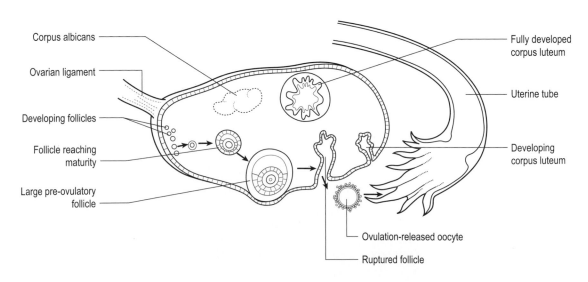

Corpus albicans

Ovarian ligament

Developing follicles

Follicle reaching maturity

Large pre-ovulatory follicle

Fully developed corpus luteum

Uterine tube

Developing corpus luteum

Ovulation-released oocyte

Ruptured follicle

Figure 4.1

3.

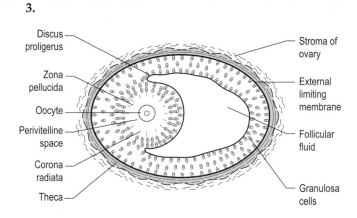

Labels (clockwise from top left):
- Discus proligerus
- Zona pellucida
- Oocyte
- Perivitelline space
- Corona radiata
- Theca
- Stroma of ovary
- External limiting membrane
- Follicular fluid
- Granulosa cells

Figure 4.2

4.

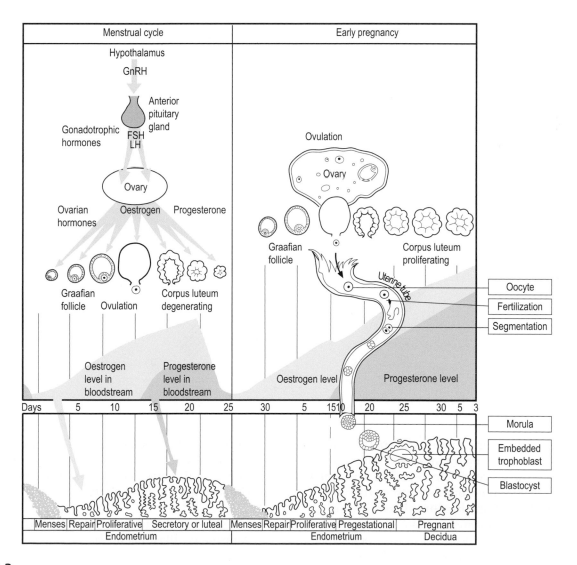

Figure 4.3

5. Menstrual phase: a, c, e, h, m, o
   Proliferative phase: d, f, l, n, p, q, s
   Secretory phase: b, g, i, j, k, r

6.

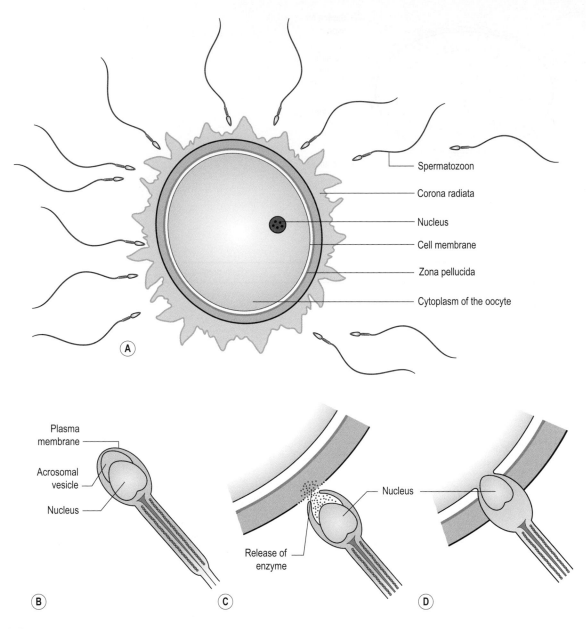

Figure 4.4

7. Once inside the uterine tubes, the sperm undergo changes to the plasma membrane resulting in the removal of the glycoprotein coat. The **acrosomal** layer of the sperm becomes reactive with the release of the enzyme **hyaluronidase.** This is known as the **acrosome** reaction. This reaction disperses the outermost layer of the oocyte called **corona radiata**, allowing access to the **zona pellucida**. The first sperm that reaches the **zona pellucida** penetrates it with the aid of several enzymes. Upon penetration, **cortical** reaction occurs, which makes the **zona pellucida** impermeable to other sperm. The **plasma membranes** of the oocyte and sperm fuse. The oocyte at this stage completes its **second** meiotic division and becomes **mature.**

8. Haploid-c; Blastocyst-e; Diploid-d; Morula-a; Blastomeres-b.

9. **i.** Ectoderm; **ii.** Autosomes; **iii.** Mesoderm; **iv.** 300 million; **v.** 200; **vi.** Endoderm; **vii.** Epiblast cells.

10. In the first few days following fertilization, the zygote undergoes mitotic cellular replication and division as it journeys along the uterine tubes. The blastocyst, formed between days 3 and 5, enters the <u>uterus</u>. The blastocyst possesses an inner cell mass (or <u>embryoblast</u>) and an outer cell mass (or <u>trophoblast</u>). Implantation of the <u>trophoblast</u> layer occurs into the endometrium, and this layer is now known as the <u>decidua</u>. The outer cell mass (or <u>trophoblast</u>) becomes the a) <u>placenta</u> and b) chorion, while the inner cell mass (or <u>embryoblast</u>) becomes the c) <u>embryo</u>, d) <u>amnion</u> and e) <u>umbilical cord</u>.

11. True: a, b, c, d, e, f, h, j, k, l.　False: g, i.

12. a.　13. e.　14. d.　15. b.　16. a.　17. d.　18. d.　19. e.

20. Correct: i, ii, iv, v, vi, viii.

21. **i.** One X-chromosome without a Y or second X (monosomy X, Turner syndrome—the only viable human monosomy); XXX, XYY, and XXY or XXXY (Klinefelter syndrome).
ii. Phenylketonuria, galactosaemia and cystic fibrosis.
iii. Achondroplasia, Marfan syndrome and Huntington disease.
iv. Duchenne muscular dystrophy, red/green colour blindness and the haemophilias.

5 The placenta

ANSWERS

1.

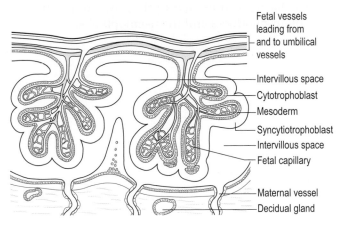

Fetal vessels leading from and to umbilical vessels
Intervillous space
Cytotrophoblast
Mesoderm
Syncytiotrophoblast
Intervillous space
Fetal capillary
Maternal vessel
Decidual gland

Figure 5.1

2.

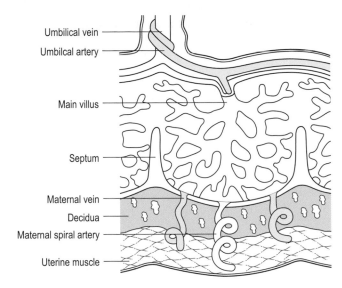

Umbilical vein
Umbilcal artery
Main villus
Septum
Maternal vein
Decidua
Maternal spiral artery
Uterine muscle

Figure 5.2

3.

Table 5.1   Early development of the placenta

a.	By 10 days, the **blastocyst** is completely buried in the decidua. The **trophoblasts** have a potent invasive capacity. The decidua secretes **cytokines** and protease inhibitors that moderate this invasion.
	↓
b.	From about 3 weeks after fertilization, proliferation of projections from the trophoblastic layer form the **chorionic villi.** This becomes more profuse in the **decidual basilis**, where there is a rich blood supply. This is known as the *chorion frondosum*, which will develop into the **placenta**.
	↓
c.	The portion of the decidua surrounding the blastocyst where it projects into the uterine cavity is known as the **decidua capsularis**. The villi under this area degenerates (because of lack of nutrition) forming the **chorion laeve** from where the chorionic membrane originates. The remaining decidua is known as the **decidua vera** (or parietalis).
	↓
d.	As the uterus is filled with the enlarging fetus, the **decidua capsularis** thins and disappears and the chorion meets the **decidua vera** (or parietalis) on the opposite wall of the uterus.
	↓
e.	The villi penetrate the **decidua** and erode the walls of the maternal blood vessels, opening them up to form a lake of maternal blood in which they float. The opening blood vessels are known as **sinuses** and the area surrounding the villi are called **blood spaces**.

4.

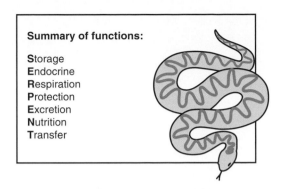

Summary of functions:

Storage
Endocrine
Respiration
Protection
Excretion
Nutrition
Transfer

Figure 5.3 The placenta also provides placental circulation.

5. Maternal blood is discharged into the intervillous space by **80 to 100** spiral arteries within the decidua basilis after **10 to 12 weeks**. Blood flows **slowly** around the villi, eventually returning to the endometrial **veins** and the maternal circulation. There are about **150 mL** of maternal blood in the intervillous spaces, which is exchanged **3 or 4** times per minute.
Fetal blood is **low** in oxygen. The fetal heart pumps the blood towards the placenta along the umbilical **arteries** and then transported along their branches to the **capillaries** of the chorionic **villi** where exchange of nutrients takes place between mother and fetus. After yielding **carbon dioxide** and waste products and absorbing **oxygen** and nutrients, the blood is returned to the fetus via the umbilical **vein**.

6. True: c, e, g, h, i.   False: a, b, d, f, j.

7. **a.** Anchoring villi and nutritive villi;   **b.** Tubercle bacillus or Treponema of syphilis;   **c.** Rubella and human cytomegalovirus;   **d.** Human chorionic gonadotrophin (HCG), progesterone; oestrogens (oestrone; oestradiol; oestriol); human placental lactogen (hPL).

8. 1-d; 2-c; 3-b; 4-e; 5-a.

9. Chorion: a, e, h, i, j, m, n.   Amnion: b, c, d, f, g, k, l.

10. During pregnancy: a, b, e, g, h.   In labour (with intact membranes): c, d, f.

11. Correct: a, c, d, f, h, i, k.   Incorrect: b, e, g, j, l, m.

12. b.   13. c.   14. c.   15. d.   16. b.   17. b.   18. c.   19. b.   20. b.

21. **A.** Circumvallate placenta—description: the membranes (amnion and chorion) have folded back on themselves on the fetal side, forming a thick ring because the chorionic plate is too small. The ring also comprises degenerated decidua vera and fibrin between the membranes. Risk factors: placental abruption, oligohydramnios, preterm birth and miscarriage
B. Battledore placenta—description: an abnormal variation where the umbilical cord attachment is sited at the placental margin, resulting in a racquet style appearance. This type of insertion may progress to a velamentous cord insertion and is associated with monochorionic twin pregnancies. Risk factors: intrauterine growth retardation and consequently low birth weight, fetal distress, cord prolapse and preterm birth.
C. Bilobed placenta (also known as a *bipartite placenta*)—description: this variation refers to a placenta separated into two roughly equal-sized lobes. Further variants may include more lobes which are termed accordingly, for example, 3 lobes=trilobed. Risk factors: bleeding during early pregnancy, polyhydramnios, retained placenta and abruption.

6 The fetus

ANSWERS

1. 0–4 weeks: f, g, n.   4–8 weeks: i.   8–12 weeks: a, c, j.   12–16 weeks: b, d, h, l.   16–20 weeks: e, k, m.

2. 20–24 weeks: d, k,m.   24–28 weeks: b, j.   28–32 weeks: g, l.   32–36 weeks: a, c, f, h, i.   36 weeks–birth: e.

3.

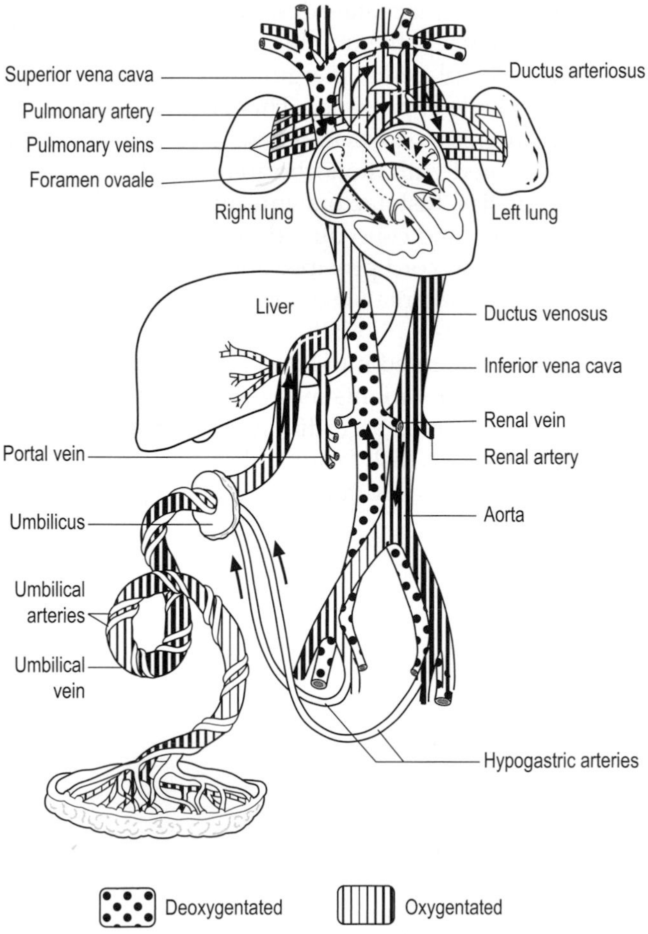

Figure 6.1

4. **a.** Ductus venosus.   **b.** Ductus arteriosus.   **c.** Foramen ovale.   **d.** Hypogastric arteries.

5. Table 6.4
   a. Oxygenated blood from the placenta travels **to** the fetus in the **umbilical vein**. The **umbilical vein** divides into two branches: one that supplies the **portal vein** in the liver, the other the **ductus venosus** joining the **inferior** vena cava.
   b. Most of the oxygenated blood that enters the **right** atrium passes across the foramen ovale to the **left** atrium and from here into the **left** ventricle, and then to the **aorta**. The head and **upper** extremities receive about half of the blood supply via the coronary and carotid arteries, and subclavian arteries, respectively. The remainder of blood travels in the **descending aorta**, mixing with **deoxygenated** blood from the **right** ventricle.
   c. Deoxygenated blood collected from the upper parts of the body returns to the **right** atrium in the **superior** vena cava. Blood that has entered the **right atrium** from the inferior and superior vena cava passes into the **right** ventricle. A small amount of blood travels to the lungs in the **pulmonary artery** for lung development.
   d. Most blood passes through the **ductus arteriosus** into the **descending** aorta. **Deoxygenated** blood travels back to the placenta via the **internal** iliac arteries, leading into the hypogastric **arteries**, which lead into the umbilical **arteries.**

6. **a.** Ligamentum venosum.   **b.** Ligamentum teres (hepatis).   **c.** Ligamentum arteriosum.   **d.** Fossa ovalis.   **e.** Obliterated hypogastric arteries; superior vesical arteries.

7. b.   **8.** d.   **9.** c.   **10.** a.   **11.** d.   **12.** c.   **13.** a.

14. Correct: a, d, e.   Incorrect: b, c, f.

Fetal skull

15. a. 14 bones. **b.** Non-compressible. **c.** The vital centres in the medulla. **d.** Key ossification centres: i. Occipital protuberance, ii. Parietal eminence, iii. Frontal eminence. **e.** Orbital ridges, nape of the neck. **f.** It relates to the process involved in laying down of the bones of the vault from the ossification centres. **g.** A suture is a cranial joint formed where two bones meet. A fontanelle is formed where two or more sutures meet.

16. a. Two frontal bones, Form the forehead and sinciput, Frontal eminence
b. Two parietal bones, Lie on either side of the skull, Parietal eminences
c. Occipital bone, Lies at the back of the head, Occipital protuberance

17. a. Coronal suture, Separates the frontal bones from the parietal bones, passing from one temple to the other.
b. Frontal suture, Runs between the two halves of the frontal bone.
c. Lambdoidal suture, Separates the occipital bone from the two parietal bones.
d. Sagittal suture, Lies between the two parietal bones.

18. a. Posterior fontanelle (or lambda); Small, triangular, shaped like the Greek letter Lambda λ; Situated at the junction of the lambdoidal and sagittal sutures; 6 weeks.
b. Anterior fontanelle (or bregma); Broad, kite-shaped, 3–4 cm long and 1.5–2 cm wide; Found at the junction of the sagittal, coronal and frontal sutures; 18 months.

19.

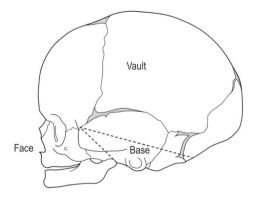

Figure 6.2

20.

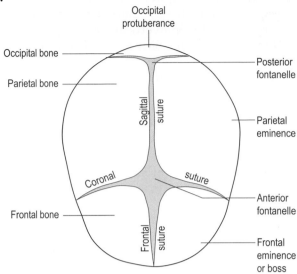

Figure 6.3

21. a. Forehead/sinciput region: this region extends from the anterior fontanelle and the coronal suture to the orbital ridges.
b. Face: this region extends from orbital ridges and the root of the nose to the junction of the chin or mentum (landmark) and the neck. The point between the eyebrows is known as the glabella (landmark).
c. Occiput region: this region lies between the foramen magnum and posterior fontanelle. The part below the occipital protuberance (landmark) is known as the suboccipital region.
d. Vertex region: this region is bounded by the posterior fontanelle, the parietal eminences and anterior fontanelle.

22.

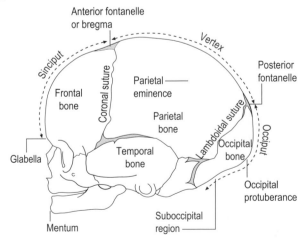

Figure 6.4

23. Table 6.12a: Suboccipitofrontal (SOF)- iii; Occipitofrontal (OF)-iv; Suboccipitobregmatic (SOB)–vi; Submentovertical (SMV)–v; Submentobregmatic (SMB)–ii; Mentovertical (MV)–i.
Table 6.12b: Suboccipitofrontal (SOF)-10 cm; Occipitofrontal (OF)-11.5; Suboccipitobregmatic-9.5 cm Submentovertical (SMV)-11.5 cm; Submentobregmatic (SMB)-9.5 cm; Mentovertical (MV)-13.5 cm.

24. a. Bregma. **b.** Bisacromial diameter-12 cm, distance between the acromion processes on the two shoulder blades. **c.** Bitrochanteric diameter-10 cm, distance between the greater trochanters of the femurs.

25.

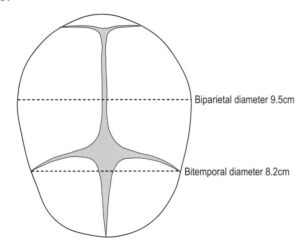

Biparietal diameter 9.5cm

Bitemporal diameter 8.2cm

Figure 6.5

26 a. Vertex presentation: when the head is well flexed, the **suboccipitobregmatic diameter (9.5 cm)** and the **biparietal diameter (9.5 cm)** present. The **suboccipitofrontal diameter (10 cm)** distends the vaginal orifice.
When the head is deflexed, the presenting diameters are the occipitofrontal **(11.5 cm)** and the **biparietal (9.5 cm)**. This often arises when the occiput is in a **posterior** position. If this remains, then the occipitofrontal diameter **(11.5 cm)** distends the vaginal orifice.
b. Face presentation: when the head is completely **extended,** the presenting diameters are the **submentobregmatic (9.5 cm)** and the **bitemporal (8.2 cm)**. The submentovertical diameter **(11.5 cm)** will distend the vaginal orifice.
c. Brow presentation: this occurs when the head is **partially** extended and the **mentovertical diameter (13.5 cm)** and **bitemporal diameter (8.2 cm)** present. Vaginal birth is unlikely.

27. a. Moulding is used to describe the change in shape of the fetal head that takes place during its passage through the birth canal.
b. The bones of the vault allow a slight degree of bending. The skull bones are soft and able to override at the sutures.

28.

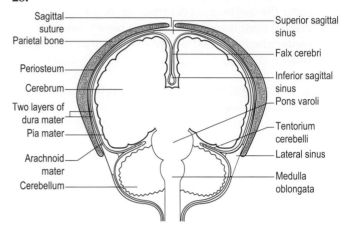

Figure 6.6

29.

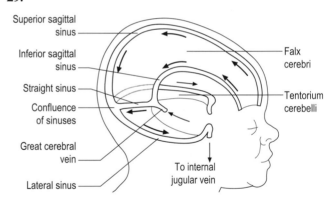

Figure 6.7

30. c.   **31.** c.   **32.** a.   **33.** c.   **34.** b.   **35.** a.

7 Anatomy and physiology: body systems revision

ANSWERS

1. **Haemopoiesis**-Blood cell formation; **Erythrocytes**–Oxygen and carbon dioxide transport function; **Leucocytes**-Defence against microorganism function; **Thrombocytes**–Has a function in haemostasis; **Pluripotent stem cell**-All blood cells descend from this bone marrow cell; **Haematocrit**-Represents the percentage of total blood volume occupied with erythrocytes; **Serum**-Blood plasma without fibrinogen and other clotting factors; **Electrolytes**–Has a function in osmotic distribution of fluid between compartments

2. **i.** pH 7.35–7.45; **ii.** 4–5 litres; **iii.** 45%; **iv.** 6%–8%; **v.** 120 days; **vi.** >99%; **vii.** 5–6 litres; **viii.** 55%

3. **Correct**: i, ii, iv, v, vii.

4.

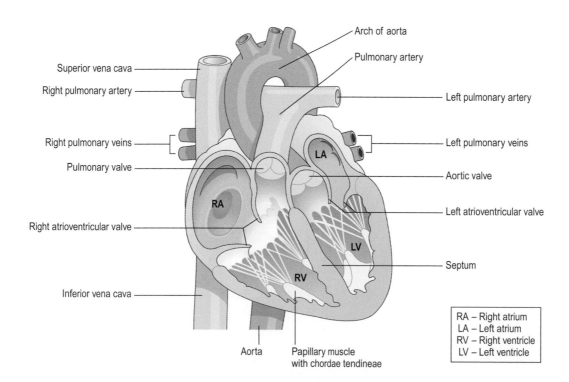

Figure 7.1

5.

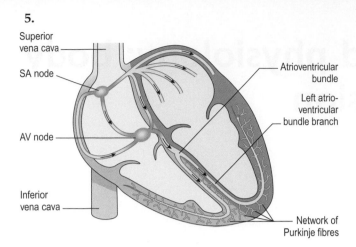

Figure 7.2

6. True: a, c, d, e, f.   False: b, g.

7.

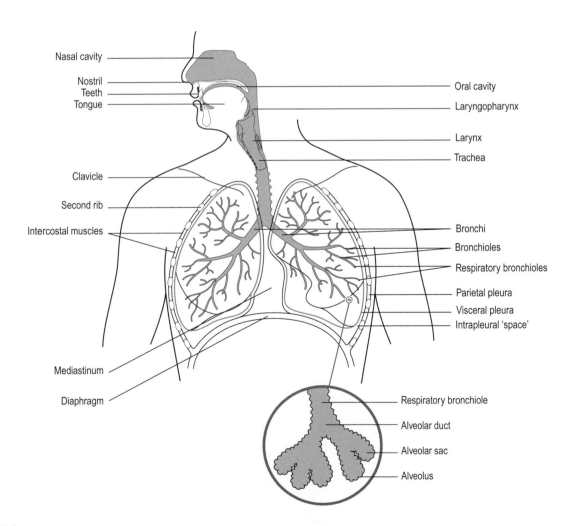

Figure 7.3

8. **Tidal volume (TV)**-Volume of air entering and leaving the lungs during a single breath.
   Residual volume (RV)-Volume of air remaining in the lungs at the end of maximal active expiration.
   Total lung capacity (TLC)-Amount of air in the lungs at the end of a maximum inspiration.
   Minute volume (pulmonary ventilation)-Total volume of air exchanged with the atmosphere in one minute.
   Functional residual capacity (FRC)-Amount of air remaining in the lungs after normal expiration.

9. **a.** vasoconstriction, **b.** stroke volume, **c.** viscosity, **d.** vasodilation, **e.** hydrostatic pressure, **f.** type O-negative blood, **g.** vasomotor tone, **h.** type AB-positive blood, **i.** heat, redness, swelling, pain.

10.

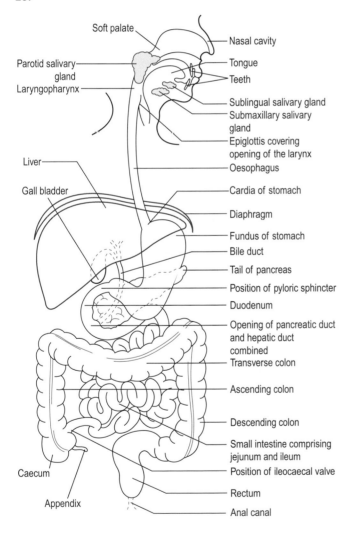

Figure 7.4

11. Correct: a, b, e, f, g, h.

12. **a.** 3.5–5.5 mmol/L.   **b.** (i) glycogenesis, (ii) glycogenolysis, (iii) gluconeogenesis.   **c.** Krebs cycle/citric acid cycle.

13.

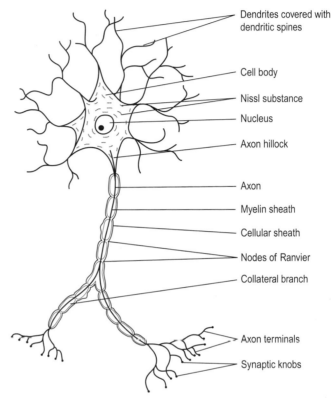

Figure 7.5

14.

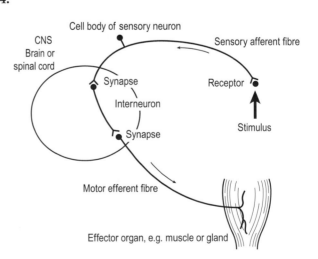

Figure 7.6.

15.

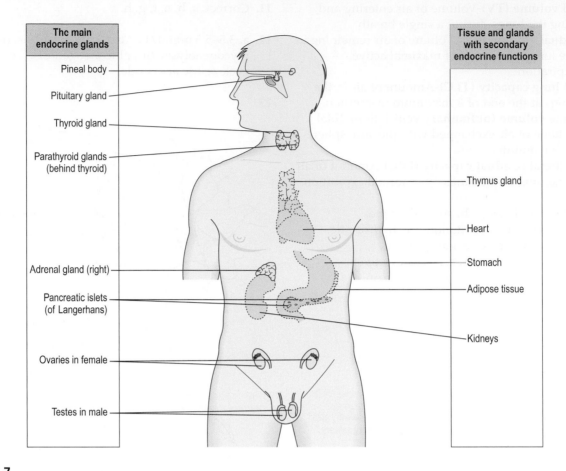

Figure 7.7

16. **Pineal gland**- Melatonin. **Pituitary gland (posterior)**-Antidiuretic hormone (ADH), oxytocin. **Pituitary gland (anterior)**-Thyroid stimulating hormone (TSH), adrenocorticotrophic hormone (ACTH), follicle stimulating hormone (FSH), luteinizing hormone (LH), growth hormone (GH), prolactin (PRL). **Thyroid gland**-Thyroxine, tri-iodothyronine.

17. True: a, b, d, e, f, g, j, k.   False: c, h, i.

8 Changes and adaptation in pregnancy

ANSWERS

1. Table 8.1a. **a.** 3–4+ weeks; **b.** 4 weeks; **c.** 4–14 weeks; **d.** 6–12 weeks; **e.** 16–20 weeks.
   Table 8.1b. **a.** 8+ weeks; **b.** 12–16 weeks; **c.** 16–28 weeks; **d.** 16 weeks; **e.** 8+ weeks; **f.** 6–12 weeks; **g.** 14 days; **h.** 9–10 days; **i.** 8+ weeks.
   Table 8.1c. **a.** 11–12 weeks; **b.** 5.5 weeks; **c.** ≥22 weeks; **d.** 4.5 weeks; **e.** 24+ weeks; **f.** 20+ weeks.

2. Table 8.2: Bladder irritability: a, g.   Nausea and vomiting: b, d, l.   Amenorrhoea: c, i, m. Quickening: e.   Presence of hCG in blood: f. Presence of human chorionic gonadotropin (hCG) in urine: k.   Pulsation of fornices: h. Early breast changes (nulliparous): n.

3. True: a, b, d, e, f, h, i, j, l.   False: c, g, k, m.

4. Table 8.4: 10 weeks' gestation: d.   12 weeks' gestation: b.   15 weeks' gestation: f.   20 weeks' gestation: a and h.   30 weeks' gestation: c. 32 weeks' gestation: i.   36 weeks' gestation: e. 38 weeks' gestation: g.

5. Chadwick's (or Jacquemeir's) sign: a, d. Osiander's sign: c.   Hegar's (or Goodnell's) sign: h. Uterine souffle: b, f, i.   Placental souffle: e, g. Funic souffle: j.

6. **a.** Cervical ripening is a more **accelerated** phase occurring in the **final** weeks of pregnancy. The process of cervical ripening involves **inflammatory** cells but is likely dependent upon **endogenously** produced **prostaglandins**.
   b. Collagen is **reduced** and the cervix becomes **thin**. The rearrangement and degradation of **collagen** fibres creates an **increase** in the space between them, **shortens** them and **increases** acidic solubility along with **reduced** capacity to **retain** water.
   c. The cervix changes to a **soft distensible** structure with **reduced** resistance to effacement and dilatation.

7. **i.** Doderlein's bacillus.   **ii.** Leucorrhoea.   **iii.** pH 3.5–6.   **iv.** Antibacterial plug.   **v.** Engagement. **vi.** Upper uterine segment.   **vii.** Progesterone. **viii.** Effacement.   **ix.** Increase vascularity and oedema.   **x.** Lower uterine segment.

8. b.   **9.** d.   **10.** a.   **11.** c.   **12.** d.   **13.** a.   **14.** e. **15.** d.

16. **A.** CVS: Heart, blood vessels and blood pressure. **B.** Cardiac output: increases by 35%–50%; Heart increases in size and is displaced upward and to the left; Heart rate: increases 10–20 beats per minute (mainly first trimester); Veins: vasodilation and impeded venous return in lower extremities; Systemic and pulmonary dramatic vasodilation to increase blood flow; Systemic blood pressure: minimal change/no reduction; Diastolic blood pressure: decrease, returning to normal by term; Pulmonary and systemic vascular resistance: decrease.

17. **A.** Haematological system: blood components. **B.** Haematology: total body water: increase; Plasma volume: marked increase 45%–50%; Red cell mass increases 18%; Platelets: slight decrease; Total blood volume increases 30%–45%; White cell count-normal levels;   **C.** Biochemistry: potassium-unchanged; Creatinine levels: lower in mid pregnancy (rises toward term); Urea levels: lower.

18. Correct: a, b, c, e, g, h.   Incorrect: d, f, i, j.

19. **a.** Inferior vena cava, the lower aorta. **b.** Dizziness, light-headedness, nausea and possible syncope.   **c.** Hypotension, bradycardia.   **d.** Loss of consciousness: caused by a decrease in blood pressure and cerebral blood flow.   **e.** Fetal compromise: compression of the aorta may lead to reduced uteroplacental and renal blood flow.

20. Increase: Oxygen (O_2) consumption; Metabolic rate; Minute volume; Tidal volume; Arterial O_2 tension; small increase in Arterial pH (PaO_2). Decrease: Functional residual capacity; Arterial CO_2 tension ($PaCO_2$).

21. True: b, c, d, e, g, h, i.   False: a, f.

22. a. Dilatation of the ureters is rarely present **below** the pelvic brim. Dilatation is possibly caused by compression by the enlarging uterus and **ovarian plexus**.
b. The early onset of ureteral dilatation suggests that smooth muscle relaxation, caused by **progesterone**, possibly plays an additional role.
c. Dilatation of the ureters is more marked on the **right** side, because of the cushioning effect of the **sigmoid** colon on the **left** and because of the uterine tendency to **dextrorotation**.

23. Maternal weight (kg): Uterus (0.9 kg) Breasts (0.4 kg)   Fat (4.0 kg)   Blood (1.2 kg) Extracellular fluid (1.2 kg). Total for maternal (7.7 kg)
Fetal weight (kg): Fetus (3.3 kg)   Placenta (0.7 kg)   Amniotic fluid (0.8 kg).

24. a. In late pregnancy, although basal insulin levels are **elevated,** maternal blood glucose levels are similar to nonpregnant levels and do not **reduce** as rapidly as usual even with **higher** circulating levels of insulin. This diabetogenic state protects the fetus, even if the mother is fasting by keeping glucose in the blood and thus available for placental transfer.
b. Normal glucose ranges during pregnancy are **3.4 to 5.5 mmol/L**. After a meal, however, the pregnant woman's levels of glucose and insulin are **higher** than those of nonpregnant women and **glycogen** is suppressed resulting in **hyper**insulinaemia, **hyper**glycaemia and insulin resistance.

25. a. (i) Progesterone; (ii) Oestrogen; (iii) Relaxin; (iv) Leptide.   **b.** Sacroiliac and sacrococcygeal joints.   **c.** Epulis.   **d.** Ptyalism.   **e.** Pica. **f.** chloasma (or melasma): Pigmentation of the face caused by melanin deposition into epidermal and dermal macrophages.   **g.** Pruritis, hyperpigmentation, some degree of skin darkening, linea nigra, striae gravidarum (stretch marks), peripheral vasodilation, acceleration of sweat gland activity, angiomas or vascular spiders (on face, neck, arms and chest), palmar erythema.

26. From early pregnancy: Development of duct system, Oestrogen.
From early pregnancy: Development of lobular formation, Progesterone.
3–4 weeks: Prickling, tingling sensation, particularly around the nipple, Increased blood supply.
6–8 weeks: Increase in size, painful, tense and nodular, delicate, bluish surface, veins become visible just beneath the skin. Hypertrophy of the alveoli. Human Placental Lactogen (hPL) and Oestrogen.
8–12 weeks: Montgomery tubercles become more prominent on the areola. Glands secrete sebum to keep nipple soft. Hypertrophy of the glands. Human Placental Lactogen (hPL) and oestrogen.
8–12 weeks: The pigmented area around the nipple (primary areola) darkens and may become more erectile. Increased melanin activity.
16 weeks: Colostrum can be expressed/the secondary areola develops with further extension of the pigmented area (often mottled in appearance), Prolactin/Oestrogen.
Late pregnancy: Colostrum may leak from the breast. The nipple becomes more prominent and mobile, Prolactin/Progesterone.

27. d.   **28.** e.   **29.** d.   **30.** d.   **31.** d.   **32.** d.   **33.** a. **34.** b.   **35.** c.   **36.** d.

9 Antenatal care and problems in pregnancy

ANSWERS

1. Correct: c, d, f, h, k.

2. Underweight: <18.5 kg/m². Normal/healthy: 18.5–24.9 kg/m². Overweight: 25.0–29.9 kg/m². Obese: ≥30 kg/m². Very obese ≥40 kg/m² (NICE PH27, 2010)

3. **a.** Ketonuria–ketones are caused by the breakdown of fat.
   b. Ketonuria may be caused by a variety of reasons, including vomiting, hyperemesis, starvation or excessive exercise.
   c. Medical: pyelonephritis, obstetric: preterm labour.
   d. Preeclampsia.
   e. Blood group, rhesus factor, full blood count.
   f. Venereal disease research laboratory (VDRL), rubella immune status, human immunodeficiency virus (HIV) antibodies (now recommended that this test is routinely offered to women), haemoglobinopathies, hepatitis B, screening tests for other blood disorders, for example, sickle cell anaemia or thalassaemias.
   g. Infections not currently recommended as routine: hepatitis c, chlamydia (women <25 years are screened through a national screening programme), cytomegalovirus, toxoplasmosis, group B streptococcus.

4. True: a, b, c, f. g. h, k, l, m, n. o.   False: d, e, i, j

5. Presentation: Refers to the part of the fetus lying at the pelvic brim or in the lower pole of the uterus; Vertex, face and brow are all cephalic presentations
   Lie: The refers to the relationship between the long axis of the fetus and long axis of the uterus
   Position: Refers to the relationship between the denominator of the presentation and the six key points on the pelvic brim
   Attitude: Refers to the relationship between the denominator of the presentation and the six key points on the pelvic brim
   Denominator: Refers to the name of the part of the presentation used when referring to fetal position

6.

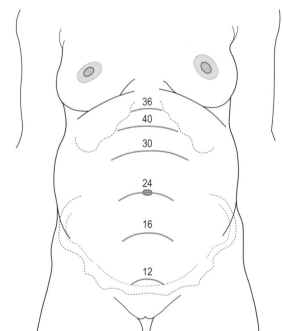

Figure 9.1

257

7.

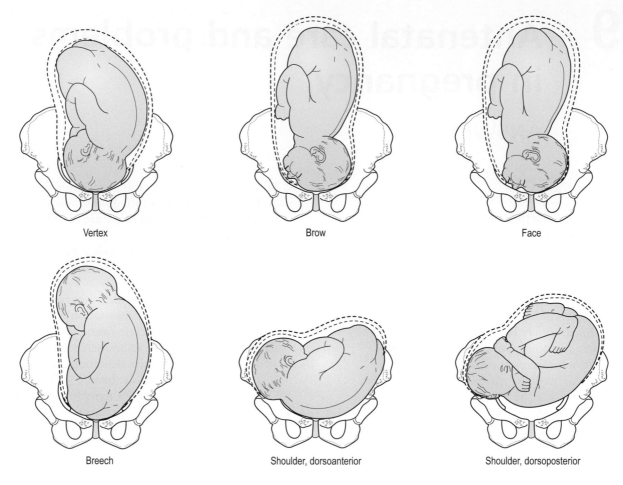

Vertex

Brow

Face

Breech

Shoulder, dorsoanterior

Shoulder, dorsoposterior

Figure 9.2

8.

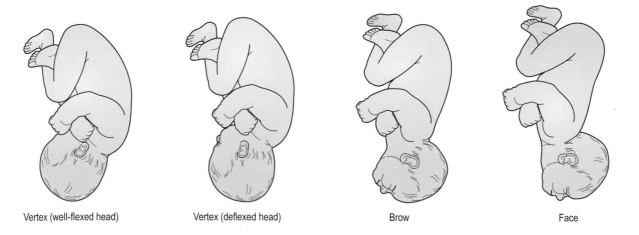

Vertex (well-flexed head)

Vertex (deflexed head)

Brow

Face

Figure 9.3

9.

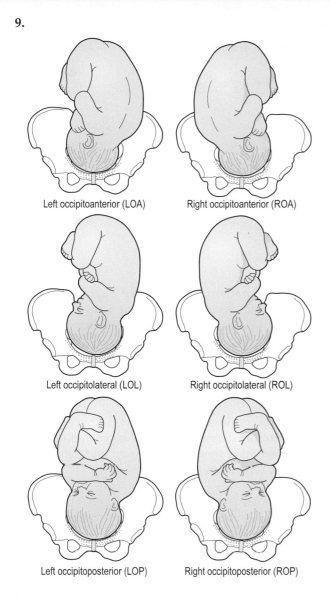

Left occipitoanterior (LOA)

Right occipitoanterior (ROA)

Left occipitolateral (LOL)

Right occipitolateral (ROL)

Left occipitoposterior (LOP)

Right occipitoposterior (ROP)

Figure 9.4

10. a. Transverse.   **b.** ≥36 weeks' gestation.
c. Biparietal 9.5 cm.   **d.** Bitrochanteric 10 cm.
e. Malposition, occipitoposterior position,
wrongly calculated gestational age,
polyhydramnios, cephalopelvic disproportion,
placenta praevia, multiple pregnancy and fetal
abnormalities.   **f.** Full bladder, pelvic
abnormalities

11. a. Transverse, longitudinal, oblique.   **b.** Flexion.
c. Mentum,   **d.** Sacrum.   **e.** Occiput.   **f.** Increasing
uterine size in comparison with the gestational age
of the fetus; Fetal movements that follow a regular
pattern from the time when they are first felt; Fetal
heart rate that is regular and variable with a rate
between 110 and 160 beats per minute.

12. a. Direct occipitoanterior (DOA): The occiput
points to the symphysis pubis; the sagittal suture
is in the anteroposterior diameter of the pelvis.
b. Left occipitoanterior (LOA): The occiput points
to the left iliopectineal eminence; the sagittal
suture is in the right oblique diameter of the
pelvis.
c. Right occipitolateral (ROL): The occiput points
to the right iliopectineal line midway between the
iliopectineal eminence and the sacroiliac joint; the
sagittal suture is in the transverse diameter of
the pelvis.
d. Right occipitoanterior (ROA): The occiput
points to the right iliopectineal eminence; the
sagittal suture is in the left oblique diameter of the
pelvis.
e. Direct occipitoposterior (DOP): The occiput
points to the sacrum; the sagittal suture is in the
anteroposterior diameter of the pelvis.
f. Left occipitoposterior (LOP): The occiput points
to the left sacroiliac joint; the sagittal suture is in
the left oblique diameter of the pelvis.
g. Left occipitolateral (LOL): The occiput points to
the left iliopectineal line midway between the
iliopectineal eminence and the sacroiliac joint; the
sagittal suture is in the transverse diameter of the
pelvis.
h. Right occipitoposterior (ROP): The occiput
points to the right sacroiliac joint; the sagittal
suture is in the right oblique diameter of the
pelvis.

13.

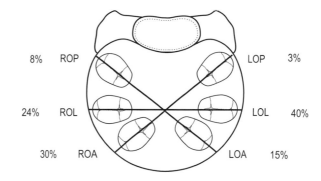

8%	ROP		LOP	3%
24%	ROL		LOL	40%
30%	ROA		LOA	15%

Figure 9.5

ROP: 8%; ROA: 30%; ROL: 24%; LOP: 3%; LOA:
15%; LOL: 40%

14. d

15. d

16. d

17. e.

18. c.

19. a

20. a. Intestinal obstruction, inflammatory bowel disease, appendicitis, UTI/pyelonephritis, acute cholestasis/cholelithiasis, gastro-oesophageal reflux/peptic ulcer disease, acute pancreatitis
b. Malaria, TB, malignant disease, psychological causes, sickle cell crisis, porphyria, rectus haematoma, arteriovenous haematoma.
c. Severe uterine torsion can become pathological.

21. Physiological: Heartburn, Soreness from vomiting, Round ligament pain, Braxton hicks contractions, Constipation, Pressure from growing fetus (vigorous/malpresenting).
Pathological: Placental abruption, Ectopic pregnancy, Abdominal pregnancy, Chorioamnionitis, Preterm labour, Hyperemesis gravidarum, Uterine/ovarian tumours, Spontaneous uterine rupture, Spontaneous miscarriage.

22. a. Recurrent miscarriage.   **b.** Ectopic pregnancy.   **c.** Implantation bleeding.   **d.** Spontaneous miscarriage.   **e.** Induced/therapeutic termination of pregnancy.   **f.** Criminal termination of pregnancy.   **g.** Inevitable miscarriage.   **h.** Missed or silent miscarriage.   **i.** Complete miscarriage.   **j.** Threatened miscarriage.   **k.** Incomplete miscarriage.   **l.** Cervical ectropion (cervical erosion).   **m.** Cervical polyps.

23. a. Genetic abnormalities.
b. Maternal general illness and maternal infection.
c. Abnormalities of the uterus, cervical incompetence.
d. Disorders of the endocrine system, endocrine factors, autoimmune factors and thrombophilic defects and alloimmune factors.
e. Uterine and adnexal tenderness, purulent vaginal loss and pyrexia.
f. Endotoxic shock, fatal hypotension, renal failure, disseminated intravascular coagulopathy and multiple petechial haemorrhages.
g. *Escherichia coli, Streptococcus faecalis, Staphylococcus albus* and *aureus, Klebsiella, Clostridium welchii* and *C. perfringens*.

24.

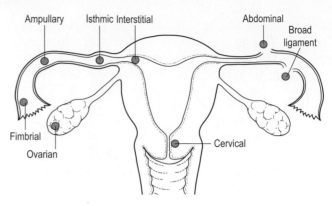

Figure 9.6

25. Classical pattern of symptoms: Vaginal bleeding, Lower abdominal pain of sudden onset starting locally, Lower abdominal pain becoming generalized as blood loss extends into the peritoneal cavity, Subdiaphragmatic irritation by blood produces referred shoulder tip pain and discomfort on breathing, May be episodes of syncope.
Clinical findings: Hypotension, Tachycardia, Abdominal distension, Guarding of abdomen with rebound tenderness, Closed and acutely tender when moved.

26. a. In molar pregnancy, the development of the placenta is **abnormal**, resulting in complete or incomplete hydatidiform mole with **no viable fetus**. The grape-like appearance of the mole is caused by **over-proliferation** of the **chorionic villi**. The condition becomes apparent in **second trimester** and most commonly presents with **bleeding**. The four associated conditions characterizing the condition include anaemia (unexplained), severe hyperemesis, preeclampsia and ovarian cysts.
b. Initially, it is usually diagnosed as a **threatened miscarriage**. The uterus is **larger** than dates in about half of the cases. If the mole remains in situ, diagnosis is confirmed by ultrasound examination revealing a '**snowstorm**' appearance and continuing raised **hCG levels**. Treatment is by **evacuation of the uterus**. Another associated disorder arising if the mole does not spontaneously miscarry is a variation of the disease progressing to **choriocarcinoma**.

27. True: b, c, e, g, i.   False: a, d, f, h.

28. Antepartum haemorrhage: Bleeding from the genital tract after the 24th week of pregnancy and before the onset of labour.

   Placenta abruption: Premature separation of a normally situated placenta occurring after the 24th week of pregnancy

   Revealed haemorrhage: Blood escapes from the placental site, separates the membranes from the uterine wall and drains through the vagina

   Concealed haemorrhage: Blood is retained behind the placenta where it is forced back into the myometrium

   Couvelaire uterus (uterine apoplexy): In haemorrhage, seepage of blood outside the normal vascular channels can cause marked damage (uterus observed as bruised, oedematous enlarged at operation)

   Placenta praevia: The placenta is partially or wholly implanted in the lower uterine segment.

   Acute emergency obstetric haemorrhage: At least two-thirds of placenta has detached with ≥2000 mL blood loss from circulation.

29. Type 1 placenta praevia: g, k, l.   Type 2 placenta praevia: a, c, e, j, m.   Type 3 placenta praevia: b, h, n.   Type 4 placenta praevia: d, f, i.

30. True: a, b, c, d, f, h.   False e, g.

31. Normal blood clotting occurs in three main stages: (1) When tissues are damaged and platelets break down, thromboplastin is released; (2) In the presence of calcium ions, thromboplastin leads to the conversion of prothrombin into thrombin; (3) Thrombin is a proteolytic (protein-splitting) enzyme that converts fibrinogen into fibrin.

   Fibrin forms a network of long-sticky strands that entrap blood cells to form a clot. The coagulated material contracts and exudes a serum, which is plasma depleted of clotting factors. The coagulation mechanism is normally held at bay by the presence of heparin which is produced in the liver.

   Fibrinolysis is the breakdown of fibrin and occurs in response to the presence of clotted blood. Coagulation will continue unless fibrinolysis takes place.

   NICE (2010) Weight management before, during and after pregnancy (Public Health guideline 27). Available: https://www.nice.org.uk/guidance/ph27

32. a. Hypertension, Sudden reduction in uterine size (e.g., membrane rupture after twin 1), High parity, Previous c/s, Trauma, Cigarette smoking
   b. Increased temperature (infection in uterus), Increased pulse and respirations, Low BP
   c. Uterus tense and painful, FHR may be normal, erratic or absent, Not too uncomfortable for the woman
   d. Renal failure, Pituitary failure
   e. Placental abruption, intrauterine fetal death, amniotic fluid embolism, intrauterine infection, preeclampsia and eclampsia.

33. True: b, c, d, e, f, h.   False: a, g, i.

34. a. Normal amniotic fluid increases in amount until 38 weeks is: 1 litre
   b. Preterm prelabour rupture of the membranes (PPROM) occurs before: 37 completed weeks
   c. Acute hydramnios usually occurs in pregnancy around: 20 weeks' gestation
   d. Two main factors frequently associated with acute hydramnios include: monozygotic twins and severe fetal abnormality
   e. Chronic hydramnios has a gradual onset usually starting at: 30 weeks' gestation
   f. Two risks associated with PPROM include: cord prolapse, antepartum haemorrhage
   g. Normal amniotic fluid at term is: 800 mL
   h. Amniotic fluid volume at term in oligohydramnios is: 300–500 mL.

35. f.   36. c.   37. a.   38. c.   39. a.

10 Conditions in pregnancy

ANSWERS

1. Common CHD in pregnancy: Atrial septal defect (ASD), Patent ductus arteriosus (PDA), Ventricular septal defect (VSD), Aortic stenosis, Pulmonary stenosis, Teratology of Fallot.
   Eisenmenger's syndrome: A large left-right shunt of blood is apparent through patent VSD, ASD and PDA. Pregnancy is not advised.
   Marfan syndrome: Autosomal-dominant (chromosome 15) disorder of connective tissue, this condition affects the musculoskeletal system, CVS and eyes. May result in aortic dilatation and rupture late in pregnancy/labour.
   Rheumatic heart disease: This condition causes inflammation and scarring of the heart valves resulting in valve stenosis with or without regurgitation.

2. **Correct**: a, b, c, e, f.

3. **a.** <11 g/dL, <110 g/L. **b.** Gastric malabsorption, multiple pregnancy, chronic blood loss, secondary causes to medical conditions. **c.** Short intervals between pregnancies, chronic infection. **d.** Tiredness, irritability, depressions, breathlessness, poor memory, muscle aches, palpitations, cardiac failure, exhaustion, poor recovery from blood loss postpartum (PP). **e.** Vitamin B. **f.** Cell growth, synthesis of ribonucleic acid (RNA) and deoxyribonucleic acid (DNA) – embryo/neural tube defects. **g.** Megaloblastic anaemia. **h.** Haemoglobinopathies.

4. Preexisting factors: Parity >3, smoking, varicose veins, age >35 years, previous VTE/ family history of VTE
   Obstetric factors: Dehydration/hyperemesis gravidarum, preeclampsia, prolonged labour
   Transient factors: Immobility, travel >4 hours, ovarian hyperstimulation syndrome, systemic infection

5. **True**: a, b, c, d, e, g. **False**, f.

6. Mild hypertension: Diastolic BP 90–99 mmHg, systolic BP 140–149 mmHg.
   Moderate hypertension: Diastolic BP 100–109 mmHg, systolic BP 150–159 mmHg.
   Severe hypertension: Diastolic BP ≥110 mmHg, systolic BP ≥160 mmHg.
   Chronic hypertension: Hypertension present at booking or <20 weeks, or if antihypertensive medication prescribed when referred (primary or secondary aetiology).
   New, gestational or pregnancy-induced hypertension: New hypertension presenting after 20 weeks without significant proteinuria.
   Preeclampsia: Diagnosed on the basis of new hypertension with significant proteinuria ≥20 weeks; A multi-system disorder affecting the placenta, kidney, brain and other organs.
   Eclampsia: Neurological condition associated with preeclampsia manifesting with onset of seizures (pregnancy/PP); Unrelated to other cerebral pathological conditions.
   Superimposed preeclampsia: Development of preeclampsia with preexisting hypertension and/or preexisting proteinuria.
   Secondary hypertension: Developed as a result of an underlying physiological condition or pathology.
   New proteinuria: Proteinuria defined as 1+ (300 mg/L or more) on dipstick testing, a protein-creatinine ratio of ≥30 mg/mmol on random sample, or urine proteinuria excretion ≥300 mg/24 hours.

7. True: a, c, d, e, g, i, j, k. False: b, f, h.

8. **a.** HELLP syndrome is a **multisystem** disorder occurring either on its own or in association with **preeclampsia**. Of all cases, **70%** will present in the antenatal period and **30%** postpartum. Antenatally, the disorder typically manifests itself between **32 and 34 weeks' gestation** and typical onset postpartum is within **48** hours of birth.
b. The disorder involves activation of the **coagulation** system. This causes increased deposits of protein **fibrin** throughout the body resulting in fragmentation of **erythrocytes**. **Fibrin** deposits on blood vessel walls initiate clumping of **platelets** resulting in blood clots and lowering of the **platelet** count. Deposits **decrease** the diameter of blood vessels, **raising** the blood pressure and **reducing** blood flow to organs. The **liver is** especially affected.
c. Haemolysis, Elevated Liver enzymes, Low Platelet count.
d. Malaise, nausea and vomiting, upper abdominal pain with tenderness, some nonspecific viral-like symptoms.
e. Abruptio placentae, disseminated intravascular coagulation, eclampsia, acute renal failure and liver haematoma and rupture, pulmonary oedema, adult respiratory distress.

9. Eclampsia: This is a **neurological** condition associated with **convulsions and coma** that cannot be attributed to other conditions, such as **epilepsy**. Eclampsia can develop from **20 weeks' gestation until 6 weeks' postpartum**.
Blood pressure: There is a sharp **rise** in BP.
Headache: This is described as being **severe** and **persistent**. It is usually located in the **frontal** region. This is caused by **cerebral vasospasm**.
Level of consciousness: The woman is typically **drowsy** and **confused**. This is caused by **cerebral vasospasm**.
Visual: Visual disturbances are caused by cerebral vasospasm. Blurring of vision and blindness.
Urinary output: Urinary output is **diminished**. Proteinuria may **increase**. This woman is in **renal** failure.
Abdominal pain: There is **liver** oedema. This causes the woman to complain of **upper** abdominal pain. The woman may also have **nausea and vomiting**.

10. **Type 1 diabetes**: Occurs when **beta** cells in the Islets of Langerhans located in the **pancreas** are destroyed, stopping the production of **insulin**.
Type 2 diabetes: Results from a **defect** in the action of **insulin**. Three main factors age, obesity and lack of physical activity.
Gestational diabetes (GDM): GDM is defined as **carbohydrate intolerance** resulting in **hyperglycaemia** of variable severity. Onset or first recognition occurs during **pregnancy**.
a. Hyperglycaemia and glycosuria
b. Excessive thirst, excessive urinary excretion and unexplained weight loss
c. Peripheral arterial disease, kidney disease, loss of vision, coronary heart disease and nerve damage

11. Table 10.11
a. Haematological-related values: Nonpregnant: 12g/dL, Pregnant: 11 g/dL, Severe anaemia: <7 g/dL. b. Normal lifespan: erythrocytes 120 days, Sickle cells 17 days. c. $150–400 \times 10^9$/L. Blood plasma glucose (metabolic) values: Normal nonpregnant range: 3–5 mmol/L, Nonpregnant (diagnosed DM): Normal fasting range: 5–7 mmol/L, Plasma glucose before meals: 4–7 mmol/L.
b. Pregnant with DM: Fasting: 5.3 mmol/L, 1 hour after meals: 7.8 mmol/L, 2 hours after meals: 6.4 mmol/L.
c. Hypoglycaemia: <2.2 mmol/L.
d. Severe hyperglycaemia: >25.0 mmol/L.

12. **a.** BMI, Previous macrosomic baby, FH of DM, ethnic family origin (high DM prevalence).
b. Oral glucose tolerance test (GTT) (2 hour – 75 g oral glucose).
c. Ketoacidosis.
d. Miscarriage, preeclampsia, preterm labour.
e. Congenital malformations, macrosomia.
f. Birth injury, stillbirth, neonatal asphyxia, Respiratory Distress Syndrome (RDS), mortality, polycythaemia, hyperbilirubinaemia.
g. Diabetic retinopathy, microvascular disease, atherosclerosis, infection.

13. Correct: a, b, c, e, g.

14. e.   **15.** b.   **16.** d.   **17.** c.   **18.** e.   **19.** a.

20. True: b, c, d, e, f, g, i, j, k, l.   False: a, h.

21. Transmitted sexually: Human immunodeficiency virus (HIV), Trichomoniasis, Group B streptococcus (GBS), Gonorrhoea, Hepatitis B virus (HBV), Chlamydia, Syphilis.
Not transmitted sexually: Hepatitis B virus (HBV), Herpes simplex virus (HSV) Type 2 HSV-2, Human cytomegalovirus (CMV), Bacterial vaginosis (BV), Genital warts.
Close sexual contact (increased sexual activity): Vulvovaginal candidiasis, Herpes simplex virus (HSV) - Type 1 HSV-1.

22. Correct: i, ii, iii, iv, v, vi, vii.

23. Monozygotic twins: uniovular twins, identical twins, develop from the fusion of one oocyte and one spermatozoon, always the same sex, have the same genes, blood group and physical features.
Dizygotic twins: fraternal twins, two oocytes fertilised by two spermatozoa, binovular twins, same or different sex.

24. a. Superfecundation.   **b.** Zygosity.
c. Superfetation.   **d.** Ultrasound scan.
e. Polyhydramnios, anaemia, exacerbation of common disorders.   **f.** Twin-to-twin transfusion syndrome, fetal malformations, conjoined twins, twin reversed arterial perfusion.
g. Malpresentation, PROM.   **h.** Cord prolapse, locked twins.

25. True: a, b, e, f, g, i.   False: c, d.

26. c.   **27.** b.   **28.** b.   **29.** d.

11 Labour: first and second stages

ANSWERS

1. True: b, d, e, f, g, h, i, k, l, n.   False: a, c, j, m.

2. **a.** First stage is associated with a progressive **rise** in cardiac output as each contraction **adds** 300–500 mL of blood **to** the circulating volume.
b. Cardiac output **rises** in first stage **10%–15% above** pregnancy values and **50% above** pregnancy levels during second stage.
c. Within **1 hour** of birth, cardiac parameters **fall** to prelabour levels and may take up to **6–8 weeks** to return to prepregnancy levels.
d. Haemoglobin levels tend to **increase** slightly in labour because of the haemoconcentration from muscular activity and dehydration.
e. Erythropoiesis (formation of RBCs) and white blood cell (WBC) count **increase** because of the stress of labour and postpartum.
f. A transitory **increase** in the activity of the coagulation system occurs during labour and **immediately** following placental separation.
g. Clot formation in the torn blood vessels on placental separation needs to be **maximized** and blood loss from haemorrhage **minimized**.
h. A **decrease** in fibrinolytic activity enhances clot formation at the placental site.
i. Placental site is **rapidly** covered by a fibrin mesh utilizing **5%–10%** of circulating **fibrinogen**.
j. Too frequent occurrence of contractions results in the **decrease** in the oxygenation of the myometrium resulting in **metabolic acidosis**.
k. Strong frequent uterine contractions **increase** in Pco_2 (because of the change to anaerobic metabolism) leading to a **fall** in pH and causing **maternal acidosis**.
l. During labour, pain cause the respiratory rate to **increase** and tidal volume to **increase**.
m. Maternal hyperventilation leads to **respiratory alkalosis**.
n. During labour, the **increase** found in maternal and fetal renin-angiotensin may be important for **reducing** uteroplacental blood flow following birth.

3. All correct a–f.   **4.** a.   **5.** b.   **6.** All correct a–d.
7. b, c, and d.   **8.** e.   **9.** b, d.   **10.** e.   **11.** a.   **12.** b.

13. Latent first stage: a period of time, not necessarily continuous, when there are painful contractions and; a period of time, not necessarily continuous when there is some cervical change, including cervical effacement and dilatation up to 4 cm.
Established first stage: regular painful contractions confirmed, there is progressive cervical dilatation from 4 cm
Second stage (Passive): finding of full dilatation of the cervix before or in the absence of involuntary expulsive contractions
Second stage (Active): baby is visible, expulsive contractions with a finding of full dilatation of the cervix or other signs of full dilatation of the cervix, active maternal effort following confirmation of full dilatation of the cervix in the absence of expulsive contractions.
Third stage: from birth of baby to the expulsion of the placenta and membranes.

14. **a.** Cervical effacement.   **b.** Spurious labour.
c. Retraction.   **d.** Lower uterine segment.
e. Show.   **f.** Upper uterine segment.
g. Operculum.   **h.** Retraction ring.   **i.** Polarity.
j. Uterine contractions.   **k.** Contraction and retraction.   **l.** Bandl's ring.

15. Correct: a, b, c, e, f, h, i.   Incorrect: d, g, j.

16. Lie: Relationship of the long axis of the fetus and the long axis of the uterus. It may be longitudinal, oblique or transverse.
Presentation: That part of the fetus which lies at the pelvic brim or in the lower pole of the uterus.
Attitude: The relationship of the fetal head and limbs to its body. It may be fully flexed, deflexed or partially/completely extended.
Denominator: Identifies the name of the part of the presentation used when referring to fetal position in relation to the pelvis.
Position: Relationship of the denominator to the six key points on the maternal pelvic brim.
Engagement: This occurs when the widest presenting transverse diameter has passed through the brim of pelvis.
Presenting part: This refers to that part of the fetus lying over the cervical os during labour.

17. Correct: a, b, d, e, f, h, j, k.   Incorrect: c, g, i, l.

18. Labia: Any sign of varicosities, oedema or vulval warts or sores.
Perineum: Any scars (previous episiotomy) or tear including scarring from cultural female genital mutilation.
Vaginal orifice: Discharge, bleeding.
Rectum: Loaded or impacted, cystocele (in multiparous women).
Cervix: Effacement and dilatation, length of the cervical canal, consistency of cervix and application to the presenting part.
Amniotic membranes: Present or absent, intact membranes, consistency of membranes, bulging, ease or difficulty in feeling membranes.
Fetal head: Descent estimation in relationship to maternal ischial spines (above or below spines), presence of moulding or caput succedaneum, position of fetal head (defined by occiput), attitude (using sutures and fontanelles located).
Other observations (if present): Colour and odour of any discharge or amniotic fluid if membranes have ruptured.

19. True: b, c, d, e, f, h, i, j, k, m.   False: a, g, l.

20. **a.** Baseline rate, presence/absence of decelerations, baseline variability, presence of accelerations.
b. Reassuring,   **c.** Nonreassuring.   **d.** Abnormal.
e. Pathological.   **f.** Suspicious.   **g.** Deceleration.
h. Bradycardia.   **i.** Normal.   **j.** Acceleration

21. b.   22. a, c, f.   23. d.   24. a, b, d.   25. a, b, c, d.
26. a, b, c, e.

27. **a.** Pain may induce changes in the **sympathetic** nervous system with release of **adrenaline (epinephrine)** into the bloodstream resulting in changes in the body systems.
b. *Respiratory system:*
Increased respiratory rate. This change may cause a **decrease** in $PaCO_2$ level with a corresponding **increase** in pH. The fetus will be affected with a subsequent **drop** in the fetal $PaCO_2$. This may be suspected by the presence of **late** decelerations on the CTG.
Hyperventilation may alter the acid–base equilibrium of the system. Resulting **alkalosis** may then affect the diffusion of **oxygen** across the placenta leading to fetal **hypoxia.**
c. *Cardiovascular system:*
Increased heart rate and blood pressure is associated with **sympathetic** response and **increase** in cardiac output. In the second stage, cardiac output **increases** by about **50%**. Pain apprehension and fear may cause a **sympathetic** response producing more of an **increase** in cardiac output.
d. *Other changes:*
- **increase** in blood glucose levels;
- **decrease** in gastric motility leading to a **delay** in stomach emptying (possible nausea and vomiting);
- **delay** in bladder emptying;
- **decrease** in cerebral and uterine blood flow because of **vasoconstriction;**
- **decrease** in blood supply to the skin (causing sweating).

28.

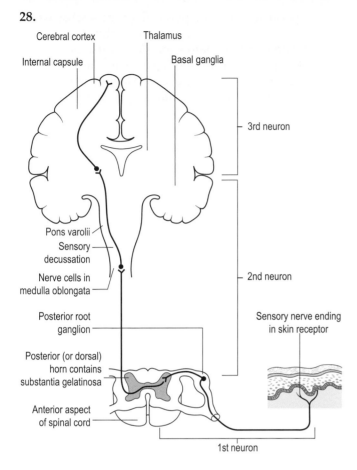

Figure 11.1

29.

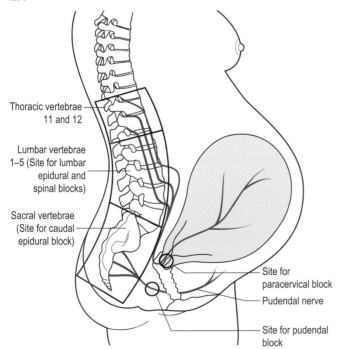

Figure 11.2

30.

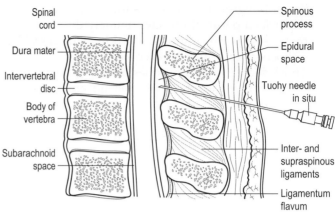

Figure 11.3

31. True: a, b. c. d. e, g, h, i, j, k, n, o, p.   False: f, l, m.

32. a. Ferguson's reflex.   **b.** Rhomboid of Michaelis.   **c.** Anal cleft line.   **d.** Fetal axis pressure.

33. a. Bladder,   **b.** Urethra.   **c.** Rectum.   **d.** Levator ani.   **e.** Perineal body.   **f.** Upright positions, squatting, all fours, standing-kneeling, using a birth ball.   **g.** Reduced pain levels and subsequent responses, less risk of: supine hypotension, reduced placental perfusion, diminished fetal oxygenation, decrease in the efficiency of uterine contractions.

34. i. The activity involving **descent** of the fetus takes place.
ii. Whichever part leads and first meets the **resistance** of the pelvic floor will **rotate** forward, until it comes under the **symphysis pubis**.
iii. Whatever emerges from the **pelvis** will pivot around the **pubic bone**.

35. i. Descent.   **ii.** Flexion.   **iii.** Internal rotation of the head.   **iv.** Extension of the head.
v. Restitution.   **vi.** Internal rotation of the shoulders.   **vii.** Lateral flexion.

36. a. Flexion.   **b.** Restitution.   **c.** Descent.
d. Internal rotation of the head.   **e.** Internal rotation of the head.   **f.** Internal rotation of the head.   **g.** Flexion.   **h.** Extension of the head.
i. Lateral flexion.   **j.** Extension of the head.
k. Internal rotation of the head.   **l.** Restitution.
m. Internal rotation of the shoulders.

37. First-degree tear: involves fourchette only.
Second-degree tear: involves fourchette and superficial perineal muscles, namely the transverse perineal muscles and in some cases the pubococcygeus may be involved.
Third-degree tear: comprises partial or complete disruption of the anal sphincter muscles. This may involve either or both external and internal anal sphincter muscles.
Fourth-degree tear: This tear involves skin of the fourchette, perineum and perineal body (superficial and deep pelvic floor muscle) as well as the external and internal anal sphincter and anal epithelium. Main superficial muscles - bulbospongiosus (bulbocavernosus) and transversus perineal muscles. Main deep pelvic floor muscles involved: iliococcygeus muscle.

38. True: a, c, d, e, g, h, i, j, k.   False: b, f,

39. c.   **40.** a.   **41.** b.   **42.** e.   **43.** e.

12 Third stage of labour

ANSWERS

1. Active management: Uterotonic drugs; controlled cord traction after signs of placenta separation, deferred cord clamping and cutting of the cord (not earlier than 1 minute from birth of healthy baby); diagnosis: 'Prolonged' if incomplete >30 minutes from birth.
Physiological management: Uterotonic drugs are not routinely used; placental delivery by maternal effort; no clamping of the cord (until pulsation has stopped): 'Prolonged' if incomplete >60 minutes from birth; also known as *expectant* management.

2. **a.** The unique characteristic of uterine muscle lies in its power of **retraction**. During the second stage, the uterine cavity progressively empties, enabling the **retraction** process to <u>accelerate</u>. At the beginning of third stage, the **placental site** has already **diminished** in area by about **75%**.
b. As this occurs, the placental becomes <u>compressed</u> and the blood in the **intervillous spaces** is forced back into the spongy layer of the <u>decidua basilis</u>. **Retraction** of the <u>oblique</u> uterine muscle fibres exerts pressure on the blood vessels so that blood does not drain back into the **maternal system**. The vessels during this process are termed '<u>tortuous</u>' as they become **tense** and **congested** with blood.
c. With the next contraction, the **distended** veins burst and a small amount of blood seeps in between the thin septa of the <u>spongy</u> layer and the placental surface, stripping the placenta from its attachment. As the surface area for placental attachment **reduces**, the relatively **non-elastic** placenta begins to detach from the uterine wall.
d. Once separation has occurred, the uterus contracts <u>strongly</u>, forcing placenta and membranes to fall into the **lower** uterine segment and finally into the <u>vagina</u> and emerging at the vulva.

3. Figure with the legend.

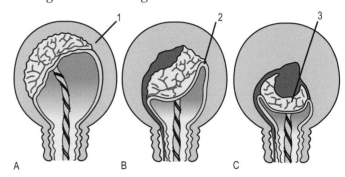

Figure 12.1 The mechanism of placental separation. (A) Uterine wall is partially retracted, but not sufficiently to cause placental separation. (B) Further contraction and retraction thicken the uterine wall, reduce the placental site and aid placental separation. (C) Complete separation and formation of the retroplacental clot. *Note*: The thin lower segment has collapsed like a concertina following the birth of the baby.

4. **a.**

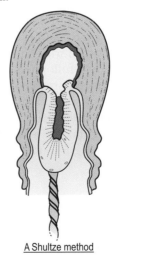

A Shultze method   B Matthews Duncan method

Figure 12.2

b. Method A: a. Schultze; b. Centrally; c. **Yes**; d. Fetal; e. **Shorter**; f. **Less**; g. Complete membranes, retroplacental clot enclosed within membranes. Method B: a. Matthews Duncan; b. Laterally (one of the borders); c. **No**; d. Maternal; e. **Longer**; f. **More**; g. Ragged membranes, no retroplacental clot.

h. The majority of placentas are situated on the **anterior or posterior wall** of the uterus. In the majority of cases, separation usually starts from the **lower** pole of the placenta and moves gradually **upwards**.

Fundal placentas separate first at both poles followed by the fundal part. The length of the third stage may be **reduced by 2 minutes** when the placenta is located at the fundus.

5. The normal volume of blood flow through a healthy placental site is **500–800** mL/min. Serious haemorrhage would occur at the time of placental separation if blood flow was not arrested within **seconds**. An interplay of the following three factors to control bleeding within the normal physiological processes is essential during this stage:

i. The **tortuous** blood vessels **intertwine through** the **oblique** uterine muscle fibres. **Retraction** of the **oblique** uterine muscle fibres in the **upper** uterine segment results in **thickening** of the muscles. This exerts pressure on the torn vessels, acting as clamps so securing a ligature action.

ii. Presence of **vigorous** uterine contraction following separation brings the **uterine** walls into apposition so that **further** pressure is exerted on the **placental site**.

iii. Haemostasis is achieved by a transitory **activation** of the coagulation and fibrinolytic systems during, and immediately following, placental separation. This protective response is especially **active** at the placental site so that clot formation in the **torn** vessels is **intensified**. Following separation, the placental site is **rapidly** covered by a **fibrin** mesh utilizing **5%–10%** of circulating **fibrinogen**.

6. Ergometrine: If ergometrine and oxytocin are combined, then 1 mL ampoule will contain 0.5 mg of this drug; If administered intramuscularly then this drug will act within 6–7 minutes; This drug is contraindicated if there is a history of hypertensive or cardiac disease.

Oxytocin: If ergometrine and oxytocin are combined then 1 mL ampoule will contain 5 IU of this drug; If this drug is administered as an IV bolus, it should be administered slowly because of profound and potentially fatal hypotensive side-effects; This drug is the synthetic form of a hormone (to stimulate smooth muscle contraction) produced in the posterior pituitary gland; If administered intramuscularly then this drug will act within 2.5 minutes.

7. **a.** Contraction occurs; large gush of blood indicates partial or complete separation.
b. Cord may lengthen; walls of vulva may bulge with descending placenta; fundus rises in the abdomen above the level of placenta; uterus becomes hard, round and mobile; placenta visible.
c. Syntocinon.
d. Syntomentrine.
e. Rapid uterine contraction enhanced by a stronger more sustained contraction lasting several hours.
f. Anterior shoulder of the baby is born.
g. Elevation of blood pressure and vomiting.

8. True: c, d, f, j. k.   False: a, b, e, g, h, i, l.

9. **i.** Polyhydramnios, multiple pregnancy.
ii. Placenta praevia.   **iii.** Placenta abruption.
iv. Couvelaire.   **v.** Precipitate labour/prolonged labour.   **vi.** Incomplete placenta/membranes/ Retained placenta.   **vii.** Full bladder.
viii. Relaxation.

10.

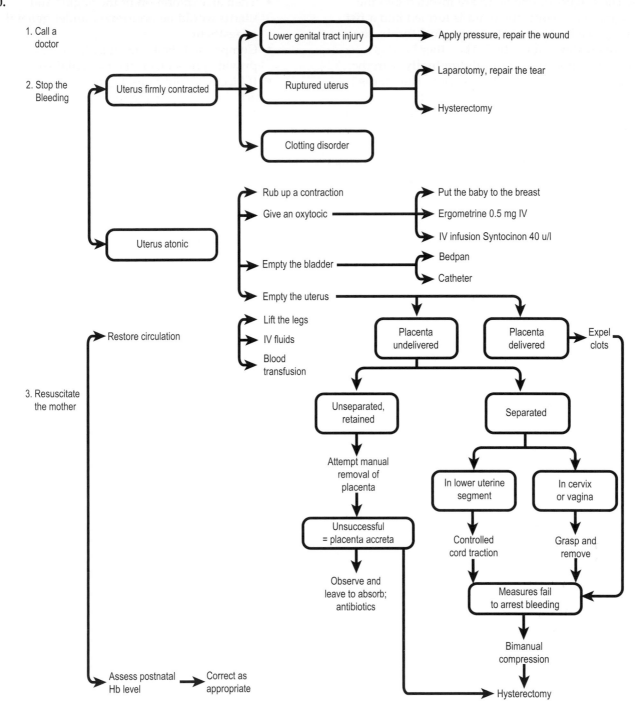

Figure 12.3

11. **a.** The fingers of one hand are inserted into the vagina like a **cone**; the hand is formed into a **fist** and placed into the **anterior** vaginal **fornix**, the **elbow** resting on the bed. The other hand is placed behind the uterus **abdominally** with the fingers pointing **toward** the cervix. The **uterus** is brought **forwards** and compressed between the **palm** of the hand positioned **abdominally** and the **fist** in the vagina.

   b. If bleeding persists:
   - The first action is to exclude a **blood clotting** disorder.
   - Then an exploration of the vagina and uterus would be performed under **general anaesthetic**.
   - Compression balloons/may be used to provide pressure on the **placental site**.
   - If bleeding continues, ligation of the **uterine** arteries or **hysterectomy** may need to be considered.

12. True: a. b. e, f, g, h, i, j.   False: c, d, k.

13 Complicated labour and birth

ANSWERS

1. True: b, c, d, e, f, g, h, i, j, k, l, m. False: a, n.

2. **a.** 24 weeks + 0 days. **b.** 41+0 and 42+0 weeks. **c.** Amniotomy. **d.** Dilation, effacement (or length), position and consistency of the cervix, the station of presenting part (in relation to ischial spines). **e.** ≥ 8. **f.** Dystocia. **g.** ≤3 hours. **h.** Macrosomia. **i.** Increased risk of need for emergency caesarean section during induced labour increased risk of uterine rupture.

3. Membrane sweep: Separates the chorionic membrane from decidua leading to release of prostaglandins and onset of labour; Involves VE with examining finger passing through the cervix to rotate against the uterine wall; This is an adjunct to IOL rather than an actual method of induction; In this VE procedure, massaging around the cervix in the vaginal fornices may achieve a similar effect if the finger cannot be admitted into the cervix; Women informed of this option at 38 week antenatal visit (offered to nulliparous at 40/41 week; 41 weeks for parous) to promote spontaneous labour and reduce formal IOL; Procedure may cause discomfort and vaginal bleeding.
Induction of labour: Uncertainties remain about how best to apply vaginal PGE2 in terms of dosage and timing; Vaginal PGE2 is the preferred method; This is appropriate method approximately 24 hours after prelabour rupture of membranes (term); Procedure involves administration of a gel, tablet or controlled-release pessary; Amniotomy, alone or with oxytocin, should not be used as this primary method; Tocolysis should be considered if uterine hyperstimulation occurs during induction of labour.

4. True: a, b, c, f, g, h, i, k. False: d, e, j.

5.

Inducibility features	0	1	2	3
Cervix: <u>Dilatation</u> (cm)	<1	1–2	2–4	>4
Cervix: <u>Consistency</u>	firm	firm	medium	soft
Cervical canal: <u>Length</u> (cm)	>4	2–4	1–2	<1
Cervix: <u>Position</u>	posterior	middle	anterior	N/A
<u>Presenting part</u>: station in cm (above or below) maternal <u>ischial spines</u>	−3	−2	−1, 0	+1, +2

6. Correct: a, b, c, e, f, g, i, j, k, l, m. Incorrect: d, h.

7. True: c, d, e, f, g, h, i, j, l, m. False: a, b, k.

8.

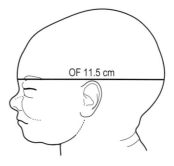

Figure 13.1 Engaging diameter of a deflexed head. + diameter

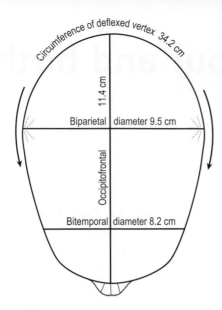

Figure 13.2 Presenting dimensions of a deflexed head. + diameter

9. Lie: longitudinal; attitude (head): deflexed; presentation: vertex; position: right occipitoposterior position; denominator: occiput; presenting part: middle part of the anterior area of the left parietal bone.
   (a) The **occipitofrontal** diameter (**11.5 cm**) lies in the **right** oblique diameter of pelvic brim.
   (b) The **occiput** points to the right sacroiliac joint and the **sinciput** to the **left** iliopectineal eminence.

10/11. Fig. 13.3: Descent and flexion: descent takes place with increasing flexion; sagittal suture lies in the right oblique diameter of the pelvis; the occiput becomes the leading part.
   Fig. 13.4: Internal rotation of the head: The occiput and shoulders have rotated 1/8th of a circle forwards; sagittal suture lies in the transverse diameter of the pelvis.
   Fig. 13.5: The occiput and shoulders have rotated 2/8th of a circle forwards; sagittal suture now lies in the left oblique diameter of the pelvis; the position is right occipitoanterior.
   Fig. 13.6: The occiput has rotated 3/8th of a circle forwards to lie under the symphysis pubis; there is a twist in the neck; sagittal suture lies in the anteroposterior diameter of the pelvis.

12. **a.** The **occiput** escapes under the symphysis pubis: Crowning.
   b. The **sinciput**, face and chin sweep the **perineum** and the head is born by a movement of **extension**: Extension.

c. The **occiput** turns 1/8th of a circle to the **right** and the head realigns with the shoulders: Restitution.
   d. The shoulders enter the pelvis in the **right** oblique diameter; the **anterior** shoulder reaches the pelvic floor first and rotates 1/8th of a circle to lie under the symphysis pubis: Internal rotation of the shoulders.
   e. At the same time the **occiput** turns a further 1/8th of a circle to the **right**: External rotation of the head.
   f. The **anterior** shoulder escapes under the symphysis pubis, the **posterior** shoulder sweeps the perineum and the body is born by **lateral flexion**: Lateral flexion.

13. Fig. 13.7: The position is **right** occipitoposterior. The <u>occiput</u> fails to rotate **forwards** in this situation. Instead the **sinciput** reaches the pelvic floor first and rotates **forwards**. The **occiput** goes into the hollow of the sacrum.

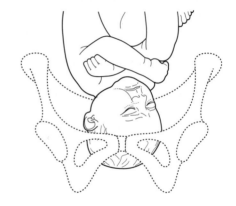

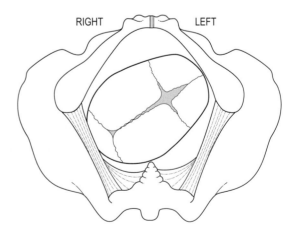

Figure 13.7 Persistent occipitoposterior position before rotation of the occiput: position right occipitoposterior.

Fig. 13.8: The position in now <u>direct</u> occipitoposterior. The baby is born facing the <u>pubic bone</u>. This is termed a '*face to pubes*' birth.

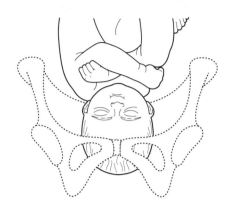

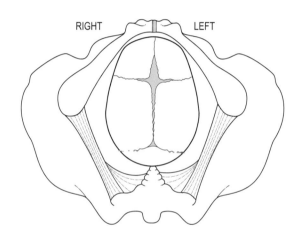

RIGHT   LEFT

Figure 13.8 Persistent occipitoposterior position after short rotation: position direct occipitoposterior.

14. Brow: Occurs when head is partially extended; May result in obstructed labour (C/S probable outcome); Mentovertical diameter (13.5 cm) and bitemporal diameter (8.2 cm) present. Vaginal birth is rare if presentation persists.
Face: Occurs when the head is completely extended. Presenting diameters: submentobregmatic (9.5 cm) and bitemporal (8.2 cm); Submentovertical diameter (11.5 cm) will distend vaginal orifice; Anencephaly can be a fetal cause; Incidence is ≤1:500; Denominator: mentum. Breech: Denominator: sacrum; Incidence at term is 3%–4%; Fetal heart heard clearly above umbilicus (in non-engagement); presenting diameter: bitrochanteric (10 cm).

15.

Label (name and length)

| Engaging diameter |
| Diameter that sweeps the perineum |

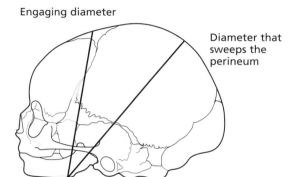

Engaging diameter

Diameter that sweeps the perineum

Figure 13.9 Diameters involved in delivery of face presentation. Engaging diameter, submentobregmatic (SMB) 9.5 cm. The submentovertical (SMV) diameter, 11.5 cm, sweeps the perineum.

16. Lie: longitudinal. Attitude: extension of the neck. Presentation: face. Position: left mentoanterior. Denominator: mentum. Presenting part: left malar bone.

17.

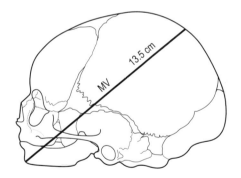

13.5 cm

MV

Figure 13.10 The mentovertical (MV) diameter, 13.5 cm, lies at the pelvic brim.

18. a.

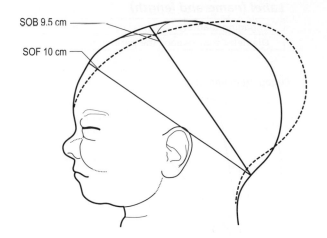

Figure 13.11 Type of moulding in a vertex presentation (SOB, suboccipitobregmatic; SOF, suboccipitofrontal).

18. b.

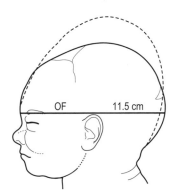

Figure 13.12 Upward moulding (dotted line) following persistent occipitoposterior position. OF, occipitofrontal.

18. c.

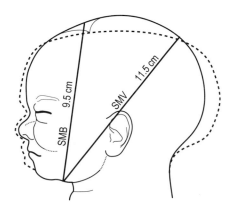

Figure 13.13 Moulding in a face presentation (dotted line). SMB, submentobregmatic; SMV, submentovertical.

d.

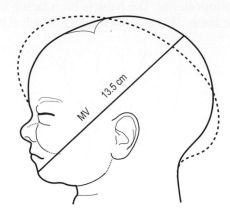

Figure 13.14 Moulding in a brow presentation (dotted line). MV, mentovertical.

19.

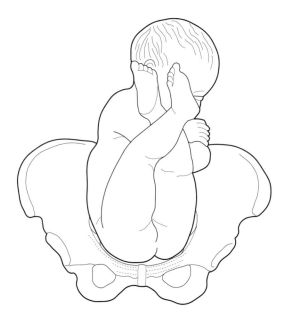

Figure 13.15 Frank breech.

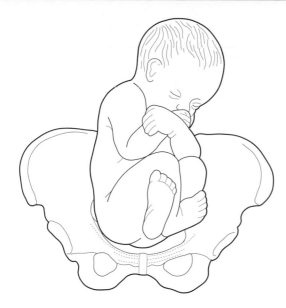

Figure 13.16 Complete breech.

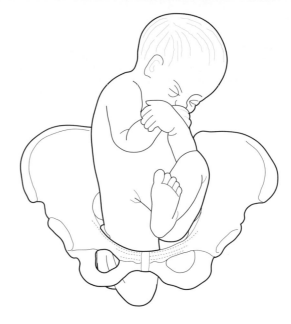

Figure 13.18 Knee presentation.

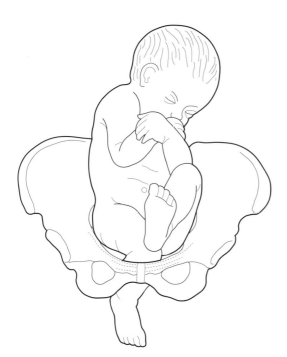

Figure 13.17 Footling presentation.

a. Frank breech
b. Complete breech
c. Footling breech
d. Knee presentation

20. Lie: longitudinal; attitude: complete flexion; presentation: breech; position: left sacroanterior; denominator: sacrum; presenting part: anterior (left) buttock.
    a. The **bitrochanteric diameter (10.0 cm)** enters the pelvis in the **left** oblique diameter of the brim. The sacrum points to the **iliopectineal eminence**.

21. **a.**

Table 13.11

	Birth of the head (breech birth)
i.	On birth of the **shoulders** the baby is allowed to hang from the vulva **without** support. The baby's weight brings the **head** onto the pelvic floor on which the **occiput** rotates.
ii.	The **sagittal** suture is now in the anteroposterior diameter of the **outlet**. If the head does not **rotate**, then two fingers should be placed on the **malar** bones and the **head** rotated. The baby can hang for up to **1 or 2 minutes**. Gradually the **neck** elongates, the hair-line appears and the **suboccipital** region can be felt.
iii.	Key methods used to achieve a controlled birth include: a) forceps applied to the after-coming head; b) Mauriceau-Smellie-Veit manoeuvre. Assistance is required for babies born with **extended** legs and **extended** arms. Controlled birth of the head is vital to avoid any sudden change in **intracranial** pressure.

21. b.

Table 13.12

i.	Mauriceau-Smellie-Veit manoeuvre is mainly used when there is delay in **descent** of the head because of **extension**. The manoeuvre promotes jaw **flexion** and shoulder **traction**.
ii.	(A) in Fig. 13.19. The hands are in position **before** the body is lifted.
iii.	(B) in Fig. 13.19. This shows extraction of the **head**.
iv.	The manoeuvre involves the baby being laid astride the **arm** with the palm supporting the **chest**. One finger is placed on **each malar bone** to flex the **head**. The middle finger may be used to apply pressure to the **chin**. Two fingers of the attendant's other hand are hooked over the **shoulders** with the middle finger pushing up the **occiput** to aid **flexion**. Traction is applied to draw the head out of the vagina and, when the **suboccipital** region appears, the body is lifted to assist the head to pivot around the **symphysis pubis**. The vault is delivered **slowly**.

21. c.

> **Extended legs**
> When the popliteal fossae appear at the vulva, **two** fingers are placed along the length of one thigh with the fingertips **in the fossa**. The leg is swept to the side of the abdomen (**abducting** the hip) and the knee is **flexed** by the pressure on its under surface and the **lower** part of the leg will emerge from the vagina. The process is repeated for the other leg.

22. Correct: a, c, d, e, g, h, i, j, k, l.   Incorrect: b, f.

23. b.   **24.** d.   **25.** c.   **26.** b.   **27.** a.   **28.** d.   **29.** d.   **30.** a, b, c, d.

31. Correct: a, b, c, e, f, g, h, j, k, l, m, n. Incorrect: d, i.

32. a, b, c, d, e.   **33.** c.   **34.** a, b, c, d, f, g.   **35.** a, b, c, d. e.   **36.** f.   **37.** a, b, c, d.   **38.** a, c, d, e.   **39.** d.   **40.** c.   **41.** e.   **42.** a.

14 Midwifery and obstetric emergencies

ANSWERS

1. True: a, b, c, e, f, h, i, k.   False: d, g, j.

2. **a.** Knee-chest position.   **b.** Exaggerated Sim's position.   **c.** Trendelenburg position.

3. Correct: b, c, d, e, f, g, h.   Incorrect: a, i.

4. General: multiparity, low birthweight (<2.5 kg), preterm labour (<37+0 weeks), fetal congenital anomalies, breech presentation, transverse, oblique and unstable lie (after 37+0 weeks), second twin, unengaged presenting part, low-lying placenta, polyhydramnios. Procedure-related: vaginal manipulation of the fetus with ruptured membranes, external cephalic version (during procedure), internal podalic version, stabilizing induction of labour, large balloon catheter induction of labour, insertion of intrauterine pressure transducer, artificial rupture of membranes with high presenting part.

5. **a.** Call for **urgent** assistance and note the **time** cord prolapse occurred.
b. If the cord lies outside the vagina, then it should be gently **replaced** to prevent **spasm**, to maintain the **temperature** and prevent **drying**.
c. The midwife may need to keep her **fingers** in the **vagina** and hold the **presenting part** off the umbilical cord, especially during a **contraction**.
d. Birth must be expedited with the greatest possible speed for a cord prolapse. What birth management would be done for the following circumstances?

- If the fetus is alive but vaginal birth is not imminent: **caesarean section** is required.
- If the presentation is cephalic the birth may be medically assisted through: **ventouse** OR **forceps**.
- If the cord prolapse is diagnosed in second stage (multiparous mother) birth may be expedited by: **episiotomy.**

6. **a.** Shoulder dystocia occurs more commonly when the **anterior** shoulder becomes trapped **behind** or on the **symphysis pubis**, while the **posterior** shoulder may be in the **hollow** of the **sacrum** or high above the **sacral promontory**.
b. Prelabour factors: Previous shoulder dystocia, Macrosomia >4.5 kg. Diabetes mellitus, Maternal BMI >30 kg/m^2. Induction of labour.
c. Intrapartum factors: Prolonged first stage, secondary arrest, prolonged second stage, oxytocin augmentation, assisted vaginal delivery.
d. Signs: Difficulty with delivery of face and chin, head remaining tightly applied to the vulva or even retracting (turtleneck sign), failure of restitution of fetal head, failure of the shoulder to descend.
e. Maternal postpartum haemorrhage, third- and fourth-degree perineal tears. Fetal: Brachial plexus injury (BPI) - Erb's palsy and Klumpke's palsy.
f. (i) The term 'adduct' means to pull or move something (e.g., arm or leg) **toward** the midline of the body.
(ii) The term 'abduct' means to pull or move something (e.g., arm or leg) **away from** the midline of the body.

7.

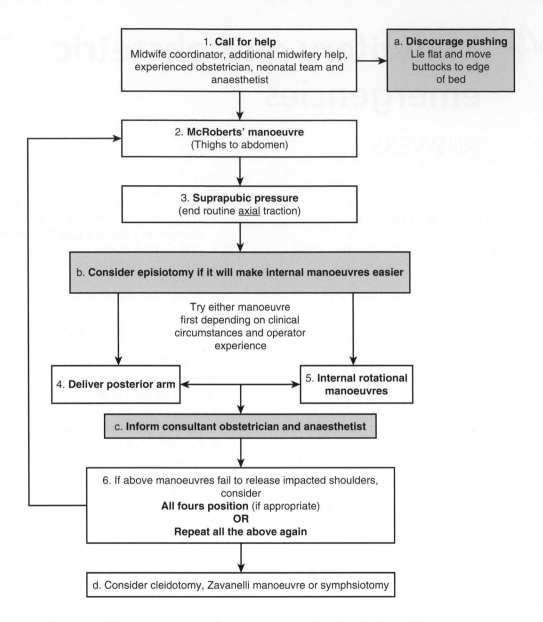

Figure 14.3 Management of shoulder dystocia – completed

8. **a.** <u>McRoberts manoeuvre</u>. This manoeuvre involves **flexion** and **abduction** of the maternal hips. It straightens the **lumbosacral** angle, **rotates** the maternal pelvis toward the mother's head and **increases** the relative anterior-posterior diameter of the pelvis. The legs should be **hyperflexed**. Apply routine traction (as in normal delivery) in an axial direction (in line with fetal spine).
b. Correct application of <u>suprapubic pressure</u>. Pressure should be exerted on the side of the fetal **back** and toward the fetal **chest**. This manoeuvre may help to **adduct** the shoulders (**reduce** the fetal bisacromial diameter) and push the **anterior** shoulder away from the **symphysis pubis** into the wider **oblique or transverse** diameter.

9. **a.** The 'all fours position' **(Gaskin manoeuvre)** may be especially helpful if the **posterior** shoulder is impacted behind the **sacral promontory**, as this position optimizes space available in the **sacral** curve and may allow the **posterior** shoulder to be delivered first.
b. Internal movements: Vaginal access uses the space available in the sacral hollow. The whole hand should be entered **posteriorly** to perform internal rotation or delivery of the **posterior** arm.

Access is made easier by repositioning the women to the end of the bed. Rotation can be most easily achieved by pressing on the anterior or posterior aspect of the **posterior** shoulder. Applying pressure on the posterior aspect of the posterior shoulder has the additional benefit of reducing the shoulder diameter by **adducting** the shoulders. Delivery can be facilitated by **rotation** into the wider **oblique** diameter or when possible by a full 180-degree rotation of the fetal trunk, or by delivery of the **posterior** arm.

If pressure on the **posterior** shoulder is unsuccessful, an attempt should be made to apply pressure on the **posterior** aspect of the anterior shoulder to **adduct** and rotate the shoulders into the **oblique** diameter.

c. Delivering the **posterior** arm reduces the diameter of the fetal shoulders by the width of the arm. The fetal wrist should be grasped and the **posterior** arm should be gently withdrawn from the vagina in a **straight line**.

d. Third-line measures are rarely required and include: **cleidotomy, symphysiotomy** and the **Zavanelli** manoeuvre.

10. Correct: b, c, d, e, f, g, h, i, j, k, l, n, o, p, q.
    Incorrect: a, i, m.

11. True: c, d, e, g.   False: a (*it may or may not expulse the fetus*), b (*it does involve tearing of the perimetrium*), f-false (*blood loss is scanty because of fibrous avascular tissue*).

12. True: a (*in a fourth-degree inversion both the uterus and vagina are inverted beyond the introitus*), c, e, f,

13. Wrigley's forceps: d. f.   Keilland's forceps: b, h.
    Neville-Barnes or Simpson's forceps: a.
    Ventouse: c, e, g.

14.

Table 14.9

Skin	→	subcutaneous fat	→	rectus sheath
	→	muscle (rectus abdominis)	→	abdominal peritoneum
	→	pelvic peritoneum	→	uterine muscle

15. Anaphylactic: May occur as a result of severe allergy or drug reaction.
    Cardiogenic: Caused by impaired ability of the heart to pump blood.
    Hypovolaemic: Results from a reduction in intravascular volume.
    Neurogenic: Results from an insult to the nervous system.

Septic or toxic: Occurs with a severe generalized infection.

16. Shock is a **complex** syndrome. It involves a **reduction** in blood flow to the **tissues.** This may result in irreversible **organ** damage and progressive **collapse** of the **circulatory** system. If left untreated it will result in **death**.
    Shock can be **acute** but prompt treatment results in **recovery** with little detrimental effect on the woman. When there is **failure** to initiate effective treatment or provide inadequate treatment this can result in a **chronic** condition ending in **multisystem** organ failure which may be **fatal.**

17. **a. Hypovolaemic:** Severe obstetric haemorrhage (antepartum haemorrhage—vasa praevia, placenta praevia, PPH).
    b. Anaphylactic: Allergy to peanuts, penicillin or other drug.
    c. Neurogenic: Acute uterine inversion.
    d. Septic or toxic: Overwhelming infection general or associated with pregnancy and childbirth, for example, infection entering through the placenta (most common potentially fatal is beta haemolytic *Streptococcus pyogenes*).
    e. Cardiogenic: Pulmonary embolism (sudden blockage of an artery in the lung); inability of heart muscle to work properly (or at all in some cases); cardiac event caused by secondary factors, for example, haemorrhage reducing blood volume.

18. **a.** The **drop** in cardiac output produces a response from the **sympathetic** nervous system through the activation of receptors in the **aorta and carotid arteries**. Blood is redistributed to the **vital organs**. There is **constriction** of the vessel in the gastrointestinal tract, kidneys, skin and lungs. The response is seen as the skin becoming **pale** and **cool**. Peristalsis **slows**, urinary output is **reduced** and exchange of gas is impaired as blood flow **diminishes**. The heart rate **increases** and the pupils of the eyes **dilate**. Sweat glands are **stimulated** and the skin becomes **moist and clammy**. Adrenaline (Epinephrine) is released from the adrenal **medulla** and aldosterone from the adrenal **cortex**. Antidiuretic hormone (ADH) is secreted from the **posterior** lobe of the pituitary gland. Their combined effect is to cause **vasoconstriction, increased** cardiac output and a **decrease** in urinary output. Venous return to the heart will **increase**, but this will not be sustained unless the fluid loss is replaced.
    b. Gas exchange is **impaired** as the physiological dead space **increases** within the lungs. Levels of carbon dioxide **rise** and arterial oxygen levels **fall**. **Ischaemia** within the lungs alters the production

of **surfactant** and as a result of this, alveoli **collapse**. Oedema in the lungs, because of **increased** permeability, **exacerbates** the existing problem of diffusion of oxygen. Atelectasis, oedema and **reduced** compliance impair ventilation and gaseous exchange, leading ultimately to respiratory **failure**.

19. **a.** Amniotic fluid embolism (AFE) occurs when amniotic fluid enters the **maternal** circulation via the <u>uterus</u> or <u>placental</u> site. Maternal collapse can progress **rapidly**. The body's initial response is pulmonary **vasospasm** causing hypoxia, **hypertension**, <u>pulmonary</u> oedema and <u>cardiovascular</u> collapse.
    b. Secondly with AFE, there is the development of **left** ventricular failure, with maternal bleeding and <u>coagulation</u> disorder and further uncontrollable <u>haemorrhage.</u>
    Mortality and morbidity are **high.** Because of maternal **hypotension,** there is uterine **hypertonus** and this will induce fetal <u>compromise</u> in response to uterine <u>hypoxia</u>.

20. **Cardiovascular system:** tachycardia; hypotension; pale clammy skin and shivering; cardiac arrest.
    Respiratory system: cyanosis, dyspnoea, respiratory distress, respiratory arrest.
    Haematological system: haemorrhage, disseminated intravascular dissemination (DIC).
    Neurological system: restlessness, panic, abnormal; convulsions.
    Fetal condition: compromised, possible death.

21. **i.** Adopt a <u>safe</u> approach to the woman. Shake and **shout** to check conscious level. Call for <u>help</u> to get appropriate assistance.
    ii. Remove any **pillows** and position the woman **supine,** on a <u>left-lateral tilt</u> to prevent <u>aortocaval</u> compression.
    iii. A – <u>Airway</u>
    Position the head in a <u>head tilt, chin lift</u>. Remove any <u>obstruction</u> in the mouth (e.g., dentures or vomit). Check for chest **movements**.
    iv. B – **Breathing**. Listen and feel for <u>breath</u>.
    v. C – <u>Circulation</u>. Check for a **pulse**.
    vi. Commence chest compressions if <u>pulse</u> absent or if <u>breathing</u> absent or abnormal.
    vii. Ratio is <u>30</u> compressions: **2** breaths.
    viii. Continue until <u>help</u> arrives or more **experienced** staff take over.
    ix. A <u>peri-mortem caesarean section</u> may be performed to assist with the resuscitation.
    N.B. Always refer to updated resuscitation guidelines.

22.

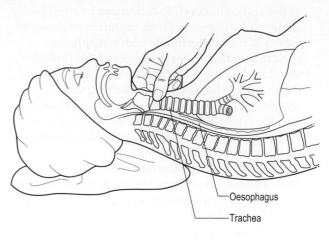

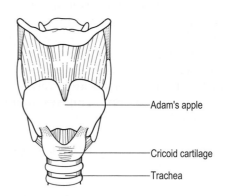

Figure 14.6

23. Cord presentation: this occurs when the umbilical cord lies in front of the presenting part with the fetal membranes still intact
    Cord prolapse: this occurs when the umbilical cord lies in front of the presenting part and the fetal membranes are ruptured
    Occult cord prolapse: this occurs when the umbilical cord lies alongside but not in front of the presenting part

24. Thrombin: Preeclampsia.
    Tone: Multiple pregnancy, Previous PPH, Fetal macrosomia, Failure to progress in second stage, Prolonged third stage of labour, General anaesthesia.
    Tissue: Retained placenta, Placenta accreta.
    Trauma: Episiotomy, Perineal laceration.

25. Hb >80 g/L, fibrinogen >2 g/L. platelet count >50 × 10^9/L, activated partial thromboplastin time (APTT) <1.5 times normal, prothrombin time (PT) <1.5 times normal.

26. a. Placental abruption, placenta praevia, uterine rupture, vasa praevia.

b. Endometritis, retained products of conception (RPOC) and subinvolution of the placental implantation site.

27. True: a, b, d, f, g, h.   False: c, e.

28. b.   **29.** c.   **30.** a.   **31.** d.   **32.** a.   **33.** c.   **34.** a.

15 The puerperium

ANSWERS

1. **a.** Immediately after birth of baby and expulsion of placenta and membranes; 6 weeks.
   b. All body systems return to their prepregnant state. **c.** Oestrogen, progesterone, human chorionic gonadotrophin, human placental lactogen. **d.** Involution. **e.** Oxytocin/posterior pituitary gland. **f.** Afterpains. **g.** Lochia.
   h. Stale blood products (erythrocytes, leucocytes), lanugo, vernix, meconium, shreds of degenerating decidua and other unwanted products from conception.

2. **a.** After birth of the baby, the separation and expulsion of placenta and membranes is assisted by the hormone **oxytocin** acting on the contraction of the **uterine muscles**. This hormone is secreted from the **posterior** (lobe) of the pituitary gland. Once placenta and membranes are expelled, this exposes ends of **major** blood vessels and the uterine **cavity** collapses **inwards**. The collapse of uterine **walls** and muscle layers of the **myometrium** simulating the action of ligatures, compress and occlude the exposed sinuses of the blood vessels. This action **reduces** blood loss.
   b. Vasoconstriction of the uterine blood supply results in the tissues receiving reduced blood supply. This leads to de-oxygenation and a state of **ischaemia** arising in the uterine tissues. The overall muscles fibres **reduce in** size through the process of **autolysis** involving autodigestion of the **ischaemic** muscle fibres by proteolytic **enzymes.** Phagocytic action of **polymorphs** and macrophages in the blood, and lymphatic systems upon the waste products of **autolysis**, which are then excreted in the urine via the **renal** system. **Coagulation** takes place through platelet aggregation and the release of thromboplastin and **fibrin.**
   c. With the exception of the placental site, the remains of the inner surface of the uterine lining regenerates **rapidly** to produce a covering of **epithelium.** Partial covering occurs within **7 to 10 days** after birth; total coverage is complete by the **21st day.** Once the placenta has separated, there is

a **reduction** in the circulating levels of pregnancy-related hormones. This leads to further physiological changes in muscle and connective tissue, as well as having a **major** influence on the secretion of **prolactin** from the anterior **pituitary** gland.
   d. To ensure that physiological processes are beginning to take place, the initial abdominal palpation is usually performed **soon after** expulsion of placenta and membranes. On abdominal palpation, the fundus should be located **centrally.** Fundal position is usually at the same level or slightly **below** the umbilicus and should feel **firm** to confirm a state of contraction.

3. Correct: a, b, e, f, g, h, i. j, k.   Incorrect: c, d, l.

4. Puerperal infection (signs/symptoms/recordings): Respiratory collapse, blood cultures may be positive, pale, may be severe breathlessness, pyrexia >38°C, tachycardia >100 beats per minute, listless, unwell with flu-like symptoms, nausea and vomiting.
   Genital tract: Blood clots may be passed, blood loss may be fresher and heavier or scanty but foul smelling (compared with previous assessment), may be tenderness on palpation, vaginal loss heavier and fresher (or scant but offensive), fundus may be deviated to one side and not progressively reducing in size, Palpation—may be subinvoluted uterus, poorly contracted/feel wide/ 'boggy'.
   Wound: Inflammation and tenderness around a wound area, virulent clear or purulent exudate, slow healing or gaping at the skin edges, pain felt deeper in the wound area.
   Renal system: Dysuria, haematuria, pain and tenderness in the renal angle (also along line of ureter, urine—cloudy, offensive with pus).
   Breasts: One segment may be flushed or reddened, one or both nipples have sore, broken or discoloured skin, feels tight and tender.

5. True: a, b, c, d, e, f, i.   False: g, h.

6. d.   **7.** f.   **8.** d.   **9.** g.   **10.** f.   **11.** d.

12.

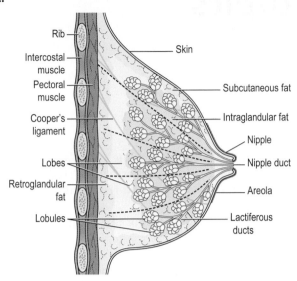

Figure 15.1

13. Table 15.5a. **a.** embryogenesis.
b. mammogenesis.   **c.** lactogenesis.   **d.** acini
cells.   **e.** myoepithelial cells.   **f.** smooth
muscle.   **g.** oxytocin.   **h.** posterior lobe of
pituitary.   **i.** lactiferous ducts.   **j.** lactiferous
tubules.   **k.** nipple. l. areola.
Table 15.5b. **a.** prolactin.   **b.** anterior lobe of the
pituitary gland.   **c.** touch.   **d.** milk removal.
e. whey protein.   **f.** autocrine inhibitory
factor (feedback inhibitor of lactation).
g. neuromuscular control.   **h.** let down or milk
ejection reflex.

14. True: a, b, d, e, j, l, m, n.   False: c, f, g, h, i, k, o.

15. a. Colostrum has a **higher** fat and protein content
than mature milk. Foremilk (at the beginning of
the feed) is of a high volume of relatively **low-fat**
milk. Hindmilk (as the feed progresses) **decreases**
in volume with an **increase** in the proportion of
fat sometimes by as much as **five** times the initial
value.

b. It is the **fat** content and not the **protein** content
that has particular significance for the **rapidly**
growing brain of the newborn. The fat content is
lowest in the morning and **highest** in the
afternoon.
c. The main carbohydrate component is provided
by **lactose** (which provides the baby with about
40% calorific requirements). This enhances the
absorption of **calcium** and promotes the growth of
lactobacilli, which **increase** intestinal acidity thus
reducing the growth of pathogenic organisms.
Whey, the dominant protein, forms soft, flocculent
curds when **acidified** in the stomach.

16. Immunoglobins: These are present to provide
protection, IgA is the most important for the baby,
IgA covers intestinal epithelium and protects
mucosal surfaces against pathogenic bacteria and
enteroviruses.
Bifidus factor: *Lactobacillus bifidus* specifically
discourages multiplication of pathogens, this
promotes the growth of gram-positive bacilli in
the gut flora.
Vitamin K: It is essential for synthesis of blood
clotting factors, this is fat soluble and present in
milk, it is present in greater concentrations in
colostrum and in the high fat hindmilk.
Lactoferrin: This binds to enteric iron, preventing
pathogenic *E.coli* from obtaining the iron needed
for them to survive.

17. a. Mastitis (noninfective).   **b.** engorgement.
c. breast abscess.   **d.** white spots.   **e.** blocked
ducts.   **f.** epithelial overgrowth.   **g.** mastitis
(infective).   **h.** sore and damaged nipples.
i. *Candida albicans* (thrush).

18. e.   **19.** b.   **20.** b.   **21.** e.   **22.** a.   **23.** a, b, c.
24. a, b, c, d, e.   **25.** a.

26. Correct: a, c, e, f, g, h, i, k, l, m, n.
Incorrect: b, d and j.

16 Miscellaneous topics

ANSWERS

1. **a.** Inner, endoderm; Middle, mesoderm; Outer, ectoderm. **b.** Pharmacokinetics. **c.** Absorption, distribution (translocation), metabolism and excretion (acronym ADME).
d. Pharmacodynamics. **e.** Teratogenic. **f.** Larger size. **g.** Smaller size.

2. **a.** Gastric motility is reduced (prolonged time in gut): may change absorption rate (oral drugs), that is, slows down, increases or no change.
b. Increased circulating plasma volume: this decreases plasma concentration.
c. Increase in blood flow to the kidneys: increase in excretion rate of the drug.
d. Increased amounts of total body water and fat: may alter distribution of the drug.
e. Some metabolic pathways in the liver increase: metabolism is quicker
f. Major changes in levels of plasma proteins to which some drugs bind: amount of the drug available is affected.

3. Box 16.2a
a. ß-blockers (<28 weeks): Reduced fetal growth.
b. Angiotensin-converting enzyme (ACE) inhibitors (2ⁿᵈ/3ʳᵈ trimester): Fetal renal failure.
c. Iodine (early-late): fetal thyroid function.
d. In 3ʳᵈ trimester, nonsteroidal antiinflammatory drugs (NSAIDs) (e.g., ibuprofen/diclofenac): Premature closure of ductus arteriosus and oligohydramnios.
e. In 1ˢᵗ trimester, commonly used antibiotic, trimethoprim: Folate metabolism interference.
Box 16.2b
a. Lithium or benzodiazepines: Cardiac defects (e.g., increased risk of Ebstein's anomaly)
b. Warfarin: Facial anomalies, CNS anomalies
c. Sodium Valproate: Neural tube defects (minor/major)
d. Phenytoin: Craniofacial abnormalities (e.g., oral deformities)
e. Retinoic acid derivatives: Craniofacial, cardiac and CNS abnormalities
f. Androgens: Masculinization of female fetus

g. Diethylstilbestrol (1st trimester): Vaginal carcinoma, urogenital abnormalities, reduced fertility (females)/increased risk of hypospadias (males).
h. Cytotoxic drugs: Most of this drug group are teratogenic.
Box 16.2c
a. Tetracyclines (e.g., tetracycline, oxytetracycline, doxycycline): Discolouration and dysplasia of fetal bones and teeth when used in 2ⁿᵈ/3ʳᵈ trimester.
b. Aminoglycosides (e.g., gentamicin, netilmicin): Risk of ototoxicity but often used in severe maternal infection.
c. Chloramphenicol: 'Gray (Grey) baby syndrome' when used in 2ⁿᵈ/3ʳᵈ trimester.
d. Nitrofurantoin: Haemolysis in fetus at term–avoid during labour/birth.
e. Quinolones (e.g., ciproflaxin, ofloxacin): Arthropathy in fetus.
f. Polar drugs (e.g., penicillin, cephalosporins): No adverse effects.

4. Correct: b, c, d, e, g, h, j, k, l, m, o, p.
Incorrect: a, f, i, n.

5. a. **6.** a. **7.** a, b, c. **8.** b. **9.** b, c, d. **10.** a, b.

11. Box 16.3a:
Defective spermatogenesis: Endocrine disorders (dysfunction of hypothalamus, pituitary, adrenal and thyroid glands), Systemic disease (e.g., diabetes mellitus), Testicular disorders (trauma/environmental).
Defective sperm transport: Obstruction or absence of seminal ducts, Impaired secretions from accessory glands.
Ineffective sperm delivery: Impotence (psychosexual problems), Drug induced problems, Physical anomalies.
Box 16.3b:
Defective ovulation: Endocrine disorders (dysfunction of hypothalamus, pituitary, adrenal and thyroid glands), Systemic disease

(e.g., renal disease), Ovarian disorders: hormonal, polycystic ovarian syndrome (PCOS), endometriosis.

Defective transport: Ovum (tubal obstruction or fimbrial adhesions), Sperm: because of thick cervical mucus or loss of tubal patency.

Defective implantation: Caused by hormone imbalance, congenital anomalies, fibroids or infection.

12. True: a, b, c, d, g, h, i.   False: e, f.

13. **a.** Carbohydrates.   **b.** Glucose.   **c.** Sucrose.
d. Starch.   **e.** Facilitated diffusion.
f. Mitochondria.   **g.** Adenosine triphosphate (ATP).   **h.** Fats.   **i.** Cholesterol.   **j.** Protein.
k. Calcium, potassium.   **l.** Iodine, zinc.
m. Vitamin C and most of vitamin B complex.
n. A, D, E and K.

14. Vitamin A: (If severe) may lead to blindness, skin disorders, tooth decay and gastrointestinal disorders.
Vitamin B6: Can cause premenstrual depression, anaemia and convulsions.
Vitamin B12 (cyanocobalamin): Can cause pernicious anaemia and neurological symptoms.
Vitamin C: Can cause poor digestion, gum disease and poor resistance to bacterial infections.

Vitamin D: May cause rickets in children and osteomalacia in adults. May be poor muscle tone, restlessness and irritability.
Vitamin E: May result in spontaneous abortion, preterm labour and still birth.
Vitamin K: Compromises blood clotting as a result of anticoagulant or antibiotic therapy.

15. Correct: a, b, f, g, h, i.   Incorrect: c, d, e.

16. **a.** Homeopathy.   **b.** Traditional Chinese medicine (TCM).   **c.** Acupuncture.   **d.** Mindfulness.
e. Reiki.   **f.** Yoga.   **g.** Reflexology.   **h.** Shiatsu.

17. Group 1 therapies: osteopathy, chiropractic, acupuncture, herbal medicine and homeopathy
Group 2 therapies: aromatherapy; Alexander technique; mindfulness, body work therapies, including massage; hypnotherapy/hypnosis; reflexology, reiki, yoga and shiatsu
Group 3 therapies: a. traditional systems–traditional Chinese medicine (TCM), Tibetan medicine; Indian Ayurvedic medicine. b. diagnostic therapies–crystal therapies, iridology.

18. True: c, d, e, f, g, h, j, k.   False: a, b, i.

17 The baby at birth

ANSWERS

1. The fetus responds to hypoxia by **accelerating** the heart rate in an effort to maintain supplies of **oxygen** to the brain. If hypoxia persists, glucose depletion will stimulate **anaerobic glycolysis**. This results in a **metabolic acidosis**. Cerebral **vessels** will dilate and some brain **swelling** may occur. **Bradycardia** develops as the fetus becomes more **acidotic** and cardiac **glycogen reserves** are depleted. The anal sphincter **relaxes** and the fetus may pass **meconium** into the liquor. Hypoxia triggers **gasping**, breathing movements which may result in the **aspiration** of **meconium-stained** liquor into the lungs.

2. Cord prolapse or compression, true knot in cord – **1.**   Maternal hypertension and vascular disease – **2.**   Placental disease, dysfunction or separation – **3.**   Fetal compromise impacting upon normal growth and development – **4.** Maternal hypoxia, cardiopulmonary disease – **5.**

3.

Table 17.2

Score	Indicator				
	Heart rate	Respiratory effort	Muscle tone	Reflex response to stimuli	Colour
0	Absent	Apnoeic	Limp	No response	Blue, pale
1	<100 beats per minute	Slow, irregular	Some flexion	Minimal grimace	Body pink, extremities blue
2	>100 beats per minute	Good or crying	Active	Cough or sneeze	Pink

4. A: Appearance (relates to colour); P: Pulse (relates to heart rate); G: Grimace (relates to response to stimuli); A: Activity (relates to tone); R: Respirations (relates to breathing).

5. **a.** Pulmonary adaptation:
Respiration is stimulated by mild **hypercapnia**, hypoxia and **acidosis**. There is a change in the rhythm of respiration from **episodic, shallow** fetal respiration to **regular, deeper** breathing. This is caused by a combination of chemical and neural stimuli, notably a **fall** in pH level, a **fall** in PaO_2 and a **rise** in $PaCO_2$. Considerable **negative** intrathoracic pressure of up to 9.8 kPa (**100** cm water) is exerted as the first breath is taken. The pressure exerted to effect **inhalation diminishes** with each breath taken until only **5 cm** of water is required to **inflate** each lung. This is caused by surfactant.
b. Surfactant is a complex of **proteins** and **lipoproteins**. In utero, the amount of surfactant **increases** until the lungs are mature at **30 to 34** **weeks'** gestation. It is produced by **type 2** epithelial cells in the lungs and lines the **alveoli** to **reduce** the **surface tension** within the **alveoli**. This permits **residual air** to remain in the **alveoli** between breaths and prevent them from **collapsing** at the **end** of each expiration. Surfactant **reduces** the work or effort of breathing.
c. Cardiovascular adaptation:
At birth, the lungs expand and pulmonary vascular resistance is **lowered**. This results in the majority of cardiac output being sent to the lungs. **Oxygenated** blood returning to the heart from the lungs **increases** the pressure within the **left** atrium. At the same time, pressure in the **right** atrium is **lowered** because blood ceases to flow through the cord. This brings about functional closure of the **foramen ovale**.
Contraction of the walls of the **ductus arteriosus** occurs almost immediately after birth. This is thought to occur because of the sensitivity of the muscle of the **ductus arteriosus** to **increased** oxygen tension and **reduction** in circulating

prostaglandins. There is usually functional closure of the **ductus arteriosus** within **8 to 10 hours** of birth with complete closure taking place within **several months**.

The remaining temporary structures of the fetal circulation—**umbilical vein, ductus venosus** and hypogastric **arteries**—close functionally within a few **minutes** after birth and constriction of the cord. Anatomical closure of fibrous tissue occurs within **2 to 3 months**.

6. **a.** 37.7°C **b.** 21°C and 25°C **c.** i. Evaporation; ii. Conduction; iii. Radiation; iv. Convection **d.** Large, head **e.** Thin **f.** Shiver **g.** Muscle activity

7.

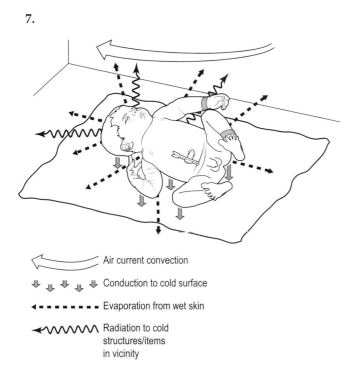

Air current convection

Conduction to cold surface

Evaporation from wet skin

Radiation to cold structures/items in vicinity

Figure 17.2

8.

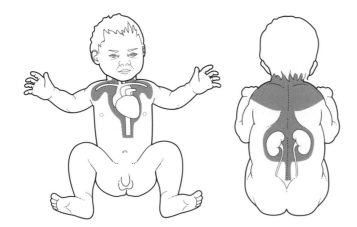

Figure 17.3

9. Cold stress causes **vasoconstriction**, thus reducing pulmonary perfusion. Respiratory **acidosis** develops as the pH and PaO_2 of the blood **decrease** and the $PaCO_2$ **increases** leading to respiratory distress exhibited by **tachypnoea**. This condition is characterized by **rapid** respirations of up to 120/min. It is common after a caesarean section. The baby may be **cyanosed** but maintains normal blood gases apart from PaO_2. There is little or no recession of the **rib cage** and there is minimum, if any, **grunt** on expiration. The **respiratory rate** may remain elevated for up to 5 days.

10. **a.** The baby is **dried** quickly. The **clock timer** is started. The **radiant heater** is switched on to prevent **hypothermia**.
b. The head should be put in the neutral position to maintain the **airway** and keep the **trachea** straightened. If necessary, a small **towel** can be put under the baby's **shoulders** to cause slight extension of the **head**. Review for signs of respiratory effort.
c. If the baby fails to respond then **assisted ventilation** is necessary. Place a correctly fitting mask to cover the **nose and mouth** and ensure a good seal. Use a 500-mL self-inflating bag to **aerate** the lungs, deliver five **sustained** inflations (each breath is for 2–3 seconds).
d. Review for **chest movement**.
If YES- this is present: continue to **ventilate** at a rate of **30 to 40** respirations per minute (ventilation breaths).
If NO- this is not present: then review the **head** position and re-commence the five **inflation** breaths. Move to **ventilation** breaths once **chest movement** is confirmed.

11. **a.** Chest compressions should be performed if the heart rate is <**60** beats per minute. **b.** The chest is depressed at a rate of **100** to **120** times per minute, at a ratio of **three** compressions to **one** ventilation and at a depth of **2 to 3** cm of the baby's chest.

12. True: a, c, d, e, g. False: b, f, h.

13. d. 14. a. 15. d. 16. b. 17. b. 18. a. 19. b.

18 The newborn baby

ANSWERS

1. **a.** The normal core temperature is generally considered to be between **36.5**°C and **37.3**°C.
   b. The respiratory rate is between **40** and **60** breaths per minute.
   c. The heart rate is between **110** and **160** beats per minute.
   d. The average haemoglobin level at term is between **15** and **23.5** g/dL, of which **50%** to **85%** is fetal haemoglobin.
   e. Meconium is passed within **24** hours of birth and is totally excreted within **48** to **72** hours
   f. The six inherited inborn errors of metabolism routinely screened for (newborn blood spot test) include: **phenylketonuria, MCADD, maple syrup urine disease, isovaleric acidaemia, glutamic aciduria type 1** and **homocystinuria.**

2. **a.** Low birthweight (LBW) babies weigh below **2500** g at birth.
   b. Very low birthweight (VLBW) babies weigh below **1500** g at birth.
   c. Extremely low birthweight (ELBW) babies weigh below **1000** g at birth.
   d. A preterm baby is one born before completion of the **37**th gestational week, regardless of birthweight.

3. True: c, d, f, g.   False: a, b, e.

4. **a.** 10 plethora,   **b.** 8 pallor,   **c.** 2 cyanosis,   **d.** 11 skin rashes,   **e.** 4 jaundice,   **f.** 6 milia,   **g.** 7 miliara,   **h.** 1 bruising,   **i.** 9 petechiae or purpura rash,   **j.** 3 erythema toxicum,   **k.** 13 thrush,   **l.** 5 herpes simplex,   **m.** 12 staphylococcal,   **n.** 14 umbilical sepsis.

5. Warning signs:
   a. Skin appearance: Pallor, central cyanosis; jaundice.   **b.** Apnoea lasting longer than 20 seconds.   **c.** Respiratory rate <30 or >60 breaths per minute.   **d.** Heart rate <110 beats per minute or >180 beats per minute (taken during spells of inactivity).   **e.** Skin temperature (axilla) <36.2°C or > 37.2°C.   **f.** Lack of spontaneous movement and responsiveness. Abnormal lying position either hypotonic or hypertonic.

6. **a.** Persistent **tachypnoea.**   **b. Cyanosis** (this is often out of proportion to the degree of respiratory distress).   **c.** Persistent **tachycardia** at rest.   **d.** Poor feeding: infants may be **breathless** and **sweaty** during feeds.   **e.** A sudden **gain** in weight leading to clinical signs of **oedema**: this is usually noted in the baby having puffy **feet** or **eyelids** and in males, the **scrotum** may be swollen.   **f.** Enlargement of the **liver.**
   g. Evidence of **cardiac** enlargement on x-ray, persisting beyond 48 hours of life.   **h.** A very loud **systolic** murmur is invariably significant.

7. True: a, c, d, i.   False: b, e, f, g, h.

8. **a.** Grunting.   **b.** Asynchrony.   **c.** Nasal flaring.
   d. Tachypnoea.   **e.** Recessions.   **f.** Apnoea.

9. A neutral **thermal** environment is defined as the ambient air temperature at which **oxygen** consumption or heat production is minimal, with body temperature **maintained** within the normal range.

10. **Caput succedaneum** refers to a diffuse oedematous swelling under the scalp and above the periosteum. It occurs during labour. It is caused by pressure on the fetal part overlying the cervical os.
    Cephalhaematoma refers to an effusion of blood under the periosteum that covers the skull bones. This occurs during vaginal birth. It is caused by friction between the fetal skull and maternal pelvic bones resulting in the periosteum being torn from the bone resulting in bleeding.

11.

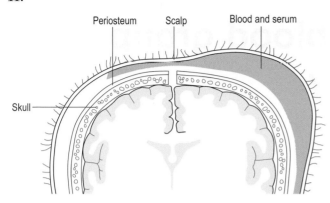

Labels: Periosteum — Scalp — Blood and serum — Skull

Figure 18.2

12.

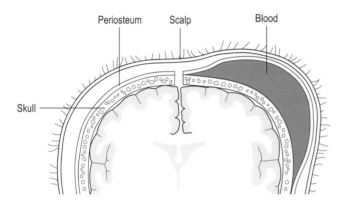

Labels: Periosteum — Scalp — Blood — Skull

Figure 18.3

13. Cephalhaematoma: a, c, g, h, j, k, m, o, p, q, r, s.
Caput succedaneum: b, d, e, f, i, l, n

14. a–Subdural haemorrhage   b–Umbilical
haemorrhage   c(i)–Brachial plexus; (ii)–Erb's
palsy, Klumpe's palsy, Total brachial palsy
d–Skin damage   e–Subarachnoid haemorrhage
f–Torticollis.

15. b.   **16.** c.   **17.** c.   **18.** e.   **19.** a.   **20.** b.   **21.** c.
22. a, d.

19 Jaundice and blood group incompatibility

ANSWERS

1. a. Haem is converted to **biliverdin** and then to **unconjugated bilirubin**.
b. Globin is broken down into **amino acids** and used by the body to make **proteins**.
c. Iron is stored in the **body** or used for new **red blood cells**.

2. a. Unconjugated bilirubin is **fat soluble** and cannot be excreted easily in bile or urine.
b. Conjugated bilirubin has been made **water soluble** in the liver and can be excreted in faeces and urine.

3.

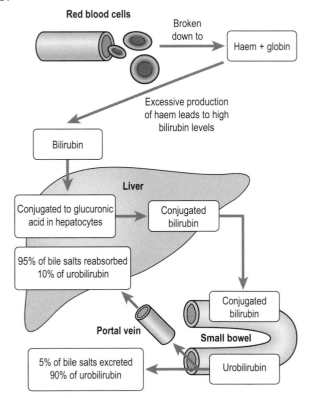

Figure 19.1

4. a. Neonatal **physiological** jaundice occurs when unconjugated (**fat** soluble) bilirubin is deposited in the **subcutaneous fat** instead of being taken to the **liver** for processing into conjugated (**water** soluble) bilirubin that can be excreted from the body in **faeces** or **urine**.
b. This is a normal transitional state affecting up to **60**% of term babies and **80**% of preterm babies who have a progressive rise in **unconjugated** bilirubin levels with jaundice on day **3**.
c. Physiological jaundice *never* appears before **24** hours of life and usually fades by **1** week, with bilirubin levels usually never exceeding **200–250** µmol/L (**12–15** mg/dL) depending on the gestational age.

5. a. iv Increased red cell breakdown. **b.** ii Decreased albumin-binding capacity. **c.** i Enzyme deficiency. **d.** ii Decreased albumin-binding capacity. **e.** iii Increased enterohepatic reabsorption. **f.** ii Decreased albumin-binding capacity.

6. a. Kernicterus (bilirubin toxicity) is an **encephalopathy** caused by deposits of **unconjugated** bilirubin in the **basal** ganglia of the **brain**.
b. Early signs can be **insidious** and include (identify as least two): **lethargy, changes in muscle tone**, a **high-pitched cry** and **irritability**.
c. Long-term clinical features can include (identify at least four): **deafness, blindness, cerebral palsy, developmental delay, learning difficulties** and **extrapyramidal disturbances**, such as **athetosis, drooling, facial grimace** and **chewing**, and **swallowing difficulties**.

7. **a.** Pathological jaundice usually occurs within the first **24** hours of life
b. A conjugated bilirubin of **250** μmol/L (or >**20**% of the total serum bilirubin) would indicate a pathological finding with further investigation required.
c. Persistence of jaundice beyond **14** days for the term infant requires investigation.

8. Conjugation: c, f, j.   Excretion: d, e, f.
Production: a, h, i, k.   Transport: b, g.

9. **a.** RhD **incompatibility** can occur when a woman with **Rh-negative** blood type is pregnant with a **Rh-positive fetus**. The placenta acts as a barrier to fetal blood entering the maternal circulation. During pregnancy or birth, fetomaternal haemorrhage (FMH) can occur when small amounts of fetal **Rh-positive** blood cross the placenta and enter the **Rh-negative** mother's blood. The woman's immune system produces **anti-D** antibodies. In subsequent pregnancies, these maternal antibodies can cross the placenta and destroy the red cells of any **Rh-positive** fetus.
b. ABO **isoimmunization** usually occurs when the mother is blood **group O** and the baby is blood **group A** (or less often **group B**). Individuals with **type O** blood develop antibodies throughout life from exposure to antigens in food, gram-**negative** bacteria or blood transfusion. The woman usually has high serum **anti-A** and **anti-B** antibody titres by the time she is pregnant for the first time. Some women produce **IgG** antibodies that can cross the placenta and attach to the red cells and destroy them.

10. True: a, d, e, g, h, i.   False: b, c, f.

11. d.   **12.** c.   **13.** a.   **14.** d.

ANSWERS

1. True: b, e, g, j, k, m.   False: a, c, d, f, h, i, l.

2. **a.** 6 Hirschsprung's disease, 7 Imperforate anus, 8 Malrotation/volvulus, 9 Meconium ileus (cystic fibrosis), 13 Rectal atresia.
   b. 3 Diaphragmatic hernia.   **c.** 12 Pyloric stenosis.   **d.** 6 Hirschsprung's disease.   **e.** 11 Pierre Robin sequence.   **f.** 4 Exomphalos.   **g.** 2 Cleft lip and palate.   **h.** 1 Choanal atresia.   **i.** 10 Oesophageal atresia.   **j.** 5 Gastroschisis.

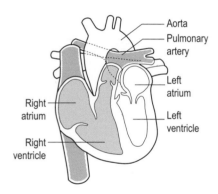

Figure 20.1

4. **i.** In this condition, the aorta arises from the **right** ventricle and the pulmonary artery arises from the **left** ventricle.
   ii. **Oxygenated** blood is circulated back through the lungs and **deoxygenated** blood is circulated back into the systemic circulation.
   iii. A **patent ductus arteriosus** needs to be maintained to provide opportunity for **oxygenated** blood to access the systemic circulation. Otherwise the baby will die.

5.

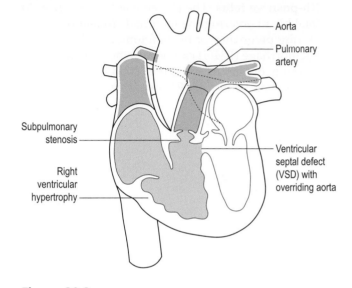

Figure 20.2

6. **i.** Pulmonary outflow is **obstructed**, **ii.** Ventricular septal defect (VSD), **iii.** Right ventricle is **hypertrophied**, **iv.** An **overriding** aorta.

7. **i.** Persistent ductus arteriosus.   **ii.** Ventricular septal defects.   **iii.** Atrial septal defects.

8. **a.** Tachypnoea.   **b.** Tachycardia.   **c.** Cyanosis.
   d. Heart murmurs.

9. a. Spina bifida results from **failure** of fusion of the **vertebral column**.
b. A meningocele refers to the protrusion of the **meninges** through the defect. It does **not** contain **neural** tissue.
c. Meningomyocele refers to the protrusion of **meninges** through the defect and it involves the **spinal cord**.
d. Encephalocele is the term used when the defect is at the **level** of the **base** of the skull.

10.

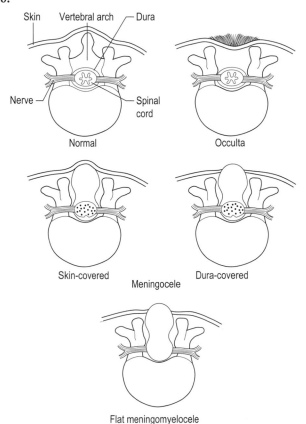

Figure 20.3

11. a. 5 Osteogenesis imperfect.   **b.** 2 Achondroplasia.   **c.** 4 Port Wine Stain.   **d.** 6 Hypospadius.   **e.** 1 Cryptochordism.   **f.** 3 Fetal alcohol syndrome/spectrum.   **g.** 9 Talipes calcaneovalgus.   **h.** 7 Potter syndrome.   **i.** 8 Talipes equinovarus.

12. Infants born to a diabetic mother have **low** blood glucose concentrations because of the excess of **insulin**. This is produced by the fetal **pancreatic gland** as a result of stimulation by **increased** maternal **glucose** concentrations. The excess of **insulin** also acts as a **growth factor** and brings about **excessive** fat and glycogen deposition. The baby usually has a macrosomic appearance.

13. True: a, c, e, f, h, i, j.   False: b, d, g.

14. a, b, e, f.

15. a. The **Moro (startle)** reflex may be absent following heavy sedation of hypoxemic ischaemic encephalopathy (HIE).
b. The **sucking** reflex may be depressed in the preterm neonate or following maternal sedation during labour.
c. Visual cues should normally replace the **rooting** reflex by 4 months age.

16. a, d, e.

17. Right-sided palsy; eye open on the paralysed side with the mouth also drawn over to the nonparalysed side.